Covid-19 in India, Disease, Health and Culture

This book is a cultural exploration of health and wellness, with a focus on impacts of Covid-19 on the population of India.

The chapters in this book present original research, systematic reviews, theoretical and conceptual frameworks, encompassing multidisciplinary, inter- and intra-disciplinary fields of study, in the context of how culture and disease sufficiently unpack and inform each other. The book includes contributions from the social sciences and the humanities, and analyses issues that range from smallpox to the history of vaccine, indigenous healing practices, the Macbeth paradigm, Zizekian encounters, mental asylum, and marginalised genders. Using the theme of intellectual interconnectedness in the times of self-isolation and social distancing, the book is a collaboration of critical thinkers who identify and visibilise the hidden global issues related to 'disease' and 'health' that have divided the world into narrow binaries – individual/society, poor/rich, proletariat/bourgeoisie, margin/centre, colonised/coloniser, servitude/liberty, and powerless/powerful. By doing so, the book emphasises the potential of holistic wellness to improve human life and humanity across the globe.

A novel contribution on the cultural factors that played an important role in contemporary times of Covid-19, this book will be of interest to researchers in the fields of Cultural Studies, Health and Society, and South Asian Studies.

Anindita Chatterjee (Phd) is an Associate Professor and the Head of the Department of English, Durgapur Government College, India. Her research interests centre on British Literature of the Romantic and the Victorian Period, Indian Writing in English, Films, Gender Studies, and Popular Culture, and she has published on Socialist Ecofeminism. She has also co-edited *Re-theorising the Indian Subcontinental Diaspora: Old and New Directions*.

Nilanjana Chatterjee (Phd) is Assistant Professor of English at Durgapur Government College, India. She is the author of *Reading Jhumpa Lahiri: Women, Domesticity and the Indian American Diaspora* (Routledge, forthcoming). Some of her ongoing projects include work on Angami Kire's formation of digital ethnic identity and on women and natural resource management in Naga folktales and stories. She has co-edited *Re-theorising the Indian Subcontinental Diaspora: Old and New Directions*.

Covid-19 in India, Disease, Health and Culture

Can Wellness be Far Behind?

Edited by
Anindita Chatterjee
Nilanjana Chatterjee

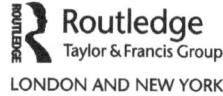

Routledge
Taylor & Francis Group

LONDON AND NEW YORK

First published 2023
by Routledge
4 Park Square, Milton Park, Abingdon, Oxon OX14 4RN

and by Routledge
605 Third Avenue, New York, NY 10158

Routledge is an imprint of the Taylor & Francis Group, an informa business

British Library Cataloguing-in-Publication Data
A catalogue record for this book is available from the British Library

Library of Congress Cataloging-in-Publication Data
Names: Chatterjee, Nilanjana, editor. | Chatterjee, Anindita, editor.
Title: Covid-19 in India, disease, health and culture : can wellness be far
behind? / edited by Nilanjana Chatterjee, and Anindita Chatterjee.
Description: Abingdon, Oxon ; New York, NY : Routledge, 2023. |
Series: Routledge contemporary South Asia series; 154 | Includes
bibliographical references and index.
Identifiers: LCCN 2022020397 (print) | LCCN 2022020398 (ebook) |
ISBN 9781032292687 (hardback) | ISBN 9781032292700 (paperback) |
ISBN 9781003300762 (ebook)
Subjects: LCSH: Public health—India—History. | Medical care. |
COVID-19 (Disease)—Social aspects—India. | COVID-19 (Disease)—
Social aspects—South Asia.
Classification: LCC RA394.6 C68 2023 (print) | LCC RA394.6 (ebook) |
DDC 306.4/613—dc23/eng/20220610
LC record available at https://lccn.loc.gov/2022020397
LC ebook record available at https://lccn.loc.gov/2022020398

ISBN: 978-1-032-29268-7 (hbk)
ISBN: 978-1-032-29270-0 (pbk)
ISBN: 978-1-003-30076-2 (ebk)

DOI: 10.4324/9781003300762

Typeset in Baskerville
by codeMantra

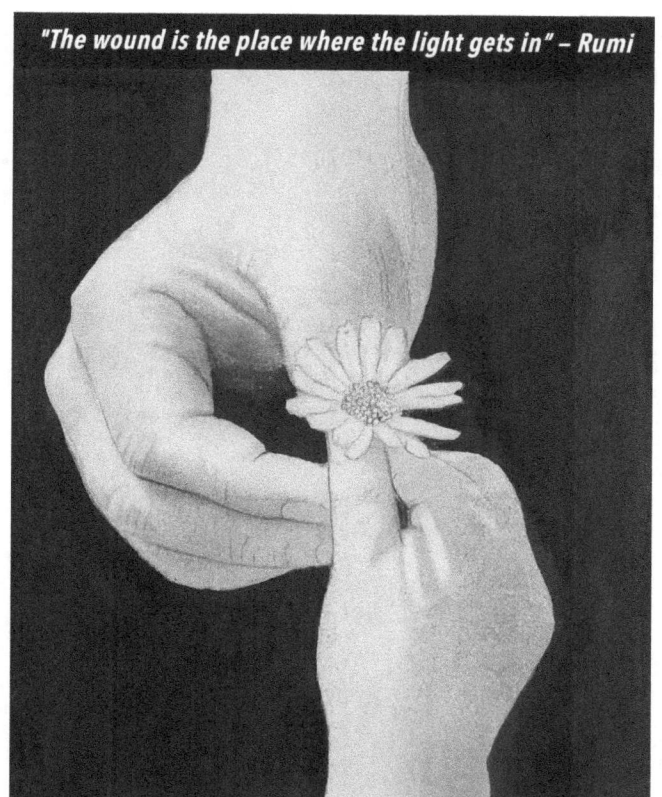

"The wound is the place where the light gets in" – Rumi

"To all the passings that deserved a better goodbye."

Contents

Acknowledgements   xiii
List of illustrations   xv
List of contributors   xvii

1 **Can Wellness Be Far Behind?: Disease, Health,
   and Culture**   1
   ANINDITA CHATTERJEE AND NILANJANA CHATTERJEE

SECTION I
Social Science Perspective   21

2 **Colonialism and Disease: Smallpox in the Aboriginal
   Population**   23
   BILL ASHCROFT

3 **Vaccine Nation and Its Miserables: Bodies and Bio-
   citizenship in the Empire**   36
   MANDIRA CHAKRABORTY

4 **Spaces of Cure or Confinement? Inside the Walls of the
   Mental Asylums of the 19th Century**   50
   ANINDITA CHATTERJEE

5 **Žižek's *Pandemic!*, the 'New Normal' Dilemma and
   Some Indian Perspectives**   62
   ANASUYA BHAR

6 **Livelihood of Internal Migrants of India during
   Covid-19 Pandemic: Concerns and Measures**   72
   DEBASIS CHAKRABORTY

7 **Federalism and Intergovernmental Coordination
during a Pandemic: A Special Reference to India**   87
CHITRA ROY

8 **Hate in the Times of Covid-19: Can We Blame the Print
Media in India?**   98
RUMELA SEN AND NUSRAT FAROOQ

9 **Neoliberal Turn in the Domain of Health Care: The
Emergence of Corporate Health Care Sector in India**   117
AMRITA BAGCHI

SECTION II
Cultural Perspective   135

10 **Disease and the Desire for Health in
Shakespeare's *Macbeth***   137
SUBHAJIT SEN GUPTA

11 **Their Mother's Gardens: Epidemic, Healing, and
Motherhood in *Year of Wonders* and *Hamnet***   157
CHANDRIMA DAS

12 **"stand aside death...today is my day": Contextualizing
the Naga Esotericism in Easterine Kire's Novels**   168
NILANJANA CHATTERJEE

13 **Dis-ease, Dis-order and the Refugee Experience:
Appraising South Asian Partition Narratives**   182
DEBASRI BASU

14 **Always in Search of her Ithaca: Women's Spiritual
Well-being in *Journey to Ithaca: A Pilgrimage in
Search of Identity* and *Eat, Pray, Love: One Woman's
Search for Everything***   194
NIBEDITA MUKHERJEE

15 **Disjunctured Subjectivities and Corporeal Well-being:
Issues of Mobility and Health in Select Transgender
Life Narratives from India**   207
RAJESH V. NAIR AND LEKSHMI R. NAIR

16 **Sustainable Eating and Wellness: Examining Nutrition Strategies in Barbara Kingsolver's** *Animal, Vegetable, Miracle: Our Year of Seasonal Eating* **and Ruth Ozeki's** *A Year of Meats* 221

SHYMASREE BASU

17 **Disease, Wellbeing, and the Idea of Health in Select Cinematic Representations of the Macbeth Metaphor** 233

ANURADHA MAZUMDER

Index 245

Acknowledgements

One (Anindita) of us had chosen Mental Health and Poetry as dissertation topic at Jadavpur University in 2010. But the intellectual seed germinated and planted itself in 2019 when the world was in a state of mourning and each one of us screamed in pain, 'I can't breathe'. It is there that the anthology started its journey. Covid-19 touched our lives in numerous ways, and we realised how everything that we had been thinking and believing as sanctified and solid was shaken to its deepest core. While the first wave came as a lesson, the second was more shocking and intense. Both of us experienced the direct impact of the virus: For Anindita, it was Pratip who was stranded in Kuwait for ten months due to the travel ban imposed during the pandemic and after he could finally meet his family, Covid touched him. For Nilanjana, it was her husband Arup (a medical professional) who had been affected even before the PPEs arrived in the hospitals. It was our immediate experience of dis-ease with disease that brought us closer and somehow, we got more personally involved with the book. The term disease became a powerful and significant motif in our lives, and we employed our suffering and uncertainties to understand the various facets of it. We were not sure if we would make it till the end, but somehow our academic connections believed in our intellectual involvement with disease and walked hand in hand on an oneiric road to wellness. We knew then that Covid-19 had (perhaps) spared none. The journey has been able to sanitise us intellectually and spiritually. It has restored our childhood faith in human kindness. One does not need excuses disclaimers and justifications for kindness. Kindness is a state of being, one is either kind or one is not.

It was a huge reassurance for us knowing in some strange sort of way that we were not alone, and it reinstated our faith in the words 'someone somewhere shares your cross, and you share theirs'. We still remember the day when our project was accepted by Routledge. It was on that day we realised how it is the way of the Universe saying that if one dares to dream one might convert it into reality someday. We sincerely thank our Guru, Prof. Bill Ashcroft for being a guiding light where 'ignorant armies clash by night'. We thank our learned Contributors, our Mentors, our Teachers from Jadavpur University, and the University of Burdwan and all the faculty members of the Department of English, Kazi Nazrul

University (Durgapur Government College is currently affiliated to KNU) for their inspiration and vision.

Our sincerest gratitude to our Principal sir, Dr. Debnath Palit for being our inspiration, stimulus, constant encouragement, and support. We extend our thanks to the Teachers' Council Secretary Dr. Swapan Kumar Ghosh, IQAC Coordinator Dr. Avijit Mondal, and all our colleagues of the DGC family. While editing this book, we have realised, it is that our boats might be different, but our journey is still the same. Therefore, this critical engagement with 'wellness' during the present autumnal West Wind might lead us to a better day of preparedness (?).

This is our way of humming Bob Dylan in the darkest of times, 'And I'll tell it and think it and speak it and breathe it…But I'll know my song well before I start singin.'

Anindita Chatterjee
Nilanjana Chatterjee

Illustrations

Figures

6.1 Trend of inter-state migration flow in India – 1991, 2001, and 2011   77
8.1 First and second Covid-19 wave in India   102
8.2 Example of Factiva Boolean keyword search screenshot for Muslim/Tablighi Event: (coronajihad or tablighi jamaat or tablighi or nizamuddin markaz or markaz) and Covid   103
8.3 Five steps in data processing   104
8.4 High-frequency words in coverage of Muslim/Tablighi event in top five newspapers   105
8.5 Most prevalent topics in coverage of Mulsim/Tablighi event in top five newspapers   107
8.6 High-frequency words in coverage of Kumbh Mela in top five newspapers   108
8.7 Most prevalent topics in coverage of Kumbh Mela in top five   108

Tables

6.1 Migrants in India in 2001 and 2011   75
6.2 Migration according to various reasons for migration (in percentage)   76
6.3 Gender-wise distribution of workers by migration stream (in percentage)   76
6.4 Proportion of migrants and non-migrants in metro cities in India (in percentage)   77
8.1 Frequency of articles on the Tablighi Jamaat event (March 15 - April 30, 2020) and the Kumbh Mela (March 15 - April 30, 2021)   99
8.2 Dates, Attendees, and Location of the Muslim and the Hindu Events   101

Contributors

Bill Ashcroft is a Professor Emeritus in the School of the Arts and Media UNSW, Australia and a founding exponent of post-colonial theory. He has co-authored *The Empire Writes Back*, which is regarded as the first text to systematically examine the area of post-colonial studies. He has authored 21 books, which have been variously translated into 5 languages. Some of his noted works include *Post-Colonial Transformation* (Routledge 2001), *Post-Colonial Futures* (2001), *Caliban's Voice* (Routledge 2008), *Intimate Horizons* (2009), and *Utopianism in Postcolonial Literatures* (Routledge 2016).

Amrita Bagchi (Phd), Assistant Professor in the Department of History at Bethune College Kolkata, completed her doctoral thesis at Jadavpur University. Her area of specialisation includes Social History of Science and Technology and Medicine. Her area of research is changing role of healthcare, equity, and right-based approach towards health. https://orcid.org/0000-0001-7284-0170.

Debasri Basu (Phd) is an Assistant Professor in WBES and is currently teaching at the Post-Graduate Department of English, Maulana Azad College, Kolkata, India. She completed her doctoral research on Partition Literature in the context of the Indian subcontinent at the University of Calcutta. Her research interests include British Literature of the Eighteenth Century, Indian Writings in English, Bengali, Hindi and English Translation, and Resistance Literature and Popular Culture. Her scholarly papers and articles have been published by Vidyasagar University, University of Burdwan, Netaji Subhas Open University, and Café Dissensus, among others. https://orcid.org/0000-0002-2158-6587.

Anasuya Bhar (Phd) is an Associate Professor and Dean of Post-graduate Studies in St. Paul's Cathedral Mission College, Kolkata. Her area of research includes Romanticism, Nineteenth-Century Bengal Studies, Gender Studies, Cultural Studies, Translation Studies, and Visual Arts. She has completed UGC-Funded MRP on 'Home and the World: The Voice of Woman in the Emerging Consciousness of Nineteenth Century Bengal'. She has various academic publications to her credit. https://orcid.org/0000-0002-3422-4702.

Shymasree Basu (Phd) is an Associate Professor in the Department of English Vidyasagar Metropolitan College, Kolkata. She completed her doctoral research at Jadavpur University in 2010. She has presented many papers, delivered lectures in several national seminars, and has several publications to her credit. https://orcid.org/0000-0002-4561-8512.

Debasis Chakraborty (Phd) is presently an Assistant Professor at the National Institute of Technology Durgapur, India. Prior to this, Dr. Chakraborty was an Assistant Professor of Economics in Durgapur Government College under the West Bengal Education Service from 2010 to 2018. He is involved in Under-Graduate-, Post-Graduate-, and Doctoral-level teaching. His areas of interests are Labour Economics, Development Economics, Migration Studies, and Urban Economics. Dr. Chakraborty has published several research papers in different international and national journals of repute. Apart from this, he has published two books on migration studies in India. https://orcid.org/0000-0002-8510-6845.

Mandira Chakraborty (Phd) is currently working as an Assistant Professor in the Department of English at Bethune College, Kolkata. She completed her doctoral thesis on 'A Study of Selected Illness Narratives' from Jadavpur University. She completed a UGC-sponsored MRP on Amitav Ghosh's 'The Calcutta Chromosome'. Her areas of specialisation are Culture Studies and Narratology. https://orcid.org/0000-0002-3632-5515.

Anindita Chatterjee (Phd) is an Associate Professor and the Head of the Department of English, Durgapur Government College, India. Her research interests centre on British Literature of the Romantic and the Victorian Period, Indian Writing in English, Films, Gender Studies, and Popular Culture, and she has published on Socialist Ecofeminism. She has also co-edited *Re-theorising the Indian Subcontinental Diaspora: Old and New Directions*.

Nilanjana Chatterjee (Phd) is Assistant Professor of English at Durgapur Government College, India. She is the author of *Reading Jhumpa Lahiri: Women, Domesticity and the Indian American Diaspora* (Routledge, forthcoming). Some of her ongoing projects include work on Angami Kire's formation of digital ethnic identity and on women and natural resource management in Naga folktales and stories. She has co-edited *Re-theorising the Indian Subcontinental Diaspora: Old and New Directions*.

Chandrima Das is an Assistant Professor in the Department of English at Durgapur Women's College. She has various academic publications to her credit. She has recently submitted her doctoral thesis at Visva-Bharati University, Santiniketan, West Bengal, India. https://orcid.org/0000-0002-0127-6872.

Nusrat Farooq is an investigative researcher in counterterrorism and violent extremism. She holds a Master of Public Admninistration from

Columbia University's School of International and Public Affairs. https://orcid.org/0000-0002-6657-6614.

Anuradha Mazumder is an Assistant Professor of English at Prafulla Chandra College, Kolkata, India. An alumnus of Presidency College, Kolkata, she completed her Masters in English Literature from Calcutta University and her M.Phil. from Jadavpur University. She is, at present, a PhD research scholar at the University of Burdwan, West Bengal. Her areas of interest include Romantic and Victorian studies as well as literature's interface with movies and popular culture. She is the author of *Jane Austen's Pride and Prejudice: With an Introduction and Explanatory Notes* (2018). https://orcid.org/0000-0002-2732-3761.

Nibedita Mukherjee (Phd) is Professor of English at Sidho-Kanho-Birsha University, Purulia, India. She specialises in Feminist Studies, South Asian Literature, and Shakespearean Drama. She has five books to her credit: *Gendering the Narrative: Gender Discourse and Indian English Fiction, Dynamics of Diasporic Identity in Commonwealth Literature, The Fictional World of Amitav Ghosh, Indian Theatre in English and Literary Feminism: Politics of Gender Identity and Authenticity,* and *The Dark Forces in Shakespeare's Plays*. She received the USA State Fellowship Award (SUSI) funded by the Dept. of State, USA. She is working with Teaching Learning Center, IIT Kharagpur as Research Collaborator and Subject Expert in a project titled 'Graphic-Novel based Pedagogy in Teaching Grammar in Schools' funded by MHRD and an ICSSR-funded project titled 'Folklores and Folkvoices: Preserving the Environmental Ethnospace'. She is also a Professor at Sidho-Kanho Birsa University. https://orcid.org/0000-0003-2638-253X.

Lekshmi R. Nair (Phd) is Associate Professor of English at Government College Kottayam, Kerala. She is an approved Research Supervisor at the Mahatma Gandhi University, Kottayam and is currently guiding four Ph.D. students. She has presented many papers, delivered lectures in several national seminars, and has several publications to her credit. https://orcid.org/0000-0002-2599-6110.

Rajesh V. Nair (Phd) is an Assistant Professor of English at the School of Letters, Mahatma Gandhi University, Kerala. He has published essays on areas such as life writing, graphic narratives, memory studies, popular culture, and gender. His current projects include an introductory book on Life Writing and essays on translation studies and street theatre. https://orcid.org/0000-0001-6118-6548.

Chitra Roy is an Assistant Professor in the Department of Political Science, Durgapur Government College. Her area of specialisation includes Political Sociology of India, Indian Politics, State Politics, Intergovernmental Relations, Indian Political Thought, and Women's Studies. https://orcid.org/0000-0002-7853-0066.

Rumela Sen (Phd) received her PhD in comparative politics from Cornell University in 2017. She is a Lecturer in the Discipline of International and Public Affairs, SIPA and is an Associate Research Scholar at Saltzman Institute of War and Peace, Columbia University. She teaches the core course Politics of Policymaking as well as courses on political development, comparative political economy, and South Asia. She recently published a book entitled *Farewell to Arms: How Rebels Retire without Getting Killed.* (2021). https://orcid. org/0000-0002-7939-027X.

Subhajit Sen Gupta (Phd) is Associate Professor in the Department of English & Culture Studies at the University of Burdwan. His research projects include the Renaissance, Drama and Performance Studies, Sports Literature, and 'Post-Independence Indian Theatre and Its Negotiations with European Drama'. A renowned scholar in Shakespeare studies, he has been extensively published in several national and international journals of repute. https://orcid.org/0000-0002-6843-8442.

1 Can Wellness Be Far Behind?

Disease, Health, and Culture

Anindita Chatterjee and Nilanjana Chatterjee

I

Academic Weapon in the Covid-19 Uncertainty

Until now, the concept of health and wellness (while "health" is a state of being, "wellness" is the state of living a healthy lifestyle) was supposed to be central to the medical paradigm. But the Covid-19 pandemic has re-revealed to humanity the inevitable fragility of human existence, necessitating inter-disciplinary and intra-disciplinary engagement with "wellness" as theory and praxis. Dipesh Chakrabarty observes, "the microbes that spread illness does not recognize sexual, gendered, racial, ethnic or class-based borders, hence the impact of pandemics are universal" (Chakraborty 2016, 378). This book therefore presents chapters on original research, systematic reviews, and theoretical or conceptual frameworks, encompassing multidisciplinary, inter-disciplinary, and intra-disciplinary fields of study, in the context of how culture and disease sufficiently unpack and inform each other. In doing so, the book strategically contextualises the concept of wellness when "nothing is to be done" in the present dystopia except waiting for the unknown (the vaccine?). Meaningful waiting, wherein time and space have completely lost their significance, calls for the unlocking of cultural isolation and re-constructing the idea of disease and illness in general, and Covid-19 crisis in particular. The study becomes relevant as over one-third of the population in developing countries lacks access to proper biomedical health care services, often relying on indigenous healing practices – traditional medicine, spiritual practice, and occultism. While disease is a perennial theme in cultural studies, wellness is a fundamental human trait, and the current pandemic has only given impetus to this discourse.

The World Health Organization defines wellness as "the optimal state of health of individuals and groups."[1] According to the World Health Organization, the notion of wellness is based on two cardinal concerns – the fullest achievement of individuals' potentials physically, psychologically, socially, spiritually, and economically, and the ability to fulfil the expectation within one's family, community, place of worship, workplace, and other settings to its best possible way. It is evident that the notion of wellness is a complex construct having multiple facets

DOI: 10.4324/9781003300762-1

and sub-dimensions. Despite being frequently used as a modern term, the word wellness has its roots located in antiquity. The tenets of wellness can be traced to the ancient civilisations of Greece, Rome, and Asia. Various aspects of the current notion of wellness can be perceived in several intellectual, religious, and medical movements that affected the United States and Europe in the nineteenth century. The modern idea of wellness as we understand it today has become popular since the 1950s. Recently, it has been proposed that the idea of spiritual wellbeing ought to be included as an important constituent along with other facets of wellness, such as mental, physical, and emotional wellnesses to represent a holistic perspective. The National Institute of Wellness considers wellness to be "an active process through which people become aware of, and make choices toward, a more successful existence" (Gomez and Fisher 2003). Wellness thus should be perceived as a multifaceted active process that culminates in a more positive, enriching, and gratifying life. When people identify the key characteristics of a good life, they include the idea of happiness, health, peace, and mental wellbeing. Subjective wellbeing thus becomes an ideal state of wellness that all desire in life, an end that living organisms crave and yearn for as a release from all the states of disease and dis-ease. While some achieve their goal, many fail to reach there; however, it can be safely asserted that despite all setbacks and failures the hope for wellness is the ultimate dream that the human life craves and aims for.

II

Wellness and Disease: A Cultural Exploration

Wellness and health, today, is the most valuable gift or wealth one could ask for in life. It includes health promotion and disease prevention. The present segment looks at the cultural determinants of health and wellness. The definition provided by the World Health Organization associates health with wellbeing and conceptualises health as a human right that requires physical and social resources to achieve and preserve. "Wellbeing" refers to a positive rather than a neutral state, framing health as a positive aspiration. This definition was adopted by the 1986 Ottawa Charter of the World Health Organization, which describes health as:

> a resource for everyday life, not the object of living. Health promotion is the process of enabling people to increase control over, and to improve, their health. To reach a state of complete physical mental and social wellbeing, an individual or group must be able to identify and to realize aspirations, to satisfy needs, and to change or cope with the environment. Health is, therefore, seen as a resource of everyday life, not the objective of living. Health is a positive concept emphasizing social and personal resources, as well as physical capacities. Therefore, health promotion is not just the responsibility of the health sector but goes beyond healthy lifestyles to wellbeing.
>
> (WHO 1986 Ottawa Charter)

In keeping with the WHO Charter, health is perceived as a fundamental human right. The Ottawa Charter emphasises certain prerequisites for health which include "peace, adequate economic resources, food and shelter, a stable ecosystem and sustainable resource use" (Nutbeam 1998, 351). Recognition of these prerequisites highlights the inextricable links between social and economic conditions, physical environment, individual lifestyle, and health. The World Health Organization's identification of the notion of health as "a state of complete physical, mental and social wellbeing and not merely the absence of disease or infirmity" (WHO 1948) is consistent with the biopsychosocial model of health, which considers all the physiological, psychological, and social factors in health and illness, and the interactions between these factors. Len Sperry defines health in terms of a balance between the "two complementary forces in the universe, the yang (positive or masculine) and yin (negative or feminine)" (Sperry 2016, 13). Disease is perceived as a rupture in this state of balance that has historically always unsettled the balance and exposed the hidden world views and cultural values that have divided the world into narrow binaries – individual/society, poor/rich, proletariat/bourgeoisie, margin/centre, colonised/coloniser, servitude/liberty, and powerless/powerful. Health can be identified theoretically in terms of certain measured values; for example, a person having normal body temperature, pulse and breathing rates, blood pressure, body weight, accuracy of vision, sensitivity of hearing, and other normal measurable characteristics might be termed normal and healthy. But that leads us to the most profound question as to what does normal mean, and how is it established? "Normal" and "abnormal" are subjective to individual perception and different societal standards which are further dependent on situation, context, age, or gender. Apart from varying from one culture to another, these two terms differ with the changing societal norms, even within a specific culture.

Encyclopaedia Britannica identifies the term disease as any harmful deviation from the normal structural or functional state of an organism, generally associated with certain signs and symptoms and differing in nature from physical injury. A diseased organism commonly exhibits signs or symptoms indicative of its abnormal state.[2] Disease implies an impairment or aberration of the normal state of a human being that interrupts, modifies, and affects the vital functions of the body. To recognise and study the hallmarks of disease, it is imperative to understand the normal condition of an organism, disease alludes to some form of disorder or breakdown of "normal" structure or function in a human, animal, or plant body especially one that produces specific/visible symptoms or that affects a specific location and is not simply a direct result of physical injury. Nevertheless, it must be noted that a sharp demarcation between disease and health is not always apparent. The pathological investigation of disease involves determining the cause of the disease (aetiology), enquiry into the process of its evolution growth and development (pathogenesis), examination of the structural changes associated with the disease process (morphological variations), and the functional consequences of the changes. In clinical terms, proper diagnosis, i.e., identification of the cause of the disease, becomes necessary to ensure a suitable line of treatment or cure. Humans and animals are all susceptible to some forms of ailment or the other which disrupts the normal "healthy" functioning of the body. Health, in clinical perspective, (almost) is an objective state. Health promoters evaluate physical or health condition as either categorically good or categorically bad and proceed towards treatment accordingly. In clinical terms, it is ethical to reinstate "health" as opposed to a diseased state because health is acclaimed as the universally desirable goal. Susan Sontag in the study "Illness as Metaphor" identifies disease as any state of discomfort which she figuratively describes as "the night-side of life, a more onerous citizenship" (Sontag 1978, 1) and everyone on the earth holds dual citizenship, in the realm of the well and in the realm of the sick.

An infection implies a foreign invasion in the body – the colonisation of a host body by a microorganism. Infections can lead to disease, which causes signs and symptoms resulting in a deviation from the normal "healthy" functioning of the host body. Unlike signs, the symptoms of disease are subjective. Symptoms are felt or experienced by the patient, but they cannot be clinically confirmed or objectively measured. Microorganisms which lead to infection or disease are identified as pathogens. Medical professionals are expected to alleviate disease and suffering, and re-establish good health. Hence the three components of the medical paradigm, namely, health, patients, and medicine, are closely intertwined and inseparable from each other. A diseased condition implies physical pain, discomfort, some form of bodily dysfunction, distress, or suffering of the afflicted individual. Over the past 20 years, the study of illness, as experienced by patients, was the conventional approach to understand sickness and health in general. However, there has been a shift towards a holistic understanding of health in recent years. Scholarly engagements with the concept of health, in the last five to six decades, have started to perceive "health" as a multidimensional concept, not limited to the level of the "physiological". The World Health Organization's definition of health in its Constitution clearly demarcates the finer nuances attached with the ideas of health and illness: health now is seen as a state of complete physical, mental, and social wellbeing, not merely as the absence of disease or infirmity. Sengupta observes:

> Studying the health sector of a nation is, on one hand, a very simple and also a very complex task. It is simple because health affects each and every person in a country, and at the micro level, every person seems to be able to be equipped to a large extent to take care of his/her health. It is complex, particularly at the macro level, because no single factor can determine good health, and health issues operate in a complex dynamic socioeconomic set-up. Health status, therefore, has been the subject of intense research by economists, sociologists, policy makers as well as the medical sciences.
>
> (Sengupta 2016, xii)

The new perception of looking at health takes into consideration its wide diversity, as it encompasses physical, psychological, intellectual, political, economic, social, emotional, and spiritual dimensions. Unlike traditional health research – which mostly focused on physical and clinical aspects of diseases, and medical treatments and rehabilitation – modern notion of health is closely interlinked to the concept of wellbeing. It constitutes the indispensable base on which human happiness is founded. Lê remarks,

> With an increasing interest in population health, particularly in the current context of globalization, the sphere of health research has been expanded to cover also social and cultural factors which not only affect health conditions of individuals and communities but also are determining health factors in some respects. Health professionals nowadays are working with patients, colleagues, and communities of diverse cultural backgrounds whose assumptions, beliefs, and practices in relation to health and wellbeing are different and diverse.
>
> (Lê 2011, ix)

Any form of discussion on disease presupposes some basic premises. Michel Foucault's *The Birth of Clinic*, for instance, mentions how the identification of the disease assumes the existence of a body:

> ... the human body defines, by natural right, the space of origin and of distribution of disease - a space whose lines, volumes, surfaces, and routes are laid down, in accordance with a now familiar geometry, by the anatomical atlas. But this order of the solid, visible body is only one way—in all likelihood neither the first, nor the most fundamental—in which one spatializes disease.
>
> (Foucault 1989, 3)

But there has been a substantial progress in this context for health is no longer confined to the premise of the body of the patient. The notion of mental health has assumed substantial importance in modern times. Mental health is a continuum, ranging from states of wellbeing to stressful life experiences to severe mental disorders. So, it is again difficult to limit, classify, and demarcate the scope of mental health. Mental health or sanity can be thought of as successful mental functioning that results in productive activities, fulfilling relationships, and the ability to cope with change and adversity. Another way of saying this is that mental health is indispensable to effective personal functioning, interpersonal and family relationships, and community life. Any form of change or deviation from a state of balance exerts an impact on mental health and it can become a major source of anxiety or stress for many in their personal and professional lives. The breaking point differs from individual to individual. Sperry observes,

> Change, by itself, whether for good or not, can be a source of stress and can negatively influence mental health. For example, technological changes

continue at an accelerating pace, and while they can be useful to many individuals, they pose a stressful challenge to others.

(Len Sperry 2016, xli)

The inextricable link between mental health and physical health has radically challenged the historical notion of mind-body duality. It is now perceived as a two-way relationship with mental health influencing physical health and vice versa. Based on his professional experience of working in a psychiatric hospital, Foucault described the influence of social structures in the history of the 'Othering' of insane people from mainstream society in *Madness and Civilization*. In his 1974 essay, "Society Must be Defended," Foucault traces the growing importance of doctors, medical practitioners, diseased bodies, and biomedicine, to make modern life more "pertinent". The present-day researchers have identified that the normal healthy state of an organism represents a condition of subtle physiological balance, or homeostasis, in terms of chemical, physical, and functional processes. In a fundamental sense, therefore, any disruption or rupture of the homeostatic control mechanisms becomes a disease/dis-ease. The notion of disease also includes disabilities, disorders, syndromes, virus infections, deaths, deviant behaviours, etc. within its scope and periphery. Diseases affect people and the family of the patient not only physically but also emotionally/mentally, as contracting and living with a disease can alter the affected person's perspective on life. Machteld Huber proposed a new definition of health as "the ability to adapt and to self-manage," which includes the ability of people to adapt to their situation as key to health (Huber et al. 2011, 1). This perspective acknowledges the subjective element of health; and thereby health becomes a flexible and relative term, differing in scope and meaning from one person to the next, depending on the context and their needs. This is considered by many to be a limitation of the broader perspective of health on the grounds that wellbeing is neither objective nor measurable, and at the same time, it is very individualistic and takes little account of the wider determinants of health. Martino believes, "Responsibility for health is now seen as individual rather than collective with little scope to promote it as a human right" (Martino 2017). The health promoters are now looking beyond alleviation of pain to enable people to live safer and more fulfilled modern lives.

Health care attitudes reflect the basic worldview and values of a culture, such as how we relate to nature, other people, time, being, society and community, children and elders, and independence and dependence. Epidemiology studies the frequency of the appearance of diseases in different groups of people and the reason behind their occurrence. Epidemiological information is used to design and evaluate strategies to prevent illness and act as a guide or manual to the management of patients in whom disease has already developed. Like the clinical results and pathology, the epidemiology of a disease is an integral part of its basic description. Illness behaviour determines who is vulnerable to illness and who agrees to become a patient – since only about one-third of the ill will see a physician. Cultural values determine how one will behave as a patient and what it means to be ill and especially to be a hospital patient. They affect decisions about a patient's treatment and, moreover, problematise the role of the decision-makers. Cultural differences create problems in communication, rapport, physical examination, treatment compliance, and follow-through. The special meaning of medicines and diet requires particular attention. The perception of physical pain and psychological distress varies from culture to culture and affects the attitudes and effectiveness of caregivers as much as that of patients. Religious beliefs and attitudes about death, which have many cultural variations, are especially relevant to hospital-based treatment. Linguistic and cultural interpreters can be essential; they are more available than realised, though there are pitfalls in their use. Finally, one must recognise that individual characteristics may outweigh the ethnic and that a good caring relationship can compensate for many cultural missteps. Sontag's *Illness as Metaphor and Aids and Its Metaphors* talks about two diseases – tuberculosis and cancer – that have been spectacularly laden by the trappings of metaphor. In Stendhal's *Armance*, the protagonist's mother refuses to use the word tuberculosis in fear that it might enhance the malady of her son. The word cancer similarly is often seen as a stigma or a disgraceful state of misery by the patient and the family which mentally unsettles the patient first before he succumbs to the malignancy physically. Sontag shows how tuberculosis was viewed in the same way as cancer is seen now – as obdurate and stubborn impediment in the course of health and wellness:

> The fantasies inspired by TB in the last century, by cancer now, are responses to a disease thought to be intractable and capricious—that is, a disease not understood—in an era in which medicine's central premise is that all diseases can be cured. Such a disease is, by definition, mysterious. For as long as its cause was not understood and the ministrations of doctors remained so ineffective, TB was thought to be an insidious, implacable theft of a life. Now it is cancer's turn to be the disease that doesn't knock before it enters, cancer that fills the role of an illness experienced as a ruthless, secret invasion—a role it will keep until, one day, its etiology becomes as clear and its treatment as effective as those of TB have become. Although the way in which disease mystifies is set against a backdrop of new expectations, the disease itself (once TB, cancer today) arouses thoroughly old-fashioned kinds of dread. Any disease that is treated as a mystery and acutely enough feared will be felt to be morally, if not literally, contagious. Thus, a surprisingly large number of people with cancer find themselves being shunned by relatives and friends and are the object of practices of decontamination by members of their household, as if cancer, like TB, were an infectious disease. Contact with someone afflicted with a disease regarded as a mysterious malevolency inevitably feels like a trespass; worse, like the violation of a taboo. The very names of such diseases are felt to have a magic power.
>
> (Sontag 1978, 10)

If doctors resort to abandon these pejorative labels to prevent inflicting further afflictions, it would also imply adding on to the secretiveness and enhancing the overwhelming power of the malady. If a disease is treated as an invincible predator, then the patients would never ever hope for wellness or cure. "The solution is hardly to stop telling cancer patients the truth, but to rectify the conception of the disease, to de-mythicize it" (Sontag 1978, 11). Since many patients feel that acquiring cancer implies an end of life for it jeopardises one's love life, one's career, one's chance of promotion, and even one's job. So, they tend to be extremely prudish, if not outright secretive, about their disease. The best way to deal with the crisis could be to inculcate positivity in the patient. It would help the patient combat the disease better.

Human history has instances of epidemic attacks over the centuries which people have overcome with their medical infrastructure and perseverance. In the summer of 430 BCE, a violent epidemic struck the Greek city of Athens. It was reported by the contemporary Athenian historian Thucydides (who himself suffered from the disease):

> Epidemics have had literary or metaphoric importance, [and] references to them have entered into popular culture and everyday speech. The epidemic in Athens in 430 B.C.E., or the Plague of Thucydides, has lived on in the world of classical studies. References to consumption dominated literary and cultural discussions in (and about) the nineteenth century, as much because of *who* suffered from it as *how many* did. And also found here is Typhoid Mary, whose "epidemic" may have only resulted in three deaths, but whose name has become a metaphor for a transmitter of any sort of trouble.
>
> (Hays 2005, x)

Malaria was a frequent malady in the ancient Roman world. It enormously increased mortality levels and sharply reduced life expectancy at all ages. In 735 (CE), smallpox epidemic began in the seaport region on the north coast of Japan. Leprosy was very widespread in medieval Europe. In many Italian cities, the last surge of these epidemics like plague and pox occurred between 1629 and 1633. In 1721, a major smallpox epidemic struck the city of Boston. A sweeping influenza pandemic passed through Europe in late 1781 and 1782. In 1817, cholera began spreading in the areas of Bengal and the Ganges River delta. Typhoid became an important endemic problem in American and European cities in the nineteenth century. When the plague struck London in 1665, Londoners lost their minds. They consulted astrologers, quacks, and the Bible. They searched their bodies for signs of the disease: lumps, blisters, and black spots. They begged for prophecies and paid for predictions. Defoe's *A Journal of the Plague Year* (1722) mentions how people prayed and yelled in fear when the plague struck. The government tried to contain the panic, and according to Daniel Defoe, the government had to "suppress the Printing of such Books as terrify'd the People" (Defoe 2010, 17). The documentation of the recent epidemics and pandemics is considerably more accurate which is partly due to the greater reliability of the statistics on population, morbidity, and mortality figures. In this context, it is significant to note that it was during the mid-nineteenth century and early twentieth century that the Western conceptions of disease and responses to disease and epidemics underwent dramatic transformations, and the West started to impose those conceptions and responses on other civilisations.

An epidemic with a larger impact is identified as a pandemic. Ebola, in 2014, was by any measure an epidemic – perhaps even a pandemic. The influenza that killed 50 million people around the world in 1918 was a pandemic. Mcmillen remarked, "A common way to think about epidemics and pandemics is as events. They come and they go" (2016, 1). But can the same perspective help understand HIV/AIDS, tuberculosis, malaria, or dengue as pandemics? Pandemics can be either discrete events or what medical practitioners like to call persistent pandemics. Tuberculosis, malaria, dengue, and HIV/AIDS, which affect the population of the globe and kill millions and millions each year, come under the category of "persistent pandemics" (Wolfe 2011, 9). The identity of several diseases underwent significant changes due to the late nineteenth-century scientific revolution in laboratory. It was the age of modern medicine. It began with Louis Pasteur in France and culminated with the work of Robert Koch in Germany. Consequently, diseases that were once explained in myriad ways were thereafter explained through the lens of science. Almost all the diseases were subjected to some form of control by modern medicines, but at the same time, they remained closely interlinked to the socio-economic conditions. This was one of the reasons why cholera disappeared from the United States more than a century ago but is still present in much of the developing world. HIV/AIDS disproportionately affects sub-Saharan Africa and the slums of Asia. Malaria is now seen as a tropical disease that infects the developing world. While some countries have been able to transcend and improvise the living conditions that do not allow infectious diseases to flourish, by offering better health care facilities, many other countries have not been able to do the same. Improvisation of the quality of life along with the advent of antibiotic medicine resulted in the decline of TB cases in the Western world. The discovery of antibiotics marked the triumphant moment of modern biomedicine which further led to a better cure of the affected patient and it resulted in lowering the mortality rate of the infected. The location of epidemic gradually shifted from the West to the global south.

While discussing the American health care system in 2017, Noam Chomsky mentioned Article 25 of the UN Declaration of Human Rights (UDHR) which states that health care is a basic human right. Chomsky pointed out how despite all egalitarian principles advocated by health care policies, around 30 million American lives still remain uninsured. Chomsky went on to write:

> I get fantastic medical care, because I'm rich and medical care is rationed by wealth. If you're rich, the system is working just right. The insurance companies, the health maintenance organizations, the pharmaceutical corporations are doing just great. Wealthy people are doing fine. If most of the population can't get decent medical care, that's not our problem. If health care costs are astronomical, too bad.
>
> (2005, 192)

If this is the condition of the United States, then one can imagine how deplorable the condition of the third world countries could be! The population density, crowded living conditions, economic inequality resulting in unequal access to medicine and drugs, and lack of proper infrastructure led to high rates of infection and greater chances of co-morbidity.

The health status of a nation has emerged unanimously as the determinant of its economic development. Sengupta, in the Indian context, observes:

> … health is an area which has received the least importance in the development plans of emerging nations including India. Investment in the health sector in India is one of the lowest in the world. India for instance, which has experienced almost 9 p.c. growth rate consistently for the last decade, has emerged as one of the nations in the world with high growth potential and has been the centre of attention by investors all over the world. However, records of health statistics in the country are lower than even some of the less developing countries of the world. The rapid growth of the private health sector makes accessibility and affordability more difficult for the rural poor, who still dominate the demographic structure of India. Though India has a very strong network of public health system, spread throughout the country, health care delivery suffers due to rampant corruption in the health sector at the service delivery point, which has a depressing effect on the health status in the country. All this is the result of inadequate application of management skills and non-professional attitude in the public health system.
>
> (2016, vii)

This is one of the primary reasons why despite adoption of some of the most innovative policies in the health sector in India, the desired and requisite health outcomes have not yet been achieved. Although there has been a considerable rise in the investment in health in the last two decades and the announcement of several health policies, the nation is still burdened with poor health indicators and so the country is saddled with the concern of emerging infectious diseases as well as chronic degenerative diseases. The new approach to health or the absence of it reflects upon changing socio-economic perspective of the nation. Health is now seen as a tangible commodity where the damage or loss of it may be insured and restored with the help of technology. Attention has shifted to those conditions which may prevent illness/disease/dis-ease – to factors that are strongly grounded in one's social and cultural surrounding. Attention is now focused on preventing or bettering those social and cultural conditions, which lead to impairment of one's health or cause suffering. In a nation where over one-third of the population lacks access to proper biomedical health care services, and relies on traditional medicine and/or self-care, health care takes on a completely different identity altogether.

Literary narratives explore real and fictional diseases, epidemics, and pandemics in their most deadly and graphic terms, foregrounding human dis-ease (and healing), fragility (and vitality), and mortality (and life). Edgar Allan Poe's 1842 tale "The Masque of the Red Death" is set in a medieval world plagued by a contagious disease that kills nearly instantly. Mary Shelley's *The Last Man*, a novel set in the twenty-first century, is the first major novel that provides a fictional account of the extinction of humanity by way of a global pandemic. The sensationalisation of fear and anxiety is not something novel or unknown to man. Sontag remarks,

> Being a spectator of calamities taking place in an--L/ other country is a quintessential modern experience, the cumulative offering by more than a century and a half's worth of those professional, specialized tourists known as journalists...Information about what is happening elsewhere, called "news," features conflict, [suffering], and violence— "If it bleeds, it leads" runs the venerable guideline of tabloids and twenty-four-hour headline news shows—to which the response is compassion, or indignation, or titillation, or approval, as each misery heaves into view.
>
> (Sontag 2003, 18)

This journalistic (including photographic and televisual) spectacularisation of the tragedies [of humanity] is commonly referred to as [the] "9/11" syndrome (Ramazani 2007, 2). The critics in the late 1990s pointed to our contemporary "wound culture's" pathological fixation on violence, fear, pain, trauma, and anxiety and, in academic circles, there was an advent of the institutionalised field of "trauma studies" which gradually went on to reach a state of saturation. It was against this backdrop that the pandemic of 2020 struck the world.

Covid-19 turned every piece of fictional imagination into reality. Novel coronavirus, as we all know now, is a new strain of flu that has devastated the planet resulting in severe respiratory illness in people, killing millions of individuals across the world, and triggering fear-related behaviours in situations of mass threat. It is being compared to the largest pandemic in history (the Spanish flu of 1918 infected one-third of the world's population). Zizek writes,

> In the last couple of years, after the SARS and Ebola epidemics, we were told again and again that a new much stronger epidemic was just a matter of time, that the question was not IF but WHEN. Although we were convinced of the truth of these dire predictions, we somehow didn't take them seriously and were reluctant to act and engage in serious preparations.
>
> (Zizek 2020, 46)

What went wrong with our system that we were caught unprepared by the Covid-19 pandemic despite scientists warning us about a pandemic for years? Wuthnow believes,

> The truth is that serious perils to the existence of humanity have become a fact of contemporary life. The threat of mass death, environmental devastation, and even human extinction is an alarming reality.
>
> (Wuthnow 2010, 8)

Medical science sees the Covid-19 virus as a threat that is external to our body – something that is attacking our cells, our respiratory systems, ourselves, our health, our lives, and our societies together and challenging our notion of wellness altogether. The deadly pandemic has taken away millions of lives in the last one and a half year across the globe. Additionally, in India due to excessive focus on Covid-19 during the first wave, several other chronic diseases were ignored like cancer, tuberculosis, dialysis, and kidney ailments. Cheena Kapoor remarks,

> Experts believe that with resources being diverting to treat COVID-19 patients, the surveillance, contact tracing, and testing for tuberculosis nearly ceased, leading to an alternate public health crisis. According to a report released in June, the COVID-19 had consumed 15,000 lives in the first three months of its outbreak. But in the same period, 20,000 people lost their lives to the TB. The Health Minister of India admitted that there had been interruptions in treatment and unavailability of other drugs, shrinkage of diagnostic tests, delays caused due to physical travel ban imposed whereby patients failed to travel to distant clinics to obtain medications.
>
> (Kapoor 2020)

Moreover, Covid-19 affected maternal health and obstetric care in some ways due to delay in seeking health care due to lockdown and fear of incurring infection which resulted in 44.7 per cent pregnancies with complications (Data based on a survey conducted. A prospective observational single-centre study was performed, including all antenatal and parturient women admitted from April to August 2020. Data were collected regarding number of admissions, deliveries, antenatal visits, reason for inaccessibility of health care, and complications during pregnancy, and compared with data from the pre-Covid-19 period from October 2019 to February 2020. Goyal Manu et al., *The effect of the Covid-19 pandemic on maternal health due to delay in seeking health care*, 2020).

However, this was not all; there was more devastation waiting for humanity. Despite the considerable drop in the number of reported infections in September 2020 in India and the consequent euphoric declaration that the country has reached the "endgame of the pandemic" and shipment of vaccines to foreign countries, India was soon caught in the grips of a devastating second wave of the virus. By mid-April, the country averaged more than 100,000 cases a day which rose to more than 350,000 cases by the beginning of May. The hope that India had successfully bent the Covid-19 infection curve was shattered to pieces. The election campaigns, casual violation of safety protocols, organisation of cricket matches, fairs festivities, and flouting of the social distancing norms proved costly for Indians. India is now again in the grips of a public health emergency. As people are desperately running around for vaccines and seeking help in all quarters, social media feeds are replete with videos of funerals of Covid-19 patients and piling dead bodies waiting, long queues for oxygen cylinders and medicines, and frantic pleas for hospital beds. Drugs are being sold on the black market and test results are taking days. The doctors and nurses are going out of their way to save the gasping patients. The idea of a welfare state is on the rise as common people are joining hands to stand by each other during this hour of crisis (Bose 2021).

Unlike the first wave of the pandemic, the impact of the second wave is heterogeneous and asynchronous. The present pandemic has given us an opportunity to look into the current health care scenario of the nation. The coronavirus pandemic has brought forth a graphic scenario of trauma, agony, victimisation, and suffering whose sentimental and clinical perception by the media led to the development of fear, panic, depression, anxiety, and need for social isolation. The context of the pandemic has certainly changed our way of looking at the world and the ideas of health, disease, illness, and wellness. The massive death toll worldwide has affected us emotionally and psychologically over the last one and half year. Writing about the pandemic Covid-19, Zizek has observed how "in the midst of the coronavirus epidemic, we are all [constantly] bombarded by calls not to touch others but to isolate ourselves and maintain a proper corporeal distance" (Zizek 2020, 1). This plea to isolate has resulted in physical and mental detachment of individuals and yet strangely enough, at the same time it has ironically united us all by a common thread of suffering as common people are coming up to help each other in times of need. Social media and digital space have been filled with news of availability of vacant ICU beds and information about oxygen cylinders with people trying to reach out to complete strangers as well. The panic has enveloped us all and none of us are immune to the threat. The wealth of health is now at stake. If we think about the virus as a threat that is external to us – something that is attacking our cells, ourselves, our health, our lives, and our societies together and destroying our idea of wellness – it will help us bond together collectively and more effectively respond to the current health crisis, and from the grim picture that surrounds us, it becomes clear how some people are no longer waiting for some abstract Godot for deliverance and salvation; instead, they are trying to find wellness through their own efforts.

Medical perception states that it is important to identify the virus as its own entity, rather than to see it as the fault of any one group. People have started to think about the pandemic virus as a real dystopia that humankind can and will collectively overcome someday. If Zizek's premonition – "There will be no return to normal, the new 'normal' will have to be constructed on the ruins of our old lives" (Zizek 2020) – is to be taken seriously, we perhaps need to take a closer look at the "new normal" moment to understand the significant position of "wellness" for humanity. Perhaps wellness is connected to but extends beyond disease for "wellness" implies a social change. It is difficult to contextualise the concept of wellness in concrete terms in these dystopic times when "nothing is to be done" except waiting for the unknown keeping in mind the uncertainty regarding the approaching third wave or looking for the availability of the vaccine. Looking at the history of epidemics one dares to hope and believe that history bears a record of how even though calamity has struck humanity from time to time and halted the progress of civilisation temporarily, it has never marred the faith in humanity and its indomitable spirit. Dis-ease/disease will never stop to test human strength and integrity, it will come from time to time and challenge human immunity system, question its established ideas of wellness and health, and dismantle the allegiance to science and medicine. The only weapon against this battle is to engage in a series of critical analyses of disease through the prism of cultural factors (human beliefs, identities, practices, values, and philosophies) to collectively stand up together as humanity in search of prevention, preparedness, and wellness – to put up a fight and dare to believe that "If Winter comes, can Spring be far behind?".

III

The Book and Its Issues

This book – using the theme of intellectual interconnectedness in the times of self-isolation and social distancing – intends to present a collaborative team of critical thinkers who seek to identify and vizibilise the hidden global issues related to "disease" and "health" that have divided the world into narrow binaries – individual/society, poor/rich, proletariat/bourgeoisie, margin/centre, colonised/coloniser, servitude/liberty, and powerless/powerful. By doing so, the authors intend to emphasise the potential of holistic (underlined) wellness to improve human life and humanity across the globe. The first segment of the project is a search for holistic wellness from the social science perspective. Ashcroft in "Colonialism and Disease: Smallpox in the Aboriginal Population" argues that disease was the most far reaching and catastrophic effect of colonial invasion, both in the Pacific and the Americas. He cites the decimation of the Aboriginal population by smallpox to suggest that throughout the colonised world, cultural, and political domination was exacerbated by the transport of diseases to indigenous populations that had no immunity nor time to develop immunity. Preparedness is a step forward to wellness, and Ashcroft prepares his global readers to look at the colonial legacy of disease as the most widespread and devastating weapon of imperialism, shaping the present state of dis-ease and disorder. In this context, if immunity gained from vaccination ensures global wellness, Mitra in "Vaccine Nation and its Miserables: Bodies and Biocitizenship in the Empire" seeks to question – immunity at what cost? She examines the history of vaccination, which has always been littered with its martyrs. She analyses the chequered history of the medical discourse connected to vaccination and the anti-vaxers who resisted it; the struggles that continue between the opposing schools of thought, the power structures operating behind the prioritisation of some bodies with respect to others and the renewed force with which the social rhetoric around "immunity" has come to blur the boundaries between Western and Oriental forms of medicine. In so doing, Mitra emphasises the ethical issues surrounding vaccination of children under the neo-liberal market forces in the age of globalisation with Big Pharma as a leading force in determining life and death issues in the times of pandemic. And yet, vaccination cannot ensure holistic wellness as it cannot always restore mental wellness. Since Mental Asylums were the preservers of mental wellness and wellbeing, A. Chatterjee in "Spaces of Confinement or

Cure? Inside the Walls of the Mental Asylums of the 19th Century" investigates the nineteenth-century public asylums of England, supposed to be the most successful effort to provide humanitarian care. Keeping in mind Kathleen Jones's *Lunacy Law and Conscience*, she argues that these institutions or corrective houses which were built with such high ideals and motives hardly lived up to its promise. For this, she explores different case studies and shows how many of these psychiatric asylums constructed as part of the social and economic reform movements were "dystopian" spaces, built as part of state-guided "sanitary" movement which sought to eliminate all forms of aberrant figures, poor, criminal, and chaotic voices from the social fabric to maintain harmony, decorum, and order. Covid-19 uncertainty, the breeding ground of the present project, can't afford to leave out Zizek's wondering aloud with the world in his handbook on pandemic. Bhar's "*Žižek's Pandemic!*, the 'New Normal' Dilemma and Some Indian Perspectives" deals with the Zizekian encounter with the Covid-19 pandemic that has laid bare the ambivalence of human control over life and death. In doing so, she looks at the Indian Covid-19 situation from a "local" perspective and thereby, restores some of the social and political issues that typify the Indian scene. The chapter concludes with a pledge for the coming together of all humanity to negotiate the pandemic. Within the dynamics of Covid-19 pandemic (during the first and the second wave), India's biopolitical crisis has implication for all global health care systems and policies. It is (absolutely) necessary to question that why was/is India most unwell in the pandemic? The book presents a series of chapters that engages in a productive dissemination of the health systems and policies in contemporary India that might help India and the world to avoid people gasping and begging for oxygen on the streets (for Covid-19 is here to stay).

Chakraborty in "Livelihood of Internal Migrants of India during Covid-19 Pandemic: Concerns and Measures" presents forthwith the unrecorded livelihood of the internal migrants of India, undoubtedly the most vulnerable class. As nationwide lockdown, in 2020, forced these destitute and marginalised people to reverse migrate to their respective native places, they came across various inhuman experiences as well as existential crises mostly due to mismanagement. Until this pandemic, little emphasis was given by the policy makers to the state of wellbeing of these internal labour migrants of India though they have been termed as the modern "city-makers." Chakraborty therefore investigates the status involving challenges and difficulties faced by the internal migrants of India during the Covid-19 pandemic and critically analyses the measures taken by both central and state governments to elevate their living standards. Roy's "Federalism and Intergovernmental Coordination during a Pandemic: A Special Reference to India" productively problematises the idea of federalism to identify the most appropriate form of governance in complex, multi-ethnic countries like India. Roy focuses on the necessities of federalism and intergovernmental cooperation in crisis management in the context of health emergency imposed by the worldwide outbreak of Covid-19. When solidarity and cooperation is very crucial for the survival of humankind, Roy examines the status of union-state relations in India in combating the Covid-19 pandemic to offer possibilities of intergovernmental cooperative relations as laid down in the Indian Constitution. Equally important is the role played by the media during the pandemic crisis in developing countries like India. Sen and Farooq in "Hate in the times of Covid-19: Can We Blame the Print Media in India?" – using primary machine learning-based textual analysis – show how in India, anxieties over coronavirus became grounds for violence, discrimination, and misinformation campaigns against the Muslims, who constitute 14.2 per cent of the population. Without engaging in a critical study of the Indian health systems, it is not possible to adequately interpret the cause of India's failure in handling the present crisis. Bagchi's chapter "Neo Liberal Turn in the Domain of Health Care: The Emergence of Corporate Health Care Sector in India" therefore highlights the neo-liberal policies in India and their subsequent impact on the private health care sector which has been corporatised significantly over the years. In this context, she notices a shift to surplus extraction without welfare, strengthening public and private sector links and subsidising the private sector, and commoditising health care in the *Liberalisation Privatisation and Globalisation* phase in India. In the package of "Reforms" of the public health care sector, the government appears to invite the entry of the private capital deliberately and skilfully within the peripheries of the public health care services. In doing so, she also questions the ethical issues of the medical profession.

Writers and filmmakers represent their many concerns about the causes, consequences, and effects of disease on humans and nature. As their concerns, approaches, and methods of representing disease differ, their understanding of health and wellness are diverse, being shaped by indigenous cultural settings, individual subject positions and imaginations, and distinct narrative strategies. Real and imagined diseases appear in plays, novels (including autobiographies), folk narratives, Partition narratives, life narratives, and films. They visibilise the undocumented eternal human concern about disease and wellness of the unheard or repressed voices of the world. Sen Gupta's "Disease and the Desire for Health in Shakespeare's *Macbeth*" is set against the backdrop of early modern England wherein puritanical living standards repeatedly identified the theatre with contagion. The public theatres, in an age less concerned about hygiene than ours, were possible sites for the manifestation and spread of bodily diseases. As several plays of the period mention or suggest specific diseases or use the rhetoric of disease and contagion to construct metaphors for the ill health of individuals or/ and the state, Sen Gupta takes up Shakespeare's *Macbeth* and critically examines not only the representations of sickness in the play but also the play's articulation of the desire for good health. This articulation, frequently ignored, is significant, like similar articulations elsewhere in Shakespeare and his contemporaries. Sen Gupta argues that the desire for health and wellness in *Macbeth*, perhaps deliberately designed by the playwright to repudiate misgivings against the theatre, could be similarly contagious and temper the rhetoric of sickness that pervades the play. In doing so, he asserts that the very complex dynamics of sickness and health in *Macbeth*, produced by the reciprocity of play and audience, with the material conditions of the early modern theatre factored in, are eventually lost in modern-day performances and acts of reading. Set in the times of the bubonic play, Das's "Their Mother's Gardens: Epidemic, Healing and Motherhood in *A Year of Wonders* and *Hamnet*" uses epidemics as a tool to decode the power relations within a society whereby the malaise in the body natural often foregrounds the dis-eases in the body politic. Das, here, explores how the themes of disease, motherhood, and healing with the help of traditional medicines are intertwined in Geraldine Brooks' *A Year of Wonders* (2001) and Maggie O' Farrell's *Hamnet* (2020). Through the perspectives and voices of Anne Frith and Agnes Shakespeare – bereaved mothers both – Das establishes and explores the tradition of herbal medicine and healing practices, the art of which is transmitted from one generation of women to another creating an exclusively matrilineal mode of knowledge. Epidemics do not discriminate based on gender, class, or race, but access to medicines and healing often does. In both the novels, Das identifies, the passage of a community from disease to wellness which is accompanied by a corollary movement from dis-eased relationships to relatively healthier ones by accommodating and acknowledging the important role played by women in societal and personal relationships in sickness and in health. A similar search for alternate healing practices – but indigenous and undocumented – is traced by N. Chatterjee in "'stand aside death…today is my day': Contextualising the Naga Esotericism in Kire's Novels" in the context of the Naga Tribe. She takes up Angami Kire's folk tales and people stories to revive and narrativise the hermetic tropes of epiphany, mystery, and initiation through Naga indigenous mythic vision and spiritual intelligence, strategically couched in Kire's metaphoric language of vivid sensuous images. In the present pandemic dystopia, Chatterjee situates Kire's esoteric references to wellness which Kire evokes in the context of historical, political, and environmental uncertainties of the Naga tribes, and connects them to the present crises, wherein individual or/and community wellbeing is/are at stake.

Partition of states has diseased human lives for centuries but has not stimulated serious academic attention. The 1947 Partition of British India – offshoot of British colonialism – carried out along religious lines, triggered an avalanche of disease in the region. Basu in "Dis-ease, Dis-order and the Refugee Experience: Appraising South Asian Partition Narratives" restores the lived lives of the people who were not killed, abducted, raped, and mutilated in the cataclysm but were helpless bearers of sickness on account of physically strenuous journeys during the migration process across newly demarcated international borders, compounded by lack of proper food and potable water. As a result, they became easy victims of a host of diseases, leading to further loss of lives. D. Basu takes up three not so popular and yet significant short stories – "The Crystal Goblet" by Ritwik Ghatak, "Ya Khuda" by Qudrat Ullah Shahab and "Hope" by Mohinder Singh Sarna – to visibilise the undocumented plight of those victims of Partition who thronged for months the refugee camps where the governments (in both India and Pakistan) proved quite inadequate in providing relief and rehabilitation. D. Basu deep studies the disease and death inflicted refugee convoys and camps to underscore the overall state of disorder in the subcontinent in the aftermath of its fateful vivisection. Marginalised genders are the worst sufferers of the present pandemic crisis. Female and transgender powerlessness and vulnerability in the society call for serious academic engagement in female and transgender wellness. N. Mukherjee in "Always in Search of her Ithaca: Women's Spiritual Wellbeing in *Journey to Ithaca: A Pilgrimage in Search of Identity* and *Eat, Pray, Love: One Woman's Search for Everything*" explores Anita Desai and Elizabeth Gilbert – two twentieth-century female writers – who write "back" to restore women who have been labelled as hysteric and mad, and in doing so, she interrogates the perceived notions of female bodies and minds. Transgenders worldwide, and especially in India, are the "sexual minorities," whose lives matter, and therefore the book presents R. Nair and L. Nair's quest for 'hijra' wellness in "Disjunctured Subjectivities and Corporeal Well-being: Issues of Mobility and Health in Select Transgender Life Narratives from India." They situate the lived lives of the legally recognised "hijras" in select Indian "Hijra" autobiographies in English and investigate the impact of the Covid-19 pandemic on their emotional and physical wellbeing.

Since food is an unfailing medicine needed for mental and physical growth and health, S. Basu in "Sustainable Eating and Wellness: Examining Nutrition Strategies in Barbara Kingsolver's *Animal, Vegetable, Miracle: Our Year of Seasonal Eating* and Ruth Ozeki's *a Year of Meats*," explores the cultural matrix of healthy eating choices. In doing so, she examines certain sustainable strategies of food and nutrition choices at individual level as well as at community level to make us mindful eaters and give us a wellness-based approach to life in the Covid-19 context. Psychiatric, Neurological, and infectious diseases in several films have been brought to public attention. But the present project presents a chapter on the cinematic representations of the sickness in individual and the society explored by film productions of the Macbethian metaphor. Mazumder in "Disease, Wellbeing, and the Idea of Health in Select Cinematic Representations of the Macbeth Metaphor" examines two twenty-first-century adaptations of Macbeth, one Indian, and the other British-French and shows how the Macbeth metaphor is used in these adaptations to allude to the elusiveness of peace and health in our life which in a way also compels us to re-think the notions of disease and health from a cultural perspective. The Macbeth metaphor reminds us that the power lies in us – we become our disease, we become our wellness. Is there a choice? The answer, dear reader, is "blowin' in the wind/ The answer is blowin' in the wind."

Notes

1 World Health Organization (1998), Health Promotion Glossary, Geneva.
2 The definition has been taken from *Encyclopaedia Britannica* accessed from https://www.britannica.com/science/infectious-disease.

References

Bose, Soutik. (2021) "Covid-19: How India Failed to Prevent a Deadly Second Wave", April 19, 2021. https://www.bbc.com/news/world-asia-india-56771766. Accessed on June 13, 2021.

Camfield, Laura and Suzanne M. Skevington. (2008) *On Subjective Well-being and Quality of Life*, London: Sage.

Chakrabarty, Dipesh. (2016) "Humanities in the Anthropocene: The Crisis of an Enduring Kantian Fable." *New Literary History*, 47(2, 3), 377–397.

Chomsky, Noam and David Barsamian. (2005) *Imperial Ambitions: Conversations on the Post–9/11 World: Interviews with David Barsamian*, New York: Metropolitan Books.

Defoe, Daniel. (2010) *A Journal of the Plague Year*, London: OUP.

Diener, Ed and Micaela Y. Chan. (2011) "Happy People Live Longer: Subjective Well Being Contributes to Health and Longevity", *Applied Psychology: Health and Well Being*, 3(1), 1–43.

Foucault, Michel. (1989) *The Birth of Clinic*, New York: Routledge.

Gomez, Rapson and John W. Fisher. (2003) "Domains of Spiritual Well Being and Development and Validation of the Spiritual Well Being Questionnaire", *Personality and Individual Differences*, 35, 1975–1991. https://www.researchgate.net/publication/256499063_Gomez_R_Fisher_JW_2003_Domains_of_spiritual_well-being_and_development_and_validation_of_the_Spiritual_Well-Being_Questionnaire_Personality_and_Individual_Differences_358_1975-1991.   Accessed   on June 14, 2022

Goyal Manu et al. (2020) "The Effect of the COVID-19 Pandemic on Maternal Health due to Delay in Seeking Health Care: Experience from a Tertiary Center", *International Journal of Gynaecology and Obstetrics*, October 31, 2020. https://doi.org/10.1002/ijgo.13457. Accessed on January 2, 2021.

Hays, Jo N. (2005) *Epidemics and Pandemics and Their Impacts on Human History*, Santa Barbara, CA: ABC Clio.

Huber, M. et al. (2011) "How Should We Define Health", *BMJ*, 26(2). https://doi.org/10.1136/bmj.d4163 .

Kapoor, Cheena. (2020) "India: Excessive Focus on Covid-19 Ignores Other Diseases", December 1, 2020. https://www.aa.com.tr/en/asia-pacific/india. Accessed on May 15, 2021.

Lê, Qunh. (2011) *Health and Well Being: A Social Cultural Perspective*, New York: Nova Science Publishers.

Lomas, Tim. (2018) *Translating Happiness: A Cross Cultural Lexicon of Well-Being*, Cambridge: The MIT Press.

Martino, Lina. (2017) *Concepts of Health and Wellbeing*, May 13, 2021. https://www.healthknowledge.org.uk/. Accessed on June 14, 2022.

Mcmillen, Christian W. (2016) *Pandemics: A Very Short Introduction*, London: OUP.

Nutbeam, Don. (1998) "Health Promotion Glossary", *Health Promotion International*, 13(4), 11–36. London: Oxford University Press.

Polychroniou, C.J. (2017) "Noam Chomsky: The US Health System Is an 'International Scandal' — and ACA Repeal Will Make It Worse", Truthout, January 12, 2017. https://truthout.org/articles/noam-chomsky-the-us-health-system. Accessed on February 6, 2021.

Ramazani, Vaheed. (2007) *Writing in Pain: Literature, History and the Culture of Denial*, New York: Palgrave.

Sengupta, Keya. (2016) *Determinants of Health Status in India*, New York: Springer.

Sontag, Susan. (1978) *Illness as Metaphor and AIDS and Its Metaphors*, New York: Picador.

Sontag, Susan. (2003) *Regarding the Pain of Others*, New York: Picador.

Sperry, Len. (2016) *Mental Health and Mental Disorders: An Encyclopedia of Conditions, Treatments and Well-Being*, Santa Barbara, CA: Greenwood.

Wolfe, Nathan. (2011) *The Viral Storm: The Dawn of a New Pandemic Age*, New York: Henry Holt and Sons.

World Health Organisation. (1986) *The 1st International Conference on Health Promotion, Ottawa, 1986.* The Ottawa Charter for Health Promotion. Accessed from https://www. who.int/teams/health-promotion/enhanced-wellbeing/first-global-conference

World Health Organisation. (1948) *The Constituition of the World Health Organisation.* Accessed from https://apps.who.int/gb/bd/PDF/bd47/EN/constitution-en.pdf

Wuthnow, Robert. (2010) *Be Very Afraid the Cultural Response to Terror, Pandemics, Environmental Devastation, Nuclear Annihilation, and Other Threats*, New York: OUP.

Zizek, Slavoj. (2020). *Pandemic!: COVID-19 19 Shakes the World*, London: OR Books.

Section I

Social Science Perspective

2 Colonialism and Disease

Smallpox in the Aboriginal Population

Bill Ashcroft

Disease has always moved with human populations. Whether through trade roots or other forms of social contact the chance of the communication of disease has always been present. Conquest and trade have long been part of human history and records of expansion and trade by land or sea date back thousands of years. But the trade and conquest initiated by European empires in the fifteenth and sixteenth centuries opened up unprecedented opportunities for the spread of disease. The introduction of new diseases in the colonized world was part of a wider pattern of plant, animal, and microbial transfers between Europe and its colonies, one that environmental historian Alfred W. Crosby dubbed the *Columbian Exchange* (2003; Nunn et al. 2010). That exchange was profoundly unequal and continued to be so as colonization advanced. But disease had a particular function in the colonial enterprise related to this unequal exchange, for it simultaneously removed the threat of indigenous resistance while paving the way for the myth of colonial philanthropy (Hewa 1995). Introduced diseases played a major part in the subjugation of colonized peoples, particularly in Australia and the Americas. The catastrophic effect of diseases on indigenous populations has led Crosby to argue that Old World pathogens were the most potent weapon of colonial invasion whether intentional or not

> ...their success provides the most spectacular example of the power of the biogeographical realities that underlay the success of European imperialists overseas. It was their germs, not these imperialists themselves, for all their brutality and callousness, that were chiefly responsible for sweeping aside the indigenes and opening the Neo-Europes to demographic takeover.
>
> (1986, 196)

Aboriginal people had their own diseases, particularly trachoma, but colonization unleashed a virtual tsunami of maladies to which they had no resistance, such as smallpox, measles, diphtheria, whooping cough, chickenpox, bubonic plague, malaria, typhoid fever, cholera, yellow fever, dengue fever, scarlet fever, amoebic dysentery, influenza, and a number of parasitic infestations (Crosby 1986, 198).

However, the story of the colonial introduction of disease into indigenous populations has much more subtle and long-lasting implications. Disease became an

DOI: 10.4324/9781003300762-3

opportunity to perpetuate the civilizing mission: having introduced diseases and nearly wiping out indigenous people, colonial powers then proceeded to "save" them through medical interventions such as vaccination, hygiene directives, and hospitalization. Disease, and particularly smallpox, was not only the most devastating consequence of colonial incursion, and not only did it serve the strategy of the civilizing mission, but can also be seen to be metonymic of colonialism in its various stages. Disease is a specific consequence that represents the whole spectrum of the colonial impact on indigenous societies. The story of smallpox in Australia offers a microcosm of the lasting effects of colonial invasion – the disappearance of whole language groups, the attempts to explain away causes, the possible weaponization of disease, and the implementation of vaccination as a strategy of control. These are just some of the ways in which disease, and the smallpox epidemic in particular, demonstrates the calamitous social and cultural effects of colonial invasion. After the initial devastation of introduced diseases, the effects of colonization continue even to the present. With the introduction of sugar, alcohol, and flour, the Aboriginal population today displays epidemic levels of diabetes, obesity, and alcoholism.

Virgin Soil

There is a heated argument in the debate about the link between colonialism and disease that revolves around the idea of indigenous societies as "virgin soil" predisposed to devastation by foreign pathogens. Few scholars would challenge the Columbian Exchange as a model but "virgin soil" is another matter because it carries overtones of eugenic attitudes about racial "weakness." Suzanne Alchon argues that the historical narrative has "swung too far in the direction of disease," minimizing the impact of "the disruption of day-to-day activities that ultimately undermined the demographic resilience" of colonized peoples (2003, 144). Several critics believe that much of the culpability of colonization has been shifted onto germs rather than the actions of invaders (Cameron et al. 2015).

Virgin soil has been employed for more than a century to describe disease outbreaks among previously unexposed populations, resulting in high morbidity and mortality. But Paul Kelton has argued that historians give germs "more agency than they deserve" (2015, 199). The result is that "the actions of the colonizers in destroying the health and well-being of the Natives become forgotten" (215). In the colonial Southeast United States – Kelton's area of expertise – some of the worst epidemics came in the wake of warfare and enslavement, both widespread in the region. Ongoing colonial violence made it difficult for Native groups to recover. David S. Jones took the critique further, characterizing virgin soil "theory" as teleological. and biologically determinist, a way of rationalizing the disproportionate suffering of Native peoples (Jones 2003, 712). He characterizes virgin soil as a construction that justifies colonial conquest and puts the blame on native peoples themselves. Instead of highlighting the "irresistible genetic and microbial forces" that reinforce a narrative of Native decline, Jones argued, historians ought to shed light on the ways that "social forces and human agency shaped" epidemiological processes. After all, such epidemics may have been caused by the "same forces of poverty, social stress, and environmental vulnerability that cause epidemics in all other times and places" (705).

The actions of colonizers cannot be hidden behind virgin soil, as Archer declares

> The destruction and subjugation of Native American peoples by newcomers and their governments was a moral catastrophe. In some cases, it was outright genocide. The perpetrators were Europeans, then Americans, who used disease and other vulnerabilities as a cudgel against Natives. Euro-Americans drove Native Americans from their homelands, exploited them in trade, played Native groups off one another, broke up families, violated treaties, imprisoned them on reservations, and hounded, cheated, and terrorized them across much of the contemporary United States. Yet for all that, the study of disease and health in the Native American past matters and needs to be integrated into our broader narratives of colonialism and North American history.
>
> (2016, 514)

From about 1770, the indigenous peoples of California, Hawaii, New Zealand, and southeast Australia – separated by thousands of miles of open sea and invaded by quite different colonizers – contracted the same new communicable diseases, with similar effects on lifespan, fertility, and infant mortality, and all reaching roughly the same population nadir (as a percentage of precontact population) in the same decade. No matter the source of the infection the overarching narrative is that colonial incursion led to extraordinary, often shattering decimation of indigenous peoples.

The virgin soil hypothesis also corresponds to the "dying race" myth prevalent in Australia in the nineteenth century. After the second epidemic of 1830 references to smallpox among Aborigines coincided with the belief that they were dying out. Most widely known was Daisy Bates' dedication to "smoothing the dying pillow" of a race doomed to extinction (Bates 1944). This term was introduced in 1860 when a Chief Protector was appointed to watch over the interests of Aboriginal people and to "smooth the dying pillow," after which similar legislation was passed in all states. In the nineteenth century, the smallpox experience seemed to suggest a natural law whereby Aborigines could contract disease from whites but not vice versa. By the end of the nineteenth century Tidswell (1898, 1060) suggested that "race tolerance" of the stronger white race had protected them from smallpox. Discussion of Aboriginal disease slid effortlessly into eugenic myths of racial susceptibility, coinciding with some astonishing racial myths developing in Britain in the late nineteenth century.[1] In a strange way the "virgin soil" theory becomes the first stage in perpetuating the discourse of the civilizing mission. Resting upon a basic fallacy of the inherent weakness of indigenous peoples, it opens the way for the perpetuation of the fallacy of the benefits of colonization and the enlightenment intervention of imperial agents.

Smallpox

Until the advent of variolation in the 1780s smallpox accounted for 10–12 per cent of all deaths in Europe. It was, until 1977 when the World Health Organization declared it eradicated, one of the world's most dreaded plagues. Smallpox is an acute, highly infectious viral disease with an incubation period of from 10 to 16 days. It is characterized by a three-day fever which is followed by a general eruption of blisters all over the body but especially on the face, arms and legs. These blisters quickly become pus-filled though, for those who recover, they begin to dry after about eight days, allowing infected people to carry the disease long distances, infecting many more. Smallpox has been by far the most catastrophic of introduced diseases. The virus was first introduced to the Americas around 1518 and "played as essential a role in the advance of white imperialism overseas as gunpowder" (Crosby 1986, 200).

Smallpox reached Europe no later than the sixth century, and by that time, the disease, caused by the variola virus, had spread across Africa and Asia. In Europe, the most common form of smallpox killed perhaps 30 per cent of its victims while blinding and disfiguring many others. But the effects were far worse in the Americas, which had no exposure to the virus prior to the arrival of Spanish and Portuguese conquistadors. It not only exterminated between a third and a half of the Arawaks on Espanola and the populations of Puerto Rico and the Caribbean, but it also decimated the Aztecs and the Incas. Smallpox "did the work of colonial genocide well in advance of the invading armies" (Crosby 1986, 201). The first *recorded* epidemic of smallpox in British or French North America erupted among the Algonkins of Massachusetts in the early 1630s: "Whole towns of them were swept away, in some not so much as one soul escaping Destruction" (Duffy 1951, 327). By the eighteenth century, it had destroyed at least half of the indigenous population between Mexico and throughout the Americas, tribe after tribe suffered near obliteration.

The Columbian Exchange was lop-sided in every way, but most unequal in the exchange of pathogens, an imbalance that worked heavily in the favor of the invaders. Tropical diseases did not travel well, particularly into the colder less humid conditions of Europe, but diseases such as smallpox, measles, influenza, and whooping cough entered Australia and the Americas, followed later by insect-borne diseases such as yellow fever and malaria. Venereal syphilis appears to have made the return voyage aboard Columbus' ships.

Aboriginal Smallpox

Smallpox spread across Australia with the advance of European settlement, bringing with it shocking death rates. It affected entire generations of the Indigenous population and survivors were in many cases left without family or community leaders. The spread of smallpox in three separate epidemics (Campbell 1983, 2002), was followed by influenza, measles, whooping cough, tuberculosis, and sexually transmitted diseases, against which Australia's Aboriginal people had no resistance and all of which brought widespread death.

According to Bennett, the epidemic at Sydney Cove in 1789 was

> one of the most significant events in Australian history...
>
> The smallpox epidemic broke out in April 1789, 15 months after the First Fleet arrived to establish a penal colony in NSW. Since most of the British colonists had been exposed to the virus at some point, they were not affected. It killed large numbers of Aborigines, locally and further afield, and had a catastrophic impact on their capacity to resist British expansion.
>
> (Bennett 2009, 39)

What is remarkable about this is that the early encounters with Aboriginal people suggest that they were envied for their physical well-being. In 1770, Joseph Banks wrote that

> On their bodies we observed very few marks of cutaneous disorders as scurf, scars of sores, etc. Their spare thin bodies indicate a temperance in eating, the consequence either of necessity or inclination, equally productive of health particularly in this respect.
>
> (Campbell 2002, 1)

Later George Worgan, naval surgeon on the First Fleet's *Sirius* also observed that the Aborigines enjoyed a high standard of health. Epidemiologist Francis Black reported, "In large measure modern advances can do no more than return to us the state of health mankind enjoyed 10,000 years ago" (Campbell 2002, 2).

The effect on the Aboriginal population was both swift and terrible. It was "more deadly, more bewildering, more devastating than we, who live in a world free of smallpox can only vaguely comprehend." (Campbell 2002, 2) David Collins, Judge Advocate of the colony recorded the experience of Arabanoo

> In 1789 they were visited by a disorder that raged among them with all the appearance and virulence of the small-pox. The number that it swept off, by their own accounts, was incredible. At that time a native [Arabanoo] was living with us; and on our taking him down to the harbor to look for his former companions, those who witnessed his expression and agony can never forget either. He looked anxiously around him in the different coves we visited; not a vestige on the sand was to be found of human foot; the excavations in the rocks were filled with the putrefying bodies of those who had fallen victims to the disorder; not a living person was any where to be met with. It seemed as if, flying from the contagion, they had left the dead to bury the dead. He lifted up his hands and eyes in silent agony for some time; at last he exclaimed, 'All dead! All dead!' and then hung his head in mournful silence, which he preserved during the remainder of our excursion.
>
> (Collins 1798, 147)

Several Aboriginal people were well known to the colonists and Bennelong reported that his friend Colbe's tribe had been reduced to just three persons and had to unite with another tribe, not only for their protection but also to avoid the extinction of their tribe. It was clear from the beginning that the outbreak was not limited to the Sydney region. Watkin Tench, a military officer with the First Fleet, hints at its rapid spread in Australia and throughout the country.

> ...a native, from his canoe, entered into conversation with us, and immediately after paddling to us with a frankness and confidence which surprised everyone. He was a man of middle age, with an open cheerful countenance, marked with the smallpox, and distinguished by a nose of uncommon magnitude and dignity.
>
> (Tench 1793)

William Bradley, after whom Bradleys Head is named, wrote:

> From the number of dead natives found in every port of the harbour... the small pox has made dreadful havoc amongst them. We...were told that scarce any [Aborigines] had been seen lately except lying dead in and about their miserable habitations whence it appears that they are deserted by their companions as soon as the disorder comes out on them, or whether they were strangers to it before is doubtful.
>
> (Wright 1987, 47)

The disease, called by Aboriginal people *gal-gal-la,* spread from the Sydney area to surrounding tribes and preceded white men across the Blue Mountains. Wherever it struck tribes were decimated. Those among whom the death rate was highest were the children and the aged – the custodians and the future custodians of law and knowledge. Even before the colonizers dispossessed the people they were battling against the collapse of society as they knew it, in a period of a few weeks, more than half of a tribe could die of a strange and awful disease never experienced before.

The most curiously persistent aspect of the epidemic has been the subtle perpetuation of the discourse of colonialism in some historians' reluctance to confirm its origin in the settlement at Sydney Cove and the emergence of a variety of explanations of its origin. We might argue that this is yet another aspect of the mythic discourse of the civilizing mission. Early in the twentieth century EC Stirling and JB Cleland suggested that the 1789 outbreak of smallpox might have originated from Asian seafarers arriving in northern Australia, the contention being that smallpox was delivered to Northern Australia by Macassan trepang fishermen. However, the chance of it making its way across Australia to Sydney Cove in 1789 is extremely remote. According to Campbell, "The balance between Aboriginal and microparasites was almost certainly undisturbed by contact with other humans, and any alien diseases they carried, until the eighteenth century" (1983, 9). Another argument against the introduction of the virus by the First Fleet concerns the ability of variolus material to survive in hot temperatures. However, the strongest, although energetically contested theory, is that variolus matter brought to the settlement by the fleet surgeon escaped either accidentally or on purpose. Warren argues that

> There is little doubt that smallpox scabs collected in 1787 handled professionally, would have retained significant viral activity for more than two years. King's 1792 request to Banks indicates King had no concerns about a voyage damaging the virus. Combined with the very low dosage for infection this demonstrates that if deployed in significant quantities (ie bottles), the First Fleet's smallpox could infect highly susceptible people such as local Aborigines around Port Jackson sometime before April 1789.
>
> (Warren 2007, 160)

The use of glass bottles as containers, presumably sealed, suggests some effort to control humidity which was deleterious to variolus matter. It remains a moot point how long the virus, in the form of dried lymph, would have remained live in such a container. Dr. James Kirkpatrick, a champion of variolation on both sides of the Atlantic, reported success in 1757 with the virus that had been dried on a thread and stored in a phial almost six years previously (Kirkpatrick 1761, 212–213). It was probably recognized that the variola virus survived longest in actual scabs.

The Weaponization of Disease

While the identification of various sources of smallpox in the colony exists, there is a more sinister possibility, that the presence of a marine detachment under attacks from Aboriginal parties and exposed by depleted arms and ammunition could have adopted a well-tried tactic and released smallpox material intentionally. This strategy is far from unknown and there is much evidence of the weaponization of disease in history (Gone 2014; Lindsay 2012; Madley 2016; Riedel 2005). One example dates back to 1348 is when the Tartars catapulted the corpses of plague victims over the walls of the citadel of the Crimean city of Caffa (now Theodosia) causing plague to flare up among the Christians. There are written records from the French-Indian war in North America in 1763 that the French considered sending smallpox-contaminated blankets and handkerchiefs to the native Indians, but it is not clear whether or not this actually happened. Nevertheless, the practice drew widespread condemnation and was banned in the Declaration of St Petersburg in 1868, the forerunner of the Hague Conference in 1907.

Certainly, the decimation of indigenous peoples worked in favor of the colonial invaders. John Winthrop, first governor of Massachusetts Bay Colony and a lawyer by training, noted on 22 May 1634, "For the natives, they are neere all dead of small Poxe, so as the Lord hathe cleared our title to what we possess" (Crosby 1986, 20). In many cases, the devastation was so great that colonial invasion could proceed with little opposition. When the French penetrated the hinterlands of the Gulf of Mexico where the Spanish had already introduced smallpox, one of the French wrote, "Touching these savages, there is a thing that I cannot omit to remark to you, it is that it appears visibly that God wishes that they yield their place to new peoples" (Crosby 1986, 215). There is evidence that early settlers in Australia distributed infected blankets along with poisoned flour to attempt to eradicate the Aboriginal population.

Warren proposes that the intentional infection of Aboriginal people was more than a remote possibility. Phillip was having trouble with Aboriginal attacks on convicts. In August 1788, Phillip's secretary, David Collins, reported that the "natives continued to molest our people whenever they chanced to meet any of them straggling and unarmed" (1798, 32). There were violent incidents over food, such as over fish, or when Aborigines threatened settlers who tried to stop them from appropriating a goat. Aborigines continued to attack convicts and during November Aborigines attacked a fishing party Watkin Tench, noted that "unabated animosity" now prevails between the Aborigines and First Fleeters (1793, 137). In the same month, an anonymous female convict, bypassing local censorship, wrote that the Aborigines "do us all the injury they can... I know not how many of our people have been killed" (Anon 1788, 747).

The grim nature of the settlement's security has given rise to the distinct possibility that other means than arms might be needed to protect the settlement. The First Fleet was supplied with a detachment of marines for protection. However, the marines' capacity proved inadequate as they ran out of ammunition and were short of manpower. Through some error, the marines left Portsmouth without armorer's tools to prepare their flintlocks and they did not leave with enough ammunition. Phillip expected to get replacements at Rio de Janeiro but this did not eventuate. In general, single-load flintlocks were no more effective than native weapons in a sudden attack. In February 1789, a party of 15 with only 3 muskets was overwhelmed by "a great number of armed men." With depleted stocks of weapons and ammunition, the settlement at least felt exposed to attack. In these circumstances says Warren "it is reasonable to consider whether some marines, worrying over their predicament and fearing a catastrophe, used bottles of smallpox to protect themselves and the settlement" (2014, 73).

By the 1770s, it appears that deploying smallpox had been an irregular military tactic for some time. Writing in the Journal of American History, Elizabeth Fenn demonstrated that British commanders used smallpox against North American Indian tribes in 1763 (Fenn 2000). Using smallpox was promoted in a military tract of the period, Major Robert Donkin's Military Collections and Remarks (1777). As Donkin served with the marines, he and some First Fleet marines possibly crossed paths in North America or elsewhere. However, any group of settlers able to take boats out of Sydney Cove could have deployed smallpox, including any informal group of senior marines without being noticed by Tench, Collins, or Phillip.

Both colonial records and Eora tradition suggest that an area around Balmoral in Sydney's Middle Harbour was ground zero for the smallpox outbreak among the Aborigines. As Warren concludes,

> Deployment may have been a private act by senior marines, possibly with assistance from a convict with access to medical supplies or, more likely, a surgeon. Given their dire predicament, the marines may have considered they had no choice than to send smallpox into the camps of their adversaries. If the Fleet had been supplied with sufficient military force and all necessary equipment, smallpox may never have been released.
>
> (2014, 79)

Medicine and health in the colonies developed from the colonist''s need to look after its own troops and civil servants to extending this largesse first to those who worked for the colonial powers and then to the whole of the population. This was not initially wholly altruistic and it was realized that health could be a tool of empire.

Vaccination

Medicine played and continues to play a significant role in the colonial strategy of conciliation and became a central feature of the civilizing mission through which the colonizers could claim to be introducing modern health practices to the indigenous people. Phillip ordered that two sick Aborigines be brought into the settlement so that "the knowledge of our humanity, and the benefits we might render them, would, it was hoped, do away the evil impressions they had received of us" (Collins 1798 n2, 53). The colonists needed to confirm the diagnosis and "The only clinical test in doubtful cases was to inoculate another person with lymph from the patient's pustules. This procedure would also serve as a first step in a general inoculation (variolation) of the susceptible population" (Bennett 2009, 43).

In general, colonial health policies arose from the desire to protect troops and civil servants from exotic diseases but it became clear that the health of the indigenous people was also important, first because they might serve as sources of infection for the colonists and, second, because disease caused economic loss in the colonial enterprise. The main purpose of the different types of health schemes developed in various countries was to ensure "health for all", but there were a number of hidden agendas including rendering the country suitable for Europeans to inhabit and to civilize the indigenous populations. In short, health was a tool of empire (Ahuja 2016). The bizarre possibility that genocidal practices by the marines existed side by side with, or preceded, medical treatment, is a paradox that lies at the heart of the colonial enterprise. Having established health systems on purely pragmatic grounds the colonial powers then turned to altruism (Hewa 1995) and devoted considerable energy to the eradication and control of diseases of importance only to the indigenous people after they, the colonists, had departed (Cox 2007).

But vaccination offers an interesting perspective on the colonial enterprise:

> Vaccination crossed and dissolved the boundary between the clean and the diseased in an altogether different logic to segregation and quarantine. Moreover, in the colonial context, the 'foreignness' of these foreign bodies was not only a biological reference but often a racial reference, as 'lymph' (as the vaccine matter was called) circulated through many populations of children, literally linking them across the globe.
>
> (Bashford 2003, 16)

The arrival of smallpox and the introduction of cowpox in southeast Australia can be seen as related episodes, historically and virologically, and as mutually informing. Both variola (smallpox) and *vaccinia* (cowpox) had to conquer the great distances of Australian space. Variolation offered some protection to people in the face of the disease, but the diffusion of the practice, involving the transport of smallpox virus in dried or scab form, always had the potential to cause new outbreaks. Unlike variola, *vaccinia* (chickenpox) was a mild infection, found only in parts of western Europe. It was nonetheless a disease; and vaccination can be regarded, in Alison Bashford's words, "as a kind of colonial contagion, as the deliberate circulation and proliferation of contagious matter along the imperial lines, and across the colonial borders of trade, travel and migration" (2003, 15). It was the European practice of variolation, however, that anticipated this role. The rapid progress of vaccination depended on prior experience with variolation, including techniques for the preservation and transport of the lymph. Vaccination has become a major public health initiative. But Bashford shows how vaccination, as an essentially "polluting procedure," did not align wholly with the concerns of the sanitary state and imperial hygiene, and how quarantine better served the needs of Australia at the time of Federation (2003, 33).

By the late eighteenth century, Europeans were making increasing use of inoculation both at home and in colonial settings (Bennett 2009, 42). But resistance to variolation arose from the fact that it involved the introduction of smallpox into previously unaffected districts. Although the British surgeons didn't usually carry samples of smallpox scabs, Watkin Tench, an officer in the marines, reports that the British surgeons on the convict transports to Botany Bay in 1787–1788 carried "variolous matter in bottles" (Tench 1793, 146). So smallpox in some form arrived in Australia with the First Fleet in 1788 both as a source of infection and a source of vaccination. The Covid-19 pandemic in the twenty-first century has confirmed the value of vaccination and the heroic efforts of biochemists to produce vaccines in record time. But there are distinct echoes of the function of vaccination to the colonial enterprise as governments applaud themselves for "protecting" their populations regardless of the incompetence and disorganization with which it has been carried out. More pertinently, the distribution of vaccines throughout the world now mirrors the inequities of colonial history with rich nations buying up available vaccines and poor nations remaining vulnerable. In May 2021, Dr. Tedros Adhanom Ghebreyesus, the head of the World

Health Organization, said that "the world is in vaccine apartheid" (May 2021). Health is still a tool of empire, and empires must re-learn the lesson that if the poor are infected all remain vulnerable.

Conclusion

Smallpox has now been eradicated, but colonialism remains, both as political policy and in its grim effects upon indigenous health and culture. In 1977, the World Health Organization declared an end to the virus, the most astounding achievement in public health in history. But the consequences of colonialism remain in indigenous societies to this day. The smallpox epidemic that decimated the Eora people in 1789 demonstrates very clearly the relationship between colonial invasion and disease. It was from the beginning a more potent weapon than gunpowder in overwhelming the indigenous inhabitants of Australia and the Americas. Whether intentionally or not it became a crucial element in colonial control, both in its disastrous effects on invaded peoples and in its confirmation of the myth of the civilizing mission. The virgin soil of people without immunity supported the racist myths of the strength of the white races. It paved the way for the civilizing mission as the colonial powers which had done so much to destroy indigenous culture proceeded to "save" the colonized with the program of vaccination and public hygiene. The course of the smallpox epidemic, its effects on indigenous populations, and eventual eradication remains a metaphor for the course of colonial appropriation. Both smallpox and colonialism have left a legacy in the health and cultural disruption of indigenous peoples that has never been repaired. But the principle of hope remains. While indigenous healers have adapted some forms of Western medicine to their traditional practices, creative writers and artists have similarly seized the means of representation by taking hold of the colonizers' language, literature, painting, and sculpture. While the grim consequences of colonialism remain in the cultural, political, and economic structure of the world, the spirit of indigenous peoples in appropriating colonial technologies confirms the resilience of decolonizing societies.

Note

1 In 1885, John Beddoe, president of the Anthropological Institute, had developed an "index of Nigrescence" that showed the people of Wales, Scotland, Cornwall and Ireland to be racially separate from the British. More specifically, he argued that those from Western Ireland and Wales were "Africanoid" in their "jutting jaws" and "long slitty nostrils," and thus originally immigrants of Africa (Szwed 1975, 20–21).

Works Cited

Ahuja, Neel. 2016. *Bioinsecurities: Disease Interventions, Empire, and the Government of Species.* Durham, NC and London: Duke University Press.
Alchon, Suzanne Austen. 2003. *A Pest in the Land: New World Epidemics in a Global Perspective.* Albuquerque: University of New Mexico Press.

Anon. 1788. Letter from a Female Convict, November 14, in *Historical Records*, vol. 2.

Archer, Seth. 2016. "Colonialism and Other Afflictions." *History Compass*, 14.10: 511–521.

Bashford, Alison. 2003. *Imperial Hygiene: A Critical History of Colonialism, Nationalism and Public Health*. London: Palgrave Macmillan Limited.

Bates, Daisy. 1944. *The Passing of the Aborigines: A Life Spent among the Natives of Australia*. London: J. Murray.

Bennett, Michael J. 2009. "Smallpox and Cowpox under the Southern Cross: The Smallpox Epidemic of 1789 and the Advent of Vaccination in Colonial Australia." *Bulletin of the History of Medicine*, 83.1 (Spring): 37–62.

Cameron, Catherine M., Paul Keltom and Alan C. Swedlund, eds. 2015. *Beyond Germs: Native Depopulation in North America*. Tucson: University of Arizona Press.

Campbell, Judy. 1983. "Smallpox in Aboriginal Australia, 1829–31." *Historical Studies*, 20.81: 536–556.

Campbell, Judy. 2002. *Invisible Invaders: Smallpox and Other Diseases in Aboriginal Australia*. Carlton: Melbourne UP.

Collins, David. 1798. *Sydney's First Four Years n. 9. pp. 146–49. Historical Records of New South Wales*, vol. 1, part 2, pp. 298–299.

Collins, David. 1975. *An Account of the English Colony of New South Wales*, 2 vols., ed. Brian H. Fletcher. Sydney: Reed in association with the Royal Australian Historical Society, 1.

Cox, Frank. 2007. "Conquest and Disease of Colonialism and Health? Special Lecture to mark the Centenary Royal Society of Tropical Medicine and Hygiene." Transcript. https://www.gresham.ac.uk/lectures-and-events/conquest-and-disease-or-colonialism-and-health.

Crosby. Alfred. 1986. *Ecological Imperialism: The Biological Expansion of Europe 900–1900*. Cambridge: Cambridge UP.

Crosby, Alfred. 2003. *The Columbian Exchange: Biological and Cultural Consequences of 1492*. Westport, CT: Praeger.

Donkin, Major Robert. 1777. *Military Collection and Remarks*. New York: H. Gaine.

Duffy, John. 1951. "Smallpox and the Indians in the American Colonies." *Bulletin of the History of Medicine*, 25: 324–341.

Fenn, Elizabeth A. 2000. "Biological Warfare in Eighteenth-Century North America: Beyond Jeffery Amherst." *Journal of American History*, 86.4: 1553f.

Ghebreyesus, Tedros Adhanom. 2021. "Director-General's opening remarks at Paris Peace Forum Spring Meeting." 17 May. https://www.who.int/director-general/speeches/detail/director-general-s-opening-remarks-at-paris-peace-forum-spring-meeting-17-may-2021.

Gone, J. P. 2014. "Colonial Genocide and Historical Trauma in Native North America: Complicating Contemporary Attributions," in A. Woolford et al. eds. *Colonial Genocide in Indigenous North America*. Durham, NC: Duke University Press: 273–291.

Hewa, Soma. 1995. *Colonialism, Tropical Disease and Medicine: Rockefeller Philanthropy in Sri Lanka*. Lanham MD: University Press of America.

Jones, D. S. 2003. "Virgin Soils Revisited." *William and Mary Quarterly*, 60.4: 703–742.

Jones, D. S. 2015. "Death, Uncertainty, and Rhetoric," in C. M. Cameron et al. eds. *Beyond Germs: Native Depopulation in North America*. Tucson: University of Arizona Press: 16–49.

Kelton, P. 2015. "Remembering Cherokee Mortality During the American Revolution," in C. M. Cameron et al. eds. *Beyond Germs: Native Depopulation in North America*. Tucson: University of Arizona Press: 198–221.

Kirkpatrick James. 1761. *The Analysis of Inoculation: Comprizing the History, Theory, and Practice of It* ..., 2nd ed. London: J. Buckland and R. Griffiths, pp. 212n–213n.

Lindsay, B. C. 2012. *Murder State: California's Native American Genocide, 1846–1873*. Lincoln: University of Nebraska Press.

Madley, B. 2016. *An American Genocide: The United States and the California Indian Catastrophe*. New Haven, CT and London: Yale University Press.

McMillen, C. W. 2008. "'The Red Man and the White Plague': Rethinking Race, Tuberculosis, and American Indians, ca. 1890–1950." *Bulletin of the History of Medicine*, 82.3: 608–645.

Nunn, Nathan and Nancy Quian. 2010. "The Columbian Exchange: A History of Disease, Food and Ideas." *Journal of Economic Perspectives*, 24.2 (Spring): 163–188.

Riedel, Stefan. 2005. "Smallpox and Biological Warfare: A Disease Revisited." *Baylor University Medical Center Proceedings*, 18: 13–20.

Szwed, J.F. 1975. 'Race and the Embodiment of Culture." *Ethnicity*, 2: 19–33.

Tench, Watkin. 1793. *Sydney's First Four Years, Being a Reprint of "A Narrative of the Expedition to Botany Bay" and "A Complete Account of the Settlement at Port Jackson"* by Captain Watkin Tench of the Marines, ed. L. F. Fitzhardinge. Sydney: Angus and Robertson in association with the Royal Historical Society, 1961.

Tidswell, F. 1898. "A Brief Sketch of the History of Smallpox and Vaccination in New South Wales." *Australasian Association for the Advancement of Science*, VII: 1060.

Warren, Christopher. 2007. "'Could First Fleet Smallpox Infect Aborigines?' – A Note." *Aboriginal History*, 31: 152–164.

Warren, Christopher. 2014. "Smallpox at Sydney Cove – Who, When, Why?" *Journal of Australian Studies*, 38:1: 68–86.

Wright, B. 1987. "Aborigines: Was It Smallpox?" *The Australian Journal of Indigenous Education*, 15.5: 52–54.

3 Vaccine Nation and Its Miserables

Bodies and Bio-citizenship in the Empire

Mandira Chakraborty

Dear Vaccine[1]

Save us, dear vaccine.
Take us seriously.
We had plans.
We were going places.
Children in kindergarten.
So many voices, in chorus.
Give us our world again!
Tiny gleaming vials,
enter our cities and towns
shining your light.
Restore us to each other.
We liked our lives.
Maybe we didn't thank them enough.
Being able to cross streets
with people we didn't know,
pressing elevator buttons,
smiling at strangers,
standing in line to pay.
We liked standing in line
more than we pretended.[2]

The Global Vaccine Poem is inspired by Naomi Shihab Nye and her global advocacy for the power of poetry, a collaborative project between the Wick Poetry Center at Kent State University & The University of Arizona Poetry Center (Nye 2020).

The word "virus" has been in circulation for hundreds of years before it started to mean a microorganism with a capacity for evolution and mutation. It was a generic term for anything that spread disease; the Latin neuter *vīrus,* meaning "poison" or any such harmful substance. This has the same root as Sanskrit "विष (viṣá)", and ancient Greek ἰός (iós, "poison, venom"). That poison can drive away poison has been a precept of Ayurvedic medicine since long back.[3]

DOI: 10.4324/9781003300762-4

Tied together with the word "virus," however, is the word "immunity" which has an equally interesting history.

In the West, the concept of immunization goes back to Greek mythology. In the Museum Boijmans Van Beuningen at Rotterdam, Netherlands, hangs Peter Paul Rubens' painting of Thetis immersing Achilles in Styx.[4] With Pluto and Proserpine on both sides of the portico and in between two caryatids Thetis immerses Achilles into the river. Pluto and Proserpina are the rulers of Hades. Thetis grasps Achilles by the heel with her left hand. Clotho, one of the Fates, helps by holding a torch to light up the space while Cerberus, the many-headed watchdog of the nether regions, lies in front. In the background, Charon ferries passengers athwart the river and is plagued by a waiting multitude on the banks, who appeal to him with open hands for passage. Ill-omened bats circle above in the air, forming an attractive frame with their wings (Biss 2014).

This painting is the first in the series from The History of Achilles, which was the last of the four tapestry commissions designed by Rubens. The last tapestry in the series shows Achilles in the throes of death due to an arrow having pierced his heel, with which his mother held him while dipping him into Styx, hence not protected. Typical of Reuben's style is also details like the fire in the sky at the left, the light emanating from the torch, and the heads of the dogs.

Immunity, like immortality, is a contentious issue. Human beings are not so much so individual organisms but an entire ecosystem of organisms, microbial partners that are involved in the development and function of essentially every organ, including the brain. We have more microorganisms in our guts than we have human cells in our bodies, and vastly more bacteriological DNA and genes than anthropoid genes. Graham Rooks[5] proposed an "old friends hypothesis" that states that a child's immunity is not developed by mere exposure to pathogens in early childhood but is a result of microbiota inherited from the mother, passed down from the early days of human evolution as a result of cooperation and communication between humans and pathogens. These are a baby's old friends, and modern lifestyle changes are causing a significant breakdown of this inherited immune system (A.W. Rook 2019). To sum it up all, the evolutionary principle depends on a continuous selection and rejection of the species of pathogens around us. In such an environment, "trust" becomes an important means of negotiation and navigation.

A virus is impossible to avoid. Beginning with civilization and the processes which saw the end of humanity's hunter-gatherer days, the very means of progress have facilitated the circulation of pathogens. Small, isolated groups have given way to large communities, and the increased mobility of humans all over the globe has enabled viruses to spread like never before. Coupled with these opportunities of never-before-possible mobility, modern industrial IT-enabled lifestyles have caused our "old friends" to disappear and us to be vulnerable.

Eula Biss, in "On Immunity: An Inoculation" says:

> Our own adaptive immune system, the branch of our immune system that develops long-lasting immunity, is thought to have borrowed its essential technology from the DNA of a virus. Some of our white blood cells combine

and recombine their genetic material like random number generators, shuffling their sequences to create an immense variety of cells capable of recognizing an immense variety of pathogens. This technology was viral technology before it was ours. Of humans and viruses, the science writer Carl Zimmer says, "There's no us and them."

(Biss 2014)

Another mother's attempts to immunize her children deserve mention; she is Lady Mary Wortley Montagu of Royalty who had variolated her own children, having observed it being done in Constantinople. Lady Mary Wortley who was the wife of the British ambassador to Turkey, provided the first report from an upper class European patient's perspective of the middle-eastern practice of variolation, or ingrafting, to prevent smallpox in a letter written on April 1, 1717, to Sarah Chiswell, a friend Lady Mary Wortley Montagu reports a community inoculation program, much like modern-day U.S. vaccine parties, where 15 or 16 children were inoculated by old women with the help of small-pox pustules in a nutshell (Boylston 2012). But scientific advancements cannot be studied out of context and do not happen in a void. Medicine, much like any other intervention, acquires a political dimension the moment personal health becomes a matter of public concern, hence subject to regulations and legislation.

The history of vaccines and vaccination starts with the first effort to prevent disease in society. It was Louis Pasteur's research in chemistry that led to Pasteur's being called the father of the "germ theory of disease," because he was the first to point out that spoilage of substances was not due to bad air but due to microorganisms present which cause the decay. Pasteur was not, however, the first to suggest methods of prevention as long before him, and even before the source of the disease was understood, prevention had already been reported in the Middle East and India.

Smallpox (like many other communicable diseases together with measles) was well known since ancient times and is believed to have originated in India or Egypt, over 3,000 years ago. Thucydides in 430 BC and Rhazes (also known as Abu Bakr) in 910 AD testified that people who had had smallpox appeared not to have it again. Preliminarily, Abu Bakr also wrote about ways in which measles and smallpox could be distinguished from each other.

During the smallpox epidemic of 1677 in North America, the first medical pamphlet which was published in Boston, "A brief rule to guide the common people of New-England how to order themselves and theirs in the small pocks, or measels" written by Thomas Thacher for instructing the masses into hygienic practices. By then smallpox had already become established in Native American populations, who had had no previous contact with the disease; it would kill an estimated 90 per cent of North America's Native peoples, before the end of the seventeenth century. Even in populations where it was established, smallpox would continue to kill an estimated 400,000 people a year in eighteenth Century Europe alone; with on average one out of every six persons who contracted smallpox dying from it (Porter 1988).

In 1768, way before Edward Jenner inoculated his gardener's son with In Boston in 1721, the Reverend Cotton Mather, best known for his involvement in the Salem Witch trials, would court controversy by pushing for a treatment told to him by his African slave Onesimus, who had been inoculated in Africa as a boy. On June 6, 1721, Mather sent reports on inoculation to local physicians, most viewing inoculation as irreverent, and not in agreement with the natural laws of medicine. Boston doctor, and great uncle of future President John Adams, Dr. Zabdiel Boylston, did successfully try the procedure on his youngest son and two slaves.

On the wall of St. George's medical school library in Tooting hangs the hide of a cow called Blossom, who allegedly gave cowpox to Sarah Nelmes, a milkmaid, thus saving her life. It was common knowledge amongst farmers and rural folk that infection by cowpox made people immune from smallpox, a deadly infectious disease in the eighteenth and nineteenth centuries that killed 20 per cent of the population and infected 60 per cent according to Voltaire. The incidence of immunity of milkmaids was noted by Edward Jenner, apprenticed in surgery and anatomy under Dr. John Hunter, who planted in him the rational spirit of Enlightenment Europe, "Don't think; try."

It was only in 1798, that smallpox vaccination was successfully demonstrated and proved to be effective by Dr. Edward Jenner, leading to smallpox's global eradication in 1980. Thus vaccination, later on, seen to be an extension of the power of the state over an individual's body, became the only route through which it became possible to prevent an epidemic. It is remarkable that Dr. Edward Jenner never patented, and indeed gave away his vaccine samples philanthropically, calling his clinic "The Temple of Vaccinia" (Varavikova 2014).

It is not required to repeat Dr. Edward Jenner's famous feat of the first vaccination nor delve into the bio-ethical issues of conducting a vaccination trial on a clearly uninformed subject, James Phipps, the eight-year-old son of Jenner's gardener, but the world today is divided into vaxxers and anti-vaxxers as it was in 1796, when Jenner introduced vaccination. His was not an isolated achievement because he was preceded by famous people like Louis Pasteur, Robert Koch, and John Hunter. It is interesting to note that Edward Jenner was not new to the concept of ousting unfavorable competition. He had been elected to the Royal Society of Medicine in 1788 following a study observing that the newly hatched cuckoo survives in the host's nest by pushing its host's eggs and other fledglings out of the nest with the help of depression on its back, contrary to the common belief that the adult cuckoo did it. This sensational discovery about brood parasitism was followed by his lifelong obsession with vaccination, using a thorn to pick a thorn as it were.

In India as well as many other countries the practice of variolation by barbers and rural medicine men was long in existence even before surgery was an established discipline in Europe. Writing a detailed account of State medicine operating as a colonial force in India, Professor David Arnold in his book "Colonizing the Body" opines that variolation, an indigenous method operating from as far back as First Century AD in India, necessarily had a religious-cultural aspect. It was not only practiced by a group of men and women who were quasi-medical but they often had religious affiliations, were Brahmins/Non-Brahmins depending on the region where they operated, invoked the goddess "Sitala," a local deity believed to inhabit the victim's body when ill, supplemented their treatments with rituals of invoking the Goddess with a final thanksgiving puja when the heat was abated and treated the sufferer with extreme reverence as a sacred object. Variolation, it appears, had very few discontents. It was a community affair, was rarely dangerous as the practitioners were experts, and was deeply rooted in faith. Vaccination, on the other hand, was imposed on the colonies by the West. Not only was it foreign, but it was also secular and at the time when it was introduced in the colonies it was not as technically advanced as it is today. The greatest disadvantage of vaccination was that the method to transmit live culture had not been perfected and the only sound method of transmitting was through arm-to-arm vaccination, most often through children, who became carriers or live petri dishes so to speak (Arnold 1993).

Much before the use of the cowpox vaccine, Catherine the Great of Russia volunteered to be variolated with smallpox pustules to escape the disease, the first person in Russia to undergo the procedure. And then she immediately declared that anyone who didn't get inoculated was an idiot. She was a pioneer indeed.

Thomas Dimsdale, a British doctor from a family of Quakers, and the Pfizer and Moderna of his day performed the procedure by slicing two or three times into the Queen's arm, grating pustules from a smallpox patient into the open wound. But Catherine, who is famed to have had 22 male lovers in the course of her rule was no frail woman. Should he accidentally kill the Empress, Dimsdale made a point to keep horses ready outside the Russian court, in case a need to escape arose. Fortunately, all went well, and Dimsdale was even named a Baron of the Russian Empire for his trouble. Variolation accidents were indeed statistically low in number and the rewards were rich.

"Vaccination was introduced at a critical moment in the history of colonialism in India," says David Arnold. For a regime but recently established by force of arms and with the struggle against the Marathas still unresolved, vaccination offered a welcome opportunity to give "fresh proof" of the East India Company's "humane and benevolent" intentions toward its subjects, "an additional mark of the fostering care of the British Government" in India. Although the protection of white soldiers and civilians was certainly an immediate consideration in the minds of the colonial authorities, it was not their only or even paramount concern as the governor of Bombay made clear in 1803. In declaring his "great joy" at the successful introduction of vaccination a few months earlier, he remarked that "the prestige that we have achieved by this one act has been the source of much goodwill from the people it is a great reward" (Arnold 1993).

The fact that calf lymph was essential in the science of vaccination failed to douse the skepticism of Indians and court their favor; as Britannia would soon learn mere mention of the holy cow did not bring them to their knees. Vaccination, for entirely different reasons, neither caught up with the Orient nor with the Occident. When Edward Jenner published his findings many Britons in the Eighteenth Century responded likewise to injecting cow-stuff into their bodies.

"The Cow-Pock—or—the Wonderful Effects of the New Inoculation!" by James Gillroy in 1802 showed Edward Jenner vaccinating patients in the small-pox and Inoculation Hospital at St. Pancras and where the patients develop features of cows (Wellcome Library no. 11752i).

Whether or not some bovine feature may be transferred to the body individual through a single needle, there is no denying the fact that there is something bovinely angelic and sacrificial about allowing oneself to be injected by the body politic. In matters of public health obedience matters. Those who are injected become immune. They become safe while becoming carriers now. Those who refuse to be injected are a threat to themselves and to society. To be or not to be a cow became the question with respect to the vaccination.

It is at the precise juncture in history that private wellness is seen as consequential to public health that liberty and individuality become a contested space and issues of assent and dissent acquire political dimensions. Then on, these issues are to be regulated by policy making and legislature. It is in the nature of infectious diseases to highlight the disputed nature of private liberty when pitted against public health. Dorothy Porter and Roy Porter write,

> The Vaccination Acts and the Contagious Diseases Acts suspended what we might call the natural liberty of the individual to contract and spread infectious disease, in order to protect the health of the community as a whole. Both sets of legislation were viewed as infractions of liberty by substantial bodies of Victorian opinion, which campaigned to repeal them. These opponents expressed fundamental hostility to the principle of compulsion and a terror of medical tyranny. The repeal organizations-above all, the Anti Compulsory Vaccination League and the National Association for the Repeal of the Contagious Diseases Acts-were motivated by different sets of social and scientific values. Nevertheless, their activities jointly highlight some of the political conflicts produced by the creation of a public health service in the nineteenth century, issues with resonances for the state provision of health care up to the present day.
>
> (Porter 1988)

In an attempt to explain the emergent logics of power in the late eighteenth and early nineteenth centuries, Michel Foucault in a series of Lectures at Collège de France in 1970 coined the term "Biopolitics" and linked it to "Biopower." Foucault analyzed biopolitics as being accompanied by two other forms of power, sovereignty, and discipline. Whereas sovereignty refers ultimately to a power to take life, and discipline to a form of power directed at training the body, biopolitics concerns the supervision of a population, which in the eighteenth century, became possible for the first time through the development of new logics and techniques that aimed to measure, quantify, classify, and evaluate the immanent characteristics of a given territory. Through the development of new statistical tools and metrics such as birth rates, death rates, census tracts, agricultural outputs and inputs, and figures concerning pestilence, disease, deviancy, and pauperism, human beings were rendered into a field of visibility and intervention, which, in turn, meant that populations and subjects came to understand themselves and their activities through these conditional and random statistical groupings (Means 2021).

It is interesting to note, as Dorothy Porter and Roy Porter write, that when compulsory vaccination was introduced in England in 1853 it followed a report of the Epidemiological Society written about the state of affairs since the passing of the first vaccination Act of 1840 by which free vaccination was to be offered to the poor by the Poor Law Guardians; the same year an extension of the same act outlawed inoculation. The management of compulsory vaccination remained in the hands of the Poor Law Guardians till 1858 after which it was moved to the Local guardians and a Medical Officer of the Privy Council. Compulsory medical intervention targeting a certain class of people based on race, class, gender, sexual orientation, ethnicity, caste, and religion has been the bane of public health policies since the beginning.

In the wake of the rollout of three kinds of vaccines at present, the last being Sputnik from Russia, the race against Covid-19 has gained momentum. In the near future, all citizens of the Vax Nation will require a Covid passport.

Medicine requires its guinea pigs; skewed power structures are conducive to scientific progress because without a willing and uninformed subject there can be no successful scientific experiment. In 1721 an enslaved African man named Onesimus–who may have been born in West Africa was variolated as a child before slave traders brought him to Boston. Once in New England, Onesimus taught his enslaver Cotton Mather the procedure, and Mather effectively persuaded doctors in the Americas of its effectiveness.

The history of medicine cannot be detached from science and its experiments; it is chronologically attuned to the history of colonization. Vaccination and its discontents exist because where there should be a relationship of trust and welfare, there exists a relationship of profiteering and exploitation. Even the Latin root of the word immunity—"munis"—means "service or duty." In the context of democracy, it simply has no meaning (Biss 2014).

On 2nd May 2011, a covert CIA operation masked as a free Hepatitis B vaccination drive for children in an attempt to collect DNA evidence linking Osama bin Laden led to the killing of the world's most wanted terrorist in Abbotabad, Pakistan. While the U.S. rejoiced over justice having been delivered, in Pakistan and adjoining regions the Talibans declared a fatwa on vaccination campaigns and the incident led to an increase in the already existing mistrust about Western charitable programs in developing countries.[6]

Vaccination can make one seriously ill and may result even in death. Such is the nature of all preventive measures in human history where the rhetoric of individual well-being is pitted against public welfare. A vaccine is not a pill which cures a disease. You have to agree to be a little ill in order to avoid being very, very ill or die. The battlefield of inoculation is strewn with the corpses of vaccine volunteers some of whom were uninformed and did not consent. This is the area where medical ethics comes into action and vaccine racism begins.

The world of pharmaceuticals is based on controlled clinical trials. Or at least it is supposed to be based on one. From there it is only one step forward to where one needs willing subjects for medical dilettantism. In Nazi Germany concentration camps were fertile grounds for human experiments of all sorts. When it comes to a developed nation looking for a medical miracle, developing or underdeveloped countries are diamond mines for conducting human trials. The same policy which can conduct espionage in the guise of charitable vaccination programs can conduct unethical human trials in the guise of charitable vaccination drives.

The utilization of prisoners, delinquents, vagabonds, lunatics and even the severely afflicted for scientific research has long been the legacy of twentieth and twenty-first century science as well. It is important to note that surveillance, quarantine, isolation, and vaccination, were all part of the colonial enterprise to curb venereal diseases like syphilis in India. Plans to prevent these diseases from going the epidemic route included the establishment of locked houses for the checking and isolation of "diseased women" who were found to be conjugating with European soldiers and sailors (Mishra 1999).

Not only was VD fatal, but it also entailed substantial amounts of expenses in replacement and recruitment as well as a fear of tainting Occidental "pure" blood with Oriental blood. Keeping in view the demand for such "lock hospitals" which were already in existence in Britain, the Governor-General in Council authorized the building of "hospitals for the reception of diseased women" at Berhampur, Cawnpur(Kanpur), Dinapur, and Fatehgarh. Initially, the Anti-vaccination lobby, at least in Britain were the skeptics who refused to credit the exact science behind vaccination. Edgar M. Crookshank, a distinguished critic of vaccination, not really an anti-vaccinationist, was a proponent of the specific etiology of disease. The first Professor of Bacteriology at King's College London, Crookshank attempted to establish the failure of Jenner's method of vaccination to diminish the epidemic nature of smallpox. In his huge, two-volume study, "Vaccination, its History and Pathology", he questioned the origin of Jenner's lymph and tried to show that the purportedly preventive material had itself been the source of a separate disease, vaccinia, and was responsible for the secondary transmission of syphilis. (Porter 1988) Thus, anti-vaccination did not draw solely upon one single technical outline for its explanations of the failure of vaccination. A re-examination of the rhetoric of the vaccination debate highlights the intricate milieu of values and beliefs at the heart of the politics of compulsory prevention of infectious disease.

While some vaccine skeptics questioned the method and the efficacy of prevention, others talked about the failure of safety protocols and demanded the repeal of the vaccine mandate because the governments never enforced a failproof roll-out system that could ensure accountability, ensuring the individual against any adverse vaccine event. Not only did the individual feel threatened and found the state's encroachment upon personal liberty offensive, at the core of the Anti-vaccination movement is a severe lack of "trust" often expressed towards the executive bodies who were entrusted with the drive of vaccination. Lack of trust and absence of a feedback loop have increased in recent times in the capitalist neo-liberalist economy when a la Foucault, biopolitics has emerged as a key element in the wake of Big Pharma.

In the era of global technology scandals involving human biologies, such as transnational drug testing, organ trade, and surrogacy often make the clinic the space for the transgression of human rights. Official or otherwise, sincere or secretive, incidents often happen in clinics in which aggressive scientific enterprise shamelessly disregards human values. Behind closed doors of state regulated and legally sanctioned spaces, policy makers allow global capital's profiteering goals to exploit the economically poor and vulnerable group (children and women) and override principles of justice. Not only that, but the global traffic in health commodities, including drugs and the biologies they interact with, when examined from the perspective, not of treatment but trial, not the clinic, but the research hospital, has been rampantly exploitative, making guinea pigs out of humans (Lahariya 2014; Rajan 2017).

This unequal and abusive space is exposed by Kaushik Sunder Rajan in "Pharmocracy: Value, Politics, and Knowledge in Global Biomedicine," a masterful study of global pharmaceutical practice as a social and civic process, and Sonia Shah, "Body Hunters: Testing the New Drugs on the World's Poorest Patients." Pharmocracy focuses on the hub of the diverse medicine trade that is India in the post-TRIPS (Trade-Related International Property Rights agreement) era, following WTO-mandated changes to India's medicine patent acts, a verdict planned to bring the Indian pharmaceutical industry—provider of cheap drugs to the world—in line with European patent rules. Matching with an increase in clinical trials in India, principles of "harmonization" guided global guidelines, with the aims of standardizing multinational medication testing and remaking patent rules to match Euro-American ones. "Trial" here is meant doubly—drug trials and legal trials. Rajan focuses on two scandals involving trials, both instances of civic grappling with the impact of new pharmaceutical paradigms. Sunder Rajan shows that India is a particularly risky location from which to contend with global pharma. In this sense, the experiential and the hypothetical are deeply intertwined.

The first instance which Sundar Rajan is reporting pertains to the philanthropic activities of the Bill Gates and Melinda Gates Foundation (BMGF) in India. BMGF funds an NGO by the name of PATH (Programme for Appropriate Technology in Health) which carry out quite a few health programs in India. PATH, which has received funds from BMGF to the tune of $2.5 billion between 1995 and May 2021, undertook the initiative to vaccinate ethnic children in Khammam with the *Human Papillomavirus* (HPV) vaccine in 2009. The trial resulted in the death of 4 tribal children (earlier Andhra Pradesh, now Telangana). The vaccination drive was conducted in four countries, namely, Uganda, Peru, Vietnam, and India. All these nations had a national immunization program and were composed of different ethnic populations. For instance, Uganda had Negroid, Peru had Hispanics, Vietnam had Mongoloids while India had Indo-Aryans, Dravidians, and tribals. Ethnicity is used as a marker for testing the safety and efficacy of certain vaccines, hence various ethnic groups were targeted. The court trials included testimonies by the victim's families who alleged a lack of informed consent. The success of the vaccination drive would have meant its inclusion in the national immunization program of the particular countries and large profit for the drug manufacturers. The objective of the project was "to generate and disseminate evidence for informed public sector introduction of HPV vaccines." During the project, PATH used the *Gardasil* vaccine by Merck & Co. to inoculate the tribal children (Rajan 2017).

Interestingly, Bill and Melinda Gates Foundation had purchased $205 million dollar worth of stocks in pharmaceutical companies, including Merck in 2002. Till the PATH project reached its conclusion, they held the shares in the company i.e., until June 2009. It, therefore, made sense for BMGF to float HPV vaccines in India through the NGO. By 2016, some 1,200 of the girls who had been subjects in the two HPV vaccine trials in India were reporting grave long-term side effects, more than 5 per cent of the total control group of 23,500. By then, the total figure of deaths had risen to seven. The Indian Parliament's Standing Committee on Health found that PATH and ICMR have been in contact since October 2006 and reported that

> It was unwise on the part of ICMR to go in the PPP (Public-Private Partnership) mode with PATH, as such as involvement gives rise to serious Conflict of interest. The Committee takes a serious view of the role of ICMR in the entire episode and is constrained to observe that ICMR should have been more responsible in the matter. The Committee strongly recommends that the Ministry may review the activities of ICMR functionaries involved in the PATH project.
>
> (Reporter 2021)

"Body Hunters" calls out the global pharmacological industry, which in its quest to develop money-spinning new drugs, has begun quietly outsourcing its clinical research to the developing world, where ethical omissions are overlooked, and distressed patients plentiful. Faced with disintegrating services, little funding and soaring health crises, developing countries often boost these very trials, even as they cause threatened resources to be diverted from providing care toward the business of enriching drug companies. She focuses on the manner in which the western pharmacological industry—'the body hunters' or Big Pharma— conducts drug trials and uses poor subjects in Third World nations in preference to subjects in their own nations.

There are good reasons for Americans to refuse to serve as subjects in clinical trials. The Tuskegee Syphilis Study (the 1970s)—where a group of poor African–Americans infected with the spirochaete causing syphilis was left untreated—and the trial of the Salk polio vaccine (1954) where 220 children given the vaccine actually developed polio are still fresh in their minds (Bard 2008).

Shah describes the development of contract research organizations (CROs). American Big Pharma grew increasingly disenchanted with American academic medical institutions for conducting their drug trials by the 1990s. Enter the CROs with their promise to obtain results for Big Pharma on schedule or even a little ahead of time, at a lower cost by tapping medical institutes in Eastern Europe, Latin America, Russia, India, South Africa, and other Asian and African countries where the sick are plentiful and costs low. CROs have been able to enroll 3,000 patients for an experimental vaccine in 9 days and 1,388 children in 12 days. Big Pharma and CROs were quick to realize that in countries where patients had no access to drugs, free drugs—no matter how experimental—were gratefully accepted, no questions asked. As Herbert Du Pont so effectively and concisely phrased it: "Anything is fair game... They can only say yes" (Bard 2008). Relocating huge drug trial businesses to countries such as India and Poland saved Big Pharma millions of dollars each year. Since the 1990s, CROs have also ensured the publication of favorable results in prestigious medical journals while killing reports on ineffective or toxic drugs.

No wonder Anti-Vaccination movements have a large following and Global outrages against drives for compulsory vaccination have been loud and clear. Not only is the issue of adverse vaccine events a third world issue but in first world countries there have been reports of vaccines causing autism in children, allegations of which have sometimes been falsified by investigations but skepticism remains. Vaccination works in many ways. As per the epidemiology of contagious diseases, vaccines often enlist a minority in the safety of the majority by a dubious doctrine called "herd immunity." The choice of the term is unfortunate, because the word "herd" may invite unintended bovine associations as well as may be invoked in a derogatory sense aligned to the term "herd mentality."

What vaccines do not cause is harder to establish than what they do cause. In the recent Covid-19 pandemic unprecedented global cooperation has seen a faster than ever vaccine rollout and worldwide vaccination programs have been completed in record time. It is interesting to note that Anti-vaccination leagues have been more active in European and American Nations, the richer the nation the fiercer the protest, than developing or underdeveloped countries where masses have been more vaccine compliant because they cannot afford to be ill in the absence of effective health infrastructure.

The term "immunity" has been fetishized in these times as never before. More than ever, immunity boosters of all kinds allopathic, homeopathic, herbal, and domestic, have been paraded as lifesaving products. Changes in lifestyle have been advocated, including walking and exercising so as to keep ill health at bay. The uncertain etiology of Covid-19 has seen the masses trying out every possible remedy in the book, including breathing lessons, sound vibrations, blowing of conch, and beating of utensils as part of a mass wellness effort. The emergence of vaccine certificates linked to Aadhaar Card and other similar identity documents has tied the question of identity and biological citizenship[7] to compliance. A possible requirement for a vaccine passport has also given rise to false hope: the requirement of vaccine passports could adversely embed social and economic inequalities that reflect the power dynamics in international relations.

Specifically, the ability to secure vaccines relates to the varying market and economic power across countries (Covid19 Vaccination Certificates and their Geopolitical Discontents 2021).

When the anthropologist Emily Martin asked an array of scientists to discuss descriptions of the immune system that depended on the metaphor of a body at war, some of them rejected the idea that this was a metaphor. It was, they insisted, "how it is." One scientist disliked the war metaphor, but only because he objected to the way war was being waged at that moment. In her study of how we think about immunity, which was conducted during the Iraq war Martin discovered that metaphors of war, *attack, defend, compromise, threaten, penetrate*, permeate our thinking about immunity. In her book "Illness as Metaphor and AIDS and its Metaphors" Susan Sontag says that military metaphors contribute to the stigmatizing of those with infectious diseases and may lead to the victimization of that individual.

> What makes the viral assault so terrifying is that contamination, and therefore vulnerability, is understood as permanent. Even if someone infected were never to develop any symptoms—that is, the infection remained, or could by medical intervention be rendered inactive—the viral enemy would be forever within. In fact, so it is believed, it is just a matter of time before something awakens ("triggers") it, before the appearance of "the tell-tale symptoms".
>
> (Sontag 1990) [8]

The Covid-19 pandemic has seen unusual vilification of the "asymptomatic" and branded the "infected" almost as a villain. In the first wave of the pandemic in India, police would come and forcibly escort infected people, entire families, away from their houses to isolation centers where Covid affected people would be hoarded like cattle. Tattoos were engraved on arms, signposts were erected at affected households, and public humiliation including beatings, streetside push-ups of offending unmasked "Covidiots," or accumulators at market places saw large scale paranoia at its height.

Michel Foucault in his lectures at College du France said that the Modern punishment State would evolve from one that "gives life/death" to "one that lets live or lets die" i.e., one that withdraws the conditions that support life. In the era of bio-citizenship,[9] the Misérables of the vaccine nation have the choice to flourish or perish. To avail of the State-funded health facility, they may either become a subject or become the equivalent of a leper stranded on the outskirts of a city in sixteenth-century Europe, watching and waiting to die.

Notes

1 The Global Vaccine Poem, launched in early April by Kent State University's Wick Poetry Centre and the University of Arizona's Poetry Centre, has grown to more than 1,700 stanzas submitted by people in all 50 states and 89 countries, as on Monday, May 18, 2021 at 12:37 PM.

2 By Naomi Shihab Nye (Young People's Poet Laureate, Poetry Foundation).

3 Similia similibus curantur: The homeopathic concept expressing the law of similars (literally, "likes are cured by likes"), the doctrine that any substance capable of producing morbid symptoms in the healthy will remove similar symptoms occurring as an expression of disease. Another reading of the concept, employed by Hahnemann, the founder of homeopathy, is similia similibus curentur, "let likes be cured by likes."

4 Thetis, a nymph according to Greek mythology, spurns the advances of the God Zeus and marries a mortal Peleus; she gives birth to Achilles who, unlike her, is mortal. She attempts to make the baby Achilles immortal, by dipping him in the River Styx (the river that runs through the underworld), while holding him by his heel. The one part of his body left untouched by the waters becomes his only point of weakness, hence the phrase 'Achilles' heel'.

5 Graham Rooks is the proponent of the "old friends" hypothesis as a substitute for the hygiene hypothesis. The Old Friends mechanism states that mammals co-evolved with an array of organisms that, because they needed to be tolerated, took on a role as inducers of immunoregulatory circuits. Such organisms include various microbiotas and commensals (gut, skin, lung, etc.) chronic infections picked up at birth; helminths that persist for life and environmental organisms from animals, mud and untreated water with which we were in daily contact in the environments in which humans evolved and lived until recently were host to these old friends. The failure of regulation of inappropriate inflammatory immune responses in people living in modern cities in high-income countries is attributable to progressive loss of contact with organisms with which we co-evolved and that play a crucial role in setting up the regulatory pathways.

6 https://www.scientificamerican.com/article/how-cia-fake-vaccination-campaign-endangers-us-all/, 2013.

7 A way of breaking with the conventional politico-economic and legal system of citizenship, biological citizenship is a way of thinking how, in the age of biomedicine, biotechnology and genomics, citizens end up thinking about subjecthood in biological terms. Connecting identity politics and biological citizenship are two closely related Foucauldian concepts of biopower and discipline as discussed in connection with Biopolitics (Nicolas Rose n.d.).

8 Foucault's concept of bio-citizenship derives from his Bio-politics.

9 The term 'biological citizenship', first used by Adriana Petryna in her study of post-Chernobyl Ukraine (HYPERLINK "https://journals.sagepub.com/doi/full/10.1177/1363459318815944"2002) and subsequently elaborated by HYPERLINK "https://journals.sagepub.com/doi/full/10.1177/1363459318815944"Rose and Novas (2005) analyze the ways in which citizens may like to be grouped in terms of genetic or biological affiliations. there was hope that this umbrella term would facilitate large-scale political activism with respect to groups in areas of public health, social welfare, and rights to state aided medical care.

References

Arnold, David. 1993. *Colonizing the Body: State Medicine and Epidemic Disease in Nineteenth Century India.* Berkeley and Los Angeles: University of California Press.

A.W.Rook, Graham. 2019. *Oxford Handbook of Evolutionary Medicine.* London: UCL.

Badrane, Sakina, Babu, Vivek and Hanadu, Sarah. 2020. *The Old Friends Hypothesis and the Covid-19 Pandemic.* Pittsburgh, 24 September.

Bard, Jennifer S. (2012). "Lack of Political Will and Public Trust Dooms Presumed Consent". *American Journal of Bioethics* 12, no. 2, 44–46.

Biss, Eula. 2014. *Immunity: An Inoculation.* Minnesota Minneapolis: Graywolf Press.

Boylston, Arthur. July 2012. "The Origins of Inoculation." *Journal of the Royal Society of Medicine* 105, no. 7, 309–13. https://doi.org/10.1258/jrsm.2012.12k044.

LEE, Tsung-Ling. 2021. "COVID-19 Vaccination Certificates and Their Geopolitical Discontents." *European Journal of Risk Regulation* 12, no. 2, 321–31. doi:10.1017/err.2021.33.

Editorial Board 2013. "How the CIA's Fake Vaccination Campaign Endangers Us All." *scientificamerican.com*. May 1. Accessed February 6, 2022. "The spies who sabotaged global health." *Scientific American* 308, no. 5, 12. https://www.scientificamerican.com/article/how-cia-fake-vaccination-campaign-endangers-us-all/

Lahariya, Chandrakant. 2014. "A Brief History of Vaccines and Vaccination in India." *Indian Journal of Medical Research* 491–511.

Means, Alexander J. 2021. "Foucault, Biopolitics, and the Critique of State Reason". *Educational Philosophy and Theory* 1–2. doi: 10.1080/00131857.2021.1871895.

Mishra, Sabya Sachi R. 1999. "Laws of Pleasure: The Making of Indian Contagious Diseases Act, 1868." *Proceedings of Indian History Congress* (Indian History Congress) 60 (DIAMOND JUBILEE): 550–561.

Nicolas Rose, Carlos Novas. n.d. "Biological Citizenship." *Researchgate.net*. Accessed February 6, 2022. https://www.researchgate.net/profile/Nikolas-Rose/publication/30528478_Biological_Citizenship/links/00b7d521788216ccc4000000/Biological-Citizenship.pdf.

Nye, Naomi Shihab. 2020. *The Global Vaccine Poem Project*. Kent: Kent State University Press.

Porter, Dorothy and Porter, Roy. 1988. "The Politics of Prevention: Anti-Vaccinationism and Public Health in Nineteenth -Century England." *Medical History* 32, no. 3, 231–252.

Rajan, Kaushik Sundar. 2017. *Pharmocracy: Value, Politics, and Knowledge in Global Biomedicine*. Durham: Duke University Press.

Reporter, Staff. 2021. "NGO Supported by Bill and Melinda Gates Foundation Was Accused of Bypassing Indian Laws, Causing Death of Tribal Children and UPA Govt Didn't Do Anything." *opindia.com*. Accessed February 5, 2022. ps://www.opindia.com/2021/10/path-bill-and-melinda-gates-foundation-bypassing-indian-laws-death-tribal-children-upa-govt-silence/. http://www.opindia.com.

Sontag, Susan. 1990. *Illness as Metaphor and AIDS and its Metaphors*. New York: Farrar, Strauss and Giroux.

Tulchinsky, Theodore H. and Varavikova, Elena A. 2014. "A History of Public Health." *The New Public Health* (Third Edition), 1–42.

4 Spaces of Cure or Confinement? Inside the Walls of the Mental Asylums of the 19th Century

Anindita Chatterjee

I

Understanding the idea of mental health and its care: The Fourth Edition of the *Diagnostic and Statistical Manual of Mental Disorders, DSM IV* defines mental disorder as a 'clinically significant behavioural or psychological syndrome or pattern that occurs in an individual. It is associated with present distress (e.g., a painful symptom) or disability (i.e., impairment in one or more important areas of functioning)'.[1] It is difficult to chart and chalk out the exact limits of the term and clinical psychology continues to ask the question as to what is the exact implication of the word 'mental' in the term 'mental disorder'. There exists great debate and conflict on the meaning, implication, consistency, and meaning of such terms as 'sanity', 'insanity', and 'mental illnesses' for it has been observed that normality and abnormality are not universal terms either. 'What is viewed as normal in one culture may be seen as quite aberrant in another. Thus, notions of normality and abnormality may not be quite as accurate as people believe they are' (Rosenhan 1973, 250).

The Summary Report on Promoting Mental Health: Concepts, Emerging Evidence, Practice published by the World Health Organization in 2019 emphasizes the different determinants of mental health and mental disorders which include not only individual attributes such as the ability to manage one's thoughts, emotions, behaviours and interactions with others, but also social, cultural, economic, political and environmental factors such as national policies, social protection, standards of living, working conditions and community support. There are many different mental disorders, with different presentations. They are generally characterized by a combination of abnormal thoughts, perceptions, emotions, behaviour and relationships with others. Health systems have not yet adequately responded to the burden of mental disorders. As a consequence, the gap between the need for treatment and its provision is [still] wide all over the world. In low- and middle-income countries, between 76 per cent and 85 per cent of people with mental disorders receive no treatment for their disorder.[2]

In its attempt to describe the concept of mental health and its promotion the *Report* tries to arrive at a degree of agreement on some common characteristics of mental health promotion as well as explore its variations across different cultures.

DOI: 10.4324/9781003300762-5

In order to arrive at an understanding of the notion of mental health care it is important to consider how conditions of mental illness have evolved historically. There has been considerable progress in the concept of treatment and therapies for mental illness over time. 'The presumed causes of mental illness too have undergone a substantial transformation over the last two centuries' (Prior 1993, 323). The fourth edition of the *American Psychiatric Association's Diagnostic and Statistical Manual of Mental Disorders (DSM IV)* begins by noting 'Although this manual provides a classification of mental disorders, it must be admitted that no definition adequately specifies precise boundaries for the concept of mental disorder' (Hershkowitz 1998, 1). Whereas societal models see madness as a product of dysfunctional interpersonal relationships, psychoanalytical models, particularly those in the Freudian tradition, (Freud 1960, 89) see it as a product of dysfunctional mental processes within the individual. Lillian Feder in *Madness in Literature,* identified madness as a form of 'deviation from the normal order and in most cases, it is subjected to control and suppression. In fact, 'all forms of deviant behavior, aberrant or bizarre thought and conducts have been regarded as "insane" throughout human experience' (Feder 1983, xii). Madness is a revolt against orderliness. Hence any attempt to define and categorize it may kill its essence. However, it remains a fact that almost all identifiable forms of madness were regarded as deviations which were subjected to incarceration and banishment from society. In a movement which Foucault describes as the 'Great Confinement', the insane and unreasonable members of the population were systematically confined during the seventeenth century.

Confinement was an institutional creation peculiar to the seventeenth century...in the history of unreason, it marked a decisive event: it was the moment when madness was perceived on the social horizon as poverty, incapacity for work, or inability to integrate with the group; and it was also the moment when madness began to be ranked among the problems of the city (Foucault 1989, 59).

It was till the end of the eighteenth century, that the 'insane', the pauper, the criminals and the poor were assembled together and ascribed a kind of similar 'abnormal' status. The notion of 'madness' as a form of illness was not clinically investigated during the early ages and there was an absence of any form of specific treatment up to the nineteenth century. David Ingleby referring to Foucault's *Madness and Civilisation* claims how 'up to the mid-19th century, the mad people had been allowed to remain in the open, [who were] either cared for by their families or set loose to roam the countryside' (Ingelby 1988, 16). Referring to Michel Foucault's *The Birth of the Clinic,* (Foucault 2003, 23), Mary Wilson Carpenter in *Health, Medicine and Society in Victorian England* identified the nineteenth century as a major turning point in the history of the medical science because it was the period that saw the birth of the 'the clinic', or the institution of treatment and cure where professional medical practitioners gathered 'not just to treat the sick but to study their diseases. By the end of the nineteenth century, the modern medical profession had emerged, organized essentially as we know it today' (Carpenter 2010, 2). Medical institutions were constructed to provide treatment to the insane. They were not mere houses of detention, but institutions which were equipped with amenities to treat madness in a clinical and scientific way.

It was during the nineteenth century that the insane inmates were 'kept in custodial care as a heterogeneous group in some sort of asylum' (Foucault 1989, 26). The clinical gaze generated a new system of medical knowledge as well as a set of new power dynamics. 'The Victorian era in England saw the formation of the medical profession as we know it now, but it was also the era in which doctors gained knowledge and authority' (Carpenter 2010, 12). With King George III on the throne 'madness' received a new stimulus in the nineteenth century in England.[3] Several kinds of humanitarian treatment began under Philippe Pinel and Samuel Tuke in these newly constructed mental hospitals.

II

Birth of Asylums in the Nineteenth Century: In 1897, during his visit to London celebrating the sixtieth anniversary of Queen Victoria's ascension to the throne, Mark Twain observed, 'British history is two thousand years old and yet in a good many ways the world has moved farther ahead since the Queen was born than it moved in all the rest of the two thousand put together' (Arnstein 1997, 591). Twain's remark captures the sense of dizzying change that characterized nineteenth-century Britain. By the beginning of the Victorian period, the Industrial Revolution had already brought about profound economic and social changes, including a mass migration of workers to industrial towns where they lived in new urban slums. The extension of the franchise resulted in widespread democratization. The century was also affected by challenges to the established religious faith. There was rapid advancement in scientific knowledge, and progress was marked in all spheres of life. The Victorian age has been noted in history for its profound progress in the fields of science, technology, literature, art, culture and social policy. Some of the most influential writers and thinkers of the modern world, including Charles Darwin and Karl Marx, lived during this time. Despite the remarkable progress and advancement in scientific and technological knowledge, the age was also fraught with doubt, crisis of faith, contradictions and uncertainty. However, it remains an accepted fact that the nineteenth century saw an 'enormous change in public perception of those who have lost their will or judgement' (Stevens 2014, 18). The new, rational approach to diagnosis and treatment was influenced by wisdom and science rather than faith and superstition. The medical practitioners no longer believed that insanity was an affliction of the soul but attempted to perceive it as an illness within the flesh and blood.

John K. Walton, in *Lunacy in the Industrial Revolution: A Study of Asylum Admissions in Lancashire*, goes on to observe how, alongside the rapid expansion and reorganization of the manufacturing industry and the high rate of urban growth in many parts of England, the first half of the nineteenth century saw a spectacular rise in the proportion of the population officially recognized as the insane. Between 1807 and 1855, the rate per 10,000 increased more than sevenfold, from 2.26 to

16.5, and although the rate of growth eased off considerably in the second half of the century, the proportions had risen further to 29.3 by 1890 (Walton 1979, 2).

'The eighteenth- and nineteenth-century public asylums', according to Leonard Smith's *Cure, Comfort and Safe Custody: Public Lunatic Asylums in Early Nineteenth Century*, 'were the direct offshoots of the voluntary subscription hospitals which formed one of the chief legacies of the Hanoverian and Georgian eras to the development of social welfare provision in Britain' (Smith 1999, 12). According to the Act for the Better Care and Maintenance of Lunatics which is also known as the Wynn's Act received the Royal Assent in Parliament on 23 June 1808, the asylums were supposed to be situated far away from the town, and the buildings, whether newly erected or adapted, were supposed to be constructed in an airy and healthy situation, with good water supply. Bedford and Nottingham were the first two asylums built under the terms of Wynn's Act in 1812, and five others came up between 1828 and 1833. The registered number of patients admitted to these asylums was small at first but there was a considerable increase in the figure over the decades. Gradually most asylums became overcrowded with patients. These newly constructed asylums were glorious buildings that demonstrated British architectural pride. Built on lavish grounds in remote rural areas, outside the city with the intention of providing the peaceful ambience for healing and producing a calm impact upon fractured, disoriented and disturbed minds, the remoteness of the asylums also kept the city away from the distressing contact with the insane.

Inside the walls of the Mental Asylums: Although the public madhouses were built with benevolent motives to provide care for all patients affected with mental problems but the treatment was beyond the means of poor patients. 'Pauper lunatics had to rely on charity and public subscriptions for funding their treatment'. (Heasman 1964, 230). Leonard Smith's study goes on to describe some of the inhuman treatment that the lunatics received during the period and how patients from superior classes who paid their own expenses enjoyed the privileges of a better life than those inmates who were in a state of financial distress. There were instances of repressive violence and coercion within the asylum premises and in many cases the inmates were treated like prisoners. 'The lunatic was [often] chained in the cellar or garret of a workhouse, fastened to the leg of a table, tied to a post in the outhouse or perhaps shut up in an uninhabited ruin'; on the other hand, if his lunacy was offensive, he was not admitted and 'left to ramble naked and half-starved through the streets and highways' (Smith' 1999, 22). Although some striking changes were introduced in mental health care practice during the late 1830s, according to Robert Allan Houston, 'it was nothing compared to their existing plight' (Houston 2006, 256). Poor inmates of asylums were often arbitrarily confined together without any classification so that they would not unsettle the harmony of the system. 'In most cases, such categorization was random and rigid, and not based on medical judgement'. (Higgs 2009, 67)

One of the pioneering institutions for the treatment of insanity was a place known as 'The Retreat' or the 'York Retreat' which operated as a non-profit charitable organization. Founded in 1796 by William Tuke, it was regarded as the first and perhaps the most successful effort to provide humanitarian care to patients, and it went on to become a model for asylums worldwide. The humane attitude and system of cure practiced at the Retreat were popularized by Samuel Tuke. At places like the Retreat, the purpose was not only to ensure proper care and management of the inmates but there was also an aim to secure their perfect cure. 'The reformers', according to Smith, sought to formulate a policy that was 'at the same time humane, conducive to the preservation of order and protective of the sensibilities of the wider public' (Smith 1999, 23).

Samuel Tuke's *Description of the Retreat* emphasized and elaborated on the principles of moral management techniques adopted during the nineteenth century in these asylums which he thought was a better way to treat insanity.

> The reformers, local worthies, medical men established the new generation of public asylums which were meant to provide moral treatment, alongside medical cure. However, it proved extremely problematic in practice to match the proclaimed aspirations. Real difficulties surrounded the implementation of techniques in a relatively large asylum although they could be successfully adopted in smaller domestic— scale madhouses and a purpose- designed asylum like the Retreat.
>
> (Smith 1999, 4)

As the century progressed, attitudes to insanity underwent substantial transformations. Included in The March-June, 1845 volume of *The Westminster Review* of London, an article entitled, "Report of the Metropolitan Commissioners in Lunacy to the Lord Chancellor," presented—a report from the Metropolitan Commissioners investigating the condition of some mental institutions in England. The report offered a precise description of various 'mental asylums', which included both 'curable' as well as 'incurable' patients. The account mentioned that the reported cases of mental illness seemed to be increasing. Presented to both the Houses of Parliament the report suggests that attitudes toward mental illness in the Victorian era were already shifting. John Conolly, a Fellow of the Royal College of Physicians in London and a physician to the Middlesex Lunatic Asylum at Hanwell, remarked in the introduction to a letter which featured in *The Westminster and Foreign Quarterly Review* in its October 1847 to January 1848 edition that the treatment of mental illness was mostly based on violence and coercion. He felt that the 'whole of the barbarous system of coercion and restraint was founded on a fallacy. Insanity, according to him, was simply a state of unsound, physical health—a state of functional disease—in the great majority of cases capable of cure, under appropriate treatment; capable also, under injudicious treatment, of being rendered permanently incurable'.[4]

Although the reformers, psychiatrists and medical men of the nineteenth century wanted to run the public asylums on scientific lines, what was actually practiced within the walls still remains a mystery. Whereas some studies focus on the progressive idea of treatment, many others bring out the picture of grim violence and viciousness within. It is difficult to retrieve the lost voices of the inmates of these asylums.

Despite the efforts undertaken by the reformers, several lunatic asylums in the nineteenth century were not so much like hospitals as they were prisons with abysmal treatment. 'The arbitrary imprisonment and confinement of men and women in public and private madhouses were a common practice in eighteenth and nineteenth century England' (Brown 2006, 426). Asylums were more custodial than therapeutic in nature and the attempts at cure 'were often more desperate than well advised' (Hunter 1957, 127). Kathleen Jones' *Lunacy, Law and Conscience* offers a vivid portrait of the conditions inside some noted mental asylums of the nineteenth century where 'flogging and cudgelling' were often used as the means of controlling insane inmates. Reports of severe 'cruel and inhuman practices, which resembled the barbaric practices of the Middle Ages, were often published' (Jones 1955, 85). Jones' study goes on to refer to the account of the wife of a pauper named William Vickers appeared who appeared before the magistrate and reformer, Godfrey Higgins, in 1813 and complained that her husband had received inhuman treatment in the asylum before he had been discharged. The reports stated that 'he was in a miserable state and could barely stand by himself and had lash marks on his back. His relatives had not been allowed to meet him for it was said that he was insensible in an apoplexy' (Jones 1955, 85). Godfrey Higgins found out several anomalies in the management of the York Asylum. He investigated into the reports of coercion, lapses and, after he failed to obtain satisfactory responses from the authorities, he communicated his observations to the press. Historical documents reveal that the asylum caught fire on December 26th of the same year and the reformers could not retrieve the records that were damaged severely by the accident. In the words of Godfrey Higgins, when 'an investigation seemed imminent, the staff resorted to panic stricken measures, burning down [some] parts of the building in order to conceal the appalling condition in which some of the patients were kept, [thus] destroying records to remove the evidence of financial peculation' (Jones 1955, 79).

Mary Huestis Pengilly's *Diary*, which was written during her stay in the Provincial Lunatic Asylum, and first published in 1882, goes on to describe the case of a 'short, fair faced, nice looking girl', who was admitted to the asylum due to some unknown mental disease.

During her stay in the asylum, she was initially treated like any other ordinary human being. She spent times reading lines from the Testament as if she were in Sunday school, frequently recited poetry and played the piano. When her father came to see her, she cried and begged him to take her home. But she was never released by the hospital authorities. Her condition deteriorated with time. She often tore off her clothes in a violent frenzy and mourned in morbid despair. The asylum authorities tied her hands with tight leather handcuffs for she suffered from frequent violent manic attacks. The handcuffs often swelled her hands and it seemed that her blood veins would burst in pressure. The author recounts how, when she pointed it out to the authorities, they completely ignored her. The hospital authorities thought it was a necessary part of the cure and the most effective means to keep her madness under control. Much to Mary Pengilly's shock, they often tied a canvas belt around the girl's waist and bound her to the back of the seat. Mary felt that such an action if practiced on her would definitely stop her breath in no time. It is needless to add that the young girl died very soon after. Mary was haunted by the trauma of torture during her stay in the asylum. The writer goes on to suggest how she thought that the girl was so not much out of her senses when she was admitted, but felt that her condition grew steadily worse with the brutal treatment that she received during her stay in the asylum.[5]

Theodore Dalrymple in his study of the *Asylums of Nineteenth Century* identified them as 'chambers of horrors, where bizarre sadistic rituals were carried out for reasons unconnected with beneficent medical endeavor'.[6] David Wright in his *Mental Disability in Victorian England: The Earlswood Asylum 1847–1901* depicts a picture of the turbulent times. The Royal Earlswood Asylum was one of the main institutions meant for the cure of insane during the nineteenth and twentieth centuries. Wright felt that all institutions meant for mentally retarded patients were 'static and dehumanizing' (Wright 2001, 8). According to Wright, despite their benevolent intentions nineteenth-century asylums were actually places of confinement 'where families [often] rid themselves of the unwanted members. It was also a resource used strategically by poor households' intent to overcome periods of impoverishment' since the institutions undertook the responsibility of looking after the 'dependent and the disabled' (Wright 2001, 197). As early as 1823, John Haslam divided the notion of 'insanity' into three broad categories on the basis of the commencement of the condition and its ability to be cured: they were—idiocy, lunacy and unsoundness of mind. Insanity, according to him, was "incurable" whereas lunacy generally began at a later stage of life and could often be temporary. Unsoundness of mind was contradistinguished from idiocy and lunacy (Wright 2001, 15).

Lindsay Granshaw and Roy Porter in *The Hospital in History* claimed that the 'mental hospitals of the early nineteenth century—served [primarily] the interests of the elite' (Granshaw 1989, 216). Kathleen Jones, in *Lunacy Law and Conscience* too made a similar observation when she remarked how these human-itarian institutions which were built with such high ideals and motives hardly lived up to its promise. 'Pauper patients who were admitted into hospitals did not require any certification and were left at the mercy of the donations from such noblemen, gentlemen and ladies who wanted to promote an institution for the relief of an unhappy part of the community' (Jones 1955, 83). In the 'Intro-duction' to *Asylums: Essays on the Social Situation of Mental Patients and Other Inmates*, Ervig Goffman identified similarities between prison houses and mental asylums of the nineteenth century classifying both of them as 'total institutions'.

A total institution may be defined as a place of residence ... where a large num-ber of like-situated individuals, cut off from the wider society for an appreciable period of time, together lead an enclosed, formally administered round of life (Goffman 1961, xiii).

Many accounts reveal how most of the early mental asylums resembled dreary prisons or where the main purpose was to prevent patients from escaping, unlike the 'modern establishments' which came up with the progress of science in the twentieth century that were designed with the well-being and comfort of the patients as main priorities. In many cases, the identification and diagnosis of insanity were arbitrary and random and 'the label was a stigma' (Sedgwick 1972, 198) that the patient had to carry and the treatment was meted out accordingly. As there was a rapid rise in the figure of institutionalized patients over the years the thrust of treatment gradually shifted from providing cure to care.

The Reform Act of 1832 expressed an urge for improvement of the life of the poorer section of society. Efforts were undertaken to provide means of freedom and comfort to the inmates so that they would not perish in the deplorable state of their confinement, but it was still not adequate to provide for all. Although there was a dearth of professional practitioners in these hospitals, it cannot be denied that there was a considerable change in the notion of the term 'hospital' during the nineteenth century. Whereas, on the one hand, we come across several accounts of repressive modes of treatment prevalent in asylums, on the other hand, at the same time, it cannot be denied that nineteenth-century Britain propagated an advancement of scientific thought which in a way was also reflected in the clinical treatment of insanity. It was within this intellectual framework that noted figures like Kraepelin, Bleuler and Schneider developed their new diagnostic theories for dealing with mental illnesses and psychiatric disorders.

III

Conclusion: The individuals who enjoyed the privileges of the modernized, bureaucratic hospitals of the twentieth century would refuse to look back on the treatment and care provided by the mental hospitals of the Victorian era. But it remains a fact that it was in the nineteenth century that for the first time 'medicine changed from treatment based largely on the patient's own account of her or his constitution to one based more on the physician's specialized knowledge of the patient's body' (Carpenter 2010, 12). The 1986 Ottawa Charter of the World Health Organization emphasized the notion of a holistic well-being which included both physical as well as mental health. The Charter emphasizes an inextricable link between mental health and physical health. It is now perceived as a two-way relationship with mental health influencing physical health and vice versa. In the light of the history of the 'Othering' of insane people from the mainstream society, we can say that the idea of the treatment of mental health has undergone a substantial transformation (Camfield 2008, 766).

Pat Thomas in his "Introduction" to *Understanding Mental Wellness* goes on to point out how 'the topic of mental health has, in recent years, become more prominent in the global health agenda, and much of the stigma and embarrassment that people once felt talking about difficult feelings and experiences has begun to disappear (Thomas 2021, 16).

Referring to the World Health Organization's mandate which asserts the importance of mental health stating that 'there is no health without mental health' Thomas shows how 'this recognition has led to increasing efforts to encourage more of us to feel comfortable talking about mental well-being and to end the stigma around mental ill health' (Thomas 2021, 17). Mental illness is no longer a label that one needs to combat or feel ashamed of or hide from the world. In fact, society has now woken up to numerous facets of depression, stress and anxiety. According to the Centre for Disease Control and Prevention the Covid-19 pandemic has had a major effect on our lives. Many of us have been facing challenges that have been stressful, overwhelming over the last two years. Pandemic has resulted in strong reactions in adults and children world-wide. 'Public health actions, such as isolation and social distancing, [which were] necessary to reduce the spread of Covid-19, [actually] made many feel isolated, depressed and lonely'.[7] A KFF Health Tracking Poll from July 2020 has found that many 'adults are now reporting specific negative impacts on their mental health and well-being, due to the increased stress and anxiety, worry and tension over the coronavirus outspread'.[8] Covid-19 pandemic and the resulting economic recession have negatively affected many people's mental health across the world and the notion of mental illness has assumed profound significance in the last two years. The prognosis of the ailment is no longer bound by predictable rules hence the treatment too is no longer conventional. Medical practitioners now see mental health as a continuum, ranging from different states of anxiety, depression, and nervous breakdowns to stressful life experiences. It is difficult to ascertain the actual face of mental illness now. Even *DSM IV* notes that although the manual provides a classification of mental disorders, 'it must be admitted that no definition adequately specifies precise boundaries for the concept of mental disorder'.[9] Medical science has now identified the evolution of the notion of mental health and clinical practitioners across the world are devising strategies to cope with it accordingly.

Modern medicine perceives insanity or mental disorder as an ailment that can be approached both clinically and scientifically. The treatment for mental health disorders is now broadly classified as 'either somatic (biological) or psychological'.

Somatic treatments include drugs, electroconvulsive therapy, and other therapies that stimulate the brain. Psychological treatments include psychotherapy (individual, group, or family and marital), behaviour therapy techniques (e.g., relaxation training or exposure therapy), and hypnotherapy (Sperry 2016, 3–xxxii).

Unlike the past, where institutions offering mental health care focused largely on reducing symptoms of ailment and aimed at returning the individuals to normalcy, in modern times, however, the treatment of mental illness focuses on increasing individuals' functioning, adaptability to treatment, resilience, and prevention of further degradation. This new dimension of treatment is identified as well-being. The future trajectory of mental health care is looking beyond the walls of confinement to provide effective help and assistance to those who need the most of it. With the main aim of health care services having altered substantially the new structure of treatment now focuses on therapy, counselling and reconciliation rather than brutal incarceration, isolation and confinement which were practiced in the asylums of the nineteenth century.

Notes

1 The *Diagnostic and Statistical Manual of Mental Disorders* is the official manual of the American Psychiatric Association. Its purpose is to provide a framework for classifying disorders and defining diagnostic criteria for the disorders listed. DSM-IV notes that mental disorders are associated with distress, disability, or a significantly increased risk of suffering death, pain, disability, or an important loss of freedom. The definition was accessed from https://www.ncbi.nlm.nih.gov/pmc/articles.

2 Accessed from the https://www.who.int/news-room/fact-sheets/detail/mental-disorders. *Mental Disorder: Key Facts from The Summary Report on Promoting Mental Health: Concepts, Emerging Evidence, Practice*, published on 28th November, 2019. The page was accessed on 22 January 2022.

3 The world remembers King George III as the 'mad king of England who ruled at the time when American colonies asserted their independence. Historians customarily viewed him a weak neurotic patient who spent his lifetime battling his mental health' and nervous disease. In 1765, he suffered mental breakdown. Information accessed from Detweiler, Robert. "Retreat from Environmentalism: A Review of the Psychohistory of George III", *The History Teacher*. Vol. 6, No. 1 (November 1972), pp. 37–46. Published By: Society for History Education. https://doi.org/10.2307/492622.

4 Conolly, John. Introduction to *The Westminster and Foreign Quarterly Review*, October 1847 to January 1848. Accessed from https://victorianweb.org/authors/bronte/cbronte/iwama8.html on May 28th, 2009.

5 Mary Huestis Pengilly, *Diary Written in the Provincial Lunatic Asylum*. A new Project Gutenberg book, which was originally published in 1882, it provides vivid records of several brutal treatments that the mentally challenged patients often received. The text was accessed from *Psychology and More* from http://www.gutenberg.org/etext/18398.

6 Dalrymple, Theodore. (2005) "In the Asylum", *City Journal*, Summer. The page was accessed from https://www.city-journal.org/html/asylum-12889.html on January 26th, 2022.

7 Stein, Dan J., Katharine A. Phillips, et al. "What Is Mental/ Psychiatric Disorder? From DSM-IV to DSM-V". Accessed from https://www.ncbi.nlm.nih.gov/pmc/articles/PMC3101504/.

8 Accessed from "Coping with Stress", https://www.cdc.gov/mentalhealth/stress-coping/cope-with-stress/. The page accessed on January 19th, 2022.

9 Panchal, Nirmita, Rabah Kamal and Cynthia Cox. (2021) "The Implications of COVID-19 for Mental Health and Substance Use". Accessed from https://www.kff.org/coronavirus-covid-19/issue-brief/the-implications-of-covid-19-for-mental-health-and-substance-us.

References

Arnstein, Walter. (1997) "History: Queen Victoria's Diamond Jubilee," *The American Scholar* Vol. 66, No. 4 (Autumn), pp. 591–597. Published by The Phi Beta Kappa Society. Accessed from https://www.jstor.org/stable/41212693 on January 9th, 2022.

Brown, Michael. (2006) "Rethinking Eary Nineteenth Century Asylum Reform," *The Historical Journal* Vol. 49, No. 2 (June), pp. 425–452. Published by CUP. Accessed from https://www.jstor.org/stable/4091622.

Camfield, Laura. (2008) "On Subjective Well-being and Quality of Life," *Journal of Health Psychology* Vol. 13, No. 764, pp. 764–775. Published by Sage. Accessed from https://10.1177/1359105308093860 on January 25th, 2022.

Carpenter, Wilson Mary. (2010) *Health, Medicine, and Society in Victorian England*. Santa Barbara, CA: ABC-CLIO-LLC.

Feder, Lillian. (1983) *Madness in Literature*. Princeton, NJ: Princeton University Press.

Foucault, Michel. (1989) *Madness and Civilisation: A History of Insanity in the Age of Reason*. Transl. from French by Richard Howard. London and New York: Routledge.

Foucault, Michel. (2003) *The Birth of the Clinic*. London: Routledge.

Freud, Sigmund. (1960) "New Introductory Lectures on Psychoanalysis," in *The Standard Edition of Complete Psychological Works of Freud*, Volumes XIII, (1913–1914), XXI, (1927–1931) XXII, (1932–1936) and Volume XX, 1925–1926, transl. by James Stratchey in collaboration with Anna Freud, pp. 89–99. London: The Hogarth Press.

Goffman, Erving. (1961) *Asylums: Essays on the Social Situation of Mental Patients and Other Inmates*. New York: Anchor Books.

Granshaw, Lindsay and Roy Porter. (1989) *The Hospital in History*. London and New York: Routledge.

Heasman, Kathleen J. (1964) "The Medical Mission and the Care of the Sick Poor in Nineteenth Century England," *The Historical Journal* Vol. 7, No. 2, pp. 230–245. Published by CUP. Accessed from https://www.jstor.org/stable/3020352 from January 26th, 2022.

Hershkowitz, Debra. (1998) *The Madness of Epics: Reading Insanity from Homer to Statius*. Oxford: Clarendon Press.

Higgs, Michelle. (2009) *Life in the Victorian Hospital*. Gloucester: The History Press.

Houston, Robert Allan. (2006) "Poor Relief and the Dangerous and Criminal Insane in Scotland, c. 1740–1840," *Journal of Social History* Vol. 40, No. 2 (Winter), pp. 453–476.

Hunter, Richard and Ida Macalpine. (1957) "William Harvey: His Neurological and Psychiatric Observations," *Journal of the History of Medicine and Allied Sciences* Vol. 12, No. 2 (April), pp. 126–139. Published by Oxford University Press. Accessed from https://www.jstor.org/stable/24619408 on January 23rd, 2022.

Ingelby, David. (1988) "Critical Psychology in Relation to Political Repression and Violence," *International Journal of Mental Health* Vol. 17, No. 4 (Winter), pp. 16–28. Published by Taylor and Francis. Accessed from https://www.jstor.org/stable/41344520 on January, 23rd 2022.

Jones, Kathleen. (1955) *Lunacy, Law and Conscience 1744–1845: The Social History of the Care of the Insane*. London: Routledge and Kegan Paul Ltd.

Link, Bruce G., Francis T. Cullen, Elmer Struening, Patrick E. Shrout and Bruce P. Dohrenwend. (1989) "A Modified Labeling Theory Approach to Mental Disorders: An Empirical Assessment," *American Sociological Review* Vol. 54, No. 3 (June), pp. 400–423. Published by American Sociological Association.

Prior, Pauline. (1993) "Mental Health Policy in Northern Ireland," *Social Policy Administration* Vol. 27, No. 4 (December), pp. 323–334. Accessed from https://doi.org/10.1111/j.1467-9515.1993.tb00548.x.

Rosenhan, David L. (1973) "On Being Sane in Insane Places," *Science* (New Series) Vol. 179, No. 4070 (January 19), pp. 250–258.

Sedgwick, Peter. (1972) "Mental Illness is Illness," *Salmagundi*, No. 20, *Psychological Man: Approaches to an Emergent Social Type* (Summer-Fall), pp. 196–224. Accessed from https://www.jstor.org/stable/40546717 on January 22nd, 2022.

Smith, Leonard. (1999) *Cure, Comfort and Safe Custody: Public Lunatic Asylums in Early Nineteenth Century*. Birmingham: Continuum International Publishing Group.

Sperry, Len. (2016) *Mental Disorders: An Encyclopedia of Conditions, Treatments, and Well-Being*. Santa Barbara, CA: Greenwood.

Stevens, Mark. (2014) *Life in the Victorian Asylum: The World of Nineteenth Century Mental Health Care*. Yorkshire: Pen and Sword Books Limited.

Thomas, Pat. (2021) *Understanding Mental Wellness: A Holistic Approach to Mental Health and Healing Natural Remedies, Foods, Lifestyle Strategies, Therapies.* New York: D K Publishing.

Walton, John K. (1979) "Lunacy in the Industrial Revolution: A Study of Asylum Admissions in Lancashire, 1848–50," *Journal of Social History* Vol. 13, No.1 (Autumn), pp. 1–22.

Wright, David. (2001) *Mental Disability in Victorian England: The Earlswood Asylum 1847–1901.* London: Oxford University Press.

5 Žižek's *Pandemic!*, the 'New Normal' Dilemma and Some Indian Perspectives

Anasuya Bhar

The difficulty in trying to look dispassionately and objectively at the world Covid situation has caused the title of this chapter to suffer not one, but a few changes even as I tried to collect my thoughts – for the pandemic is still very much alive and changing. One always suffers from the pitfalls of not having an adequate aesthetic and historical distance to look, with adequate detachedness, at a contemporary situation. A malady or disease brings with it the additional problem of not knowing, hence, not being able to prognosticate about it. There is a possibility, therefore, of there being a newer development to what one writes at present, a newer version, as it were. The Coronavirus has mutated into several newer strands, and one still does not know if the 'omicron' is its final manifestation. There is then, an uncanny sense of still living in the presence of the pandemic or gathering oneself from the spoils of it.

In India, especially in Kolkata, from where I hail and from where I write, the third wave of the Covid-19 pandemic has, perhaps, hit its worst, with every family having more than one positive patient, tested, or otherwise. Nevertheless, we seem to have overridden the original 'panic' and trusted ourselves to some kind of a resilience inevitable. The only positive aspect of the third wave in this part of the world is that, although the positivity rate is very high, the death rate is relatively low. The challenge is now to adapt oneself to the disease, live with it and try one's best to combat it. This chapter seeks to look at the social, political and personal implications of the Covid-19 pandemic, more particularly in the Indian context. In doing so it seeks to draw on Slavoj Žižek's recently published books on the *Pandemic* (2020), especially with the condition that the philosopher identifies as the 'new normal'. In looking at the Indian perspective on the pandemic, this chapter seeks to apprise readers of the 'local' problems and limitations to a 'global' crisis. This juxtaposition of the local alongside the global also identifies the ongoing pandemic as 'glocal', the way many contemporary issues and ideologies are assimilated and apprehended in several parts of the world.

The Covid World

The world was hurled into the sudden shock of a contagious viral disease in the early months of 2020. From some time in the same year, a new phrase, the 'new

DOI: 10.4324/9781003300762-6

normal', crept into our lives consequent of certain lifestyle changes ushered in by Covid-19. The most noticeable among them were the wearing of masks, maintaining physical distance and cultivating some kind of a 'don't touchism', and also the frequent washing of hands. In a tropical country like ours, washing is common and frequent; some regions even practice washing of hands with the frequency of an obsession, the act spelling everything from cleanliness to ritualistic exclusivism. It seemed more difficult to maintain distance between people in a country where overcrowding and cramming for space are normal. The wearing of masks caught on, reluctantly but more acceptably, with time. In fact, several business houses began designing fashionable face masks, until the mask became a style statement. One is here, unfailingly, reminded of Žižek's rather interesting observation that the face mask now concentrates all our attention to one's eyes, making it the most emotive feature on the face, in the absence of 'touch' (Žižek 2020b, vol. 1, 10). The social codes were changing, with many parts of the world preferring the 'namaskar' to shaking of hands. Most countries were practicing force-able closure and shut down policies, which would discourage people from stepping out of their homes. In a never-before situation most countries, including our own, executed complete 'lockdown' on their citizens, which made life stand still and added a degree of surrealism to our familiar spaces, now vacant. In fact, one also noticed the free movement of several wild animals in spaces unfrequented by humans. For a time, perhaps, even the humans were humbled, in acceptance of the co-existence of 'other' life forms.

Žižek's *Pandemic!*

The term 'new/neo normal', however, seemed to be a neologism and also some kind of trivia, in the beginning. The Covid phenomenon gradually rose to top priority news coverage in both the print and audio-visual media and throughout the day one was subjected to news of the affected the world over. Slavoj Žižek's book *Pandemic! Covid-19 Shakes the World* (2020) was possibly among the earliest efforts to rise above the smartness of savvy journalese, in an effort to look objectively at a global crisis. Being too early to theorize, the Slovenian philosopher (b. 1949) nevertheless speaks of the shock and the gradual encroachment and prioritization, of the pandemic in our daily lives. However, the rapidly changing pattern of the disease, along with other ancillary problems of social, economic, and political relevance, prompted him to also write a quick sequel to the book, titled *Pandemic! 2 Chronicles of a Time Lost* (2020). What Žižek's books have done is that they have laid the foundation for the philosophy of the Coronavirus disease. They have identified some of the key aspects of our lives and summed them up into holistic chapters, while the endless print and visual reportage captured life in minutiae and in its utmost diversity. In many ways, Žižek's books have already paved the way for the social historian, the cultural commentator, and the literary critic. The pandemic has and will spawn much literature and art, and Žižek's ideas may give birth to several other forms of creation.

Between the writing of the first and the second volumes of Žižek's books, the world has indeed changed, busting almost all the myths with which the pandemic began. Almost all of us had presumed that the changes, the closure, and the consequent stasis were a temporary and short-lived affair and were certainly and imminently to be superseded by what we usually considered to be our 'normal' lifestyles. Žižek, too, speaks about this. In the interim period, many of us wanted to savor the forced leisure in cultivating what we otherwise could not do in our work/live-a-day rush: housework, looking after family and aged parents, parenting, cuisine, and much more (Bhar 2020a), but always with the hope and understanding, that we would return, to our previous lives.[1] Many academics and authors, however, utilized the time for newer books and publications. As time progressed, however, we realized that all of us were certainly *not* 'in the same boat', and that different crises defined each country in the wake of a ruthless disease.

Covid-19 and India

In India, the Covid-19 pandemic was initially not considered to be much of a threat with other overwhelmingly critical malaises like poverty, homelessness, overcrowding, unemployment, hunger, and the prevalence, as well as the history of other diseases like malaria, dengue or even cancer. India has already a substantial history of epidemics – namely, that of cholera, malaria, and the plague, the last fearful instance of it being at the end of the nineteenth century when the country was still reeling under the British colonial yoke.[2] The Indians are more or less resilient to disease, in a stoical and forbearing manner. Hence, the threat of Covid-19 was actually denied and flouted initially. It seemed to happen 'elsewhere' and 'faraway' as our television sets reported. It perhaps took the first case, to jolt us out of our stupor.

Nevertheless, if we are to theorize about the onset of a disease, what is the rationale for its acceptance? How do we negotiate with the shock of sudden curbs on our personal freedom, consequent to a viral disease that threatened to cause a pandemic? What about the panic and the rashness, the ruthlessness and selfishness that typifies the human struggle for survival? In a very interesting study made by Elisabeth Kübler-Ross in her book *On Death and Dying*, and mentioned by Žižek,[3] the trajectory of acceptance of a terminal disease is traced. Spread across five points, the trajectory begins with an initial bout of 'denial' as in 'this cannot be happening to me', followed by a bout of 'anger' as in 'how can this happen to me?' This may be followed by a bout of 'bargaining' with the contingency of the disease itself. This may be likened to a conditional tug-of-war situation: 'let me live till my children graduate' and the likes. When one realizes that the disease is here to stay, and when one feels the pull of the disease, then one naturally falls in its clutches, in an enormous bout of 'depression'. Lastly, one is left with a resigned 'acceptance' of the disease. Kübler-Ross's theory may very effectively be superimposed on any sense of illness or personal loss, and quite truly to the Covid-19 pandemic. The waves of the disease have reached different countries at different times and until the alarming rate of deaths and consequent suffering it brought, each nation lived in a state of denial.

In India, the disease arrived through foreign travel. It was possibly first detected in a native individual arriving from Italy to New Delhi. Similar cases of infected persons returning home soon spread across the states. Initially, there was not only denial but also anger, until one realized that international travel must be shut down and even inter-state travel, must be severely regulated. Importantly enough, the railways were also shut down very early with the onset of the 'complete lockdown' in April 2020. More than being concerned about the fate of the disease, India was suffering from the pangs of the migrant laborers. They bore the maximum brunt of the shock of the Covid-19 arrival because they belonged to the 'unorganized sector' with neither the protection of work nor pay. The closure led to not only the cut in wages but also a denial of the living accommodation of the laborers; soon they were left with no alternative, but to return to their homes, sometimes across the vast stretches of the country. With the railways shut and practically no other forms of transport available, they perforce had to walk for miles in the summer heat and succumbed to hunger, fatigue, and suffering of a yet different kind, far away and unknown to the threats of Covid-19, which seemed, strangely, a rather urban, metropolitan malady. The migrant crises left thousands without work or wages. Many died (the death toll reaching around 1,000 by September 2020 (Mohanty 2020)), leaving a batch of orphans, who found no justification for this state of affairs. The Covid-19 panic had already its first line of casualty, quite independent of itself. The indefinite closure sunk the country's economy into the doldrums.

The urban and domiciled people suffered in events less contingent or less catastrophic. The closure gave rise to online trading and the cities got habituated to getting everything at their doorstep, for a price. Schools and all other educational centers have been closed ever since, giving way to 'online education' to its fullest extent, covering all aspects and all levels of the pedagogic program: from the kindergarten to the doctoral level, including taking classes, giving tests and assignments and supervising research activities. However, what one overlooked in our country was the strong digital divide, as a consequence of the economic divide in this 'developing country'. Among the earliest caution about the digital divide in our country was sounded by the reputed historian, and Vice Chancellor of Jadavpur University, Prof. Suranjan Das (Chowdhury 2020). There are thousands who have had no access to desktop computers, laptops, or smartphones, or who have had to share one between multiple siblings; thousands of children have had to drop out of education where their parents have been deprived of incomes or the children have been rendered orphans. Crimes against women, children and all the marginalized sectors of the society have increased, prompted by hunger, lust, and poverty.

Superseding these ancillary crises, however, the first wave of the Covid-19 pandemic did make its mark in the Indian cities in the second quarter of 2020. There were deaths but the numbers were manageable: what characterized the mindset was one of widespread and universal fear and panic. There was fear and consequent panic as the nature of the viral disease was unknown. There was no sure line of treatment and the vaccine was still at a level of conjecture. The precautionary measures took a heavy toll on the people, worldwide, and mostly among the aged, who were too old to adapt themselves to the new ways of online and digitized technologies. In our country, with the non-availability or paucity of medical facilities during the Covid-19 lockdown, many were reluctant to go for regular medical check-ups fearing contagion of the virus. Many others died due to lack of treatment. Hence, under the common rubric of the Covid-19 pandemic, many other deaths occurred due to negligence; some others were dubbed as a result of morbid 'co-morbidities'. The fear of a Covid death intensified itself with the cruel, isolated, and reckless aftermath, complete with the anonymity of body bags. 2020 saw the loss of many notable greats in India and Bengal, across several fields: in the world of sports, academia, performing arts, and many others, apart from the thousands of common victims (Bhar 2020b).

The second wave of the Covid-19 outbreak represented itself as several times more powerful and more sinister than the first, in the first quarter of 2021. Even while many took the vaccine, the rate of positivity was relatively much higher, attacking not the aged but the young and the middle aged. In an unprecedented occurrence, there was a severe shortage of oxygen in the country and the dead piled up in fearful numbers, with them jostling for cremation or burial. The nation woke up to frightening pictures of mass pyres (*News18.com* 2021) in an unprecedented national crisis, with the heads of the state keeping silent. This was accompanied by a characteristic shortage, and faking of vaccines in some parts of the country, where humanity was superseded by an ugly political machinery. The rapid and uncontrollable spread of the second wave in India was accelerated by the General Assembly Election campaigns in various states and facilitated by mass gatherings during religious events like Holi and the Spring festivals across the nation (*Aljazeera* 2021; Chatterjee and Thakur 2021). These spelt an end to inter-state travel bans and led to a huge conglomeration of the masses. It is well known, how in India, just two things decide the fate of the people: religion and politics. Every other aspect of the state machinery needs to contemplate on these two issues, and the spread of Covid-19 here proved no exception to the usual.

The second wave of Covid-19 in India devastated families in thousands, and kept most others in constant fear for days, with bolted doors, in lifeless silence and trauma. There was no faith even in the air we breathed in.

The Personal in the Pandemic

How did the Covid-19 pandemic affect the 'person' or the 'personal'? And how did the pandemic affect the Indians, in particular? With the spread of the pandemic, first, it seemed that the personal was being attacked – a patient's personal whereabouts, his travel history, his social circle, and his friends, acquaintances – everything and everybody seemed to be under some kind of a surveillance system. Second, each individual was denied the gestures of personal affection and love with the ban on touch. The practice of physical distancing also posed a serious hazard to sexual relations, even between married couples. While Slavoj Žižek observes how the purchase of sex toys even among couples, led to self-gratification (Žižek 2020, vol. 2, 51–55), there is also the other eventuality in India, where there has been an increase in the number of births in the past two years. There has also been a notable drop in the sex trade here where workers are suffering due to a drop in the number of customers, as a consequence of the lockdown and the attendant fear of contagion. Many have also been pushed to committing suicide and several have been thrust into chronic depression. In fact, all professions which depend on physical touch are hit in a bad way, for instance, the beauty and the cosmetic industry (Seshu et al., 2021). The other section to suffer badly is the queer community, against whom were so many bans, which only effectively, multiplied their woes. From not being able to meet one's partner (sometimes separated by countries), to not being able to claim any health benefits for him/her, the pandemic only meted out harsher treatment to the community by increasing the rigidities and prejudices usually practiced against them (Chauhan et al., 2021).

The characteristic 'work from home' ethics, beginning from 2020, did away with the physical and spatial divisions of work, office, and home. One of the most noticeable and obvious changes in the 'work from home' dynamics is the redefinition of space and the lack of boundaries. Previously, for instance, we could talk of our homes as spaces where we didn't allow our offices to encroach. But now, our offices, schools, colleges, universities, political arena, or even our doctor's chambers have all been encroached in what we usually referred to as our 'homes', sometimes even intimate spaces such as our bedrooms or even our beds. The new lifestyle, while it constantly harps on isolation and social distancing, also cuts short on our privacy and individual freedom. While we are at home, we are constantly expected to be 'available' for 'official' work, while the usual domestic chores suffer neglect and abandonment. On the other hand, with the 'abnormal' and ever-extending work hours, our leisure or personal hours suffer. This writer had ventured to express, quite helplessly, in a few lines, the efficacy and lack of 'borders' or even thresholds in our lives, when there seemed to be only one continuum to define it:

Borders

The thresholds have now gone
Between home, world and beyond
There is only one continuum
In which to survive, thrive, confine –
The borders of the mind
Of etiquette, decorum, are now dissolved
Into one seamless whole
When existence itself is
All the proof one holds.[4]

There is, indeed, a tone of helplessness in the confinement and the utter face-tiousness of a world of make-believe, virtually. Notwithstanding the attendant and looming fear of disease and well-being in mind, the expediency of working from home has led to other contingencies as well. With the lack of personal space and a healthy separation, many couples have not been able to bear the constant stress of being with each other or tolerating the proximities of largely different professions. The sanctity of the home space being vitiated many have decided to go their separate ways leading to families breaking up. There has also been an increase in events of domestic violence, due to the unhealthy proximity of family members (Vutsinas 2020). Women and children have been, as with cases of all social changes, the largest casualties in this instance as well. In India, matters assume further complications in a set-up of 'joint families' where many kin and multiple generations with their individual families cohabit in the same house-hold. In such homes, the concept of 'personal space' is a thing of dream, under all circumstances. Nevertheless, even in such cramped houses students of all levels are expected to participate in online classes, or adults to fulfill all necessities of online meetings and other job requirements.

The 'New Normal' Dilemma

In spite of the many pitfalls, it is, however, true that the online facilities have allowed us to connect with distant speakers across the world in real time. The academic fraternity has benefited immensely by conducting extensive webinars across the world and both students and teachers have gained from the knowledge of interna-tional experts. In fact, the practice seems a welcome one to encourage international collaborations of a different kind. Nevertheless, we are now excessively depend-ent on our electronic devices, namely, our phones, computers, and tablets. All our needs have been looked after by the 'artificial intelligence' of these machines. We can watch films, play games, see our friends, communicate instantly and even sat-isfy our physical needs by virtual titillation. Does that mean that human inter-communication would go out of fashion? Or, is this the yard-stick of the 'new normal' – machines replacing human proximity and touch? Slavoj Žižek hints at this horrifying eventuality in his books on the *Pandemic*. We run the risk of literally making 'one little room, an everywhere'[5] in a horribly grotesque, mechanical, and feigned reality of self-sufficiency. In fact, the world has even got accustomed to online marriage broadcasts or even online funeral services. In a way, the readiness with which we can easily dispense with human presence and human company in our lives, and substitute it with virtual presences is not only frightening but also a wry reminder of the impending selfishness of humans. On the flip side, perhaps we can do without our friends and family around us. Perhaps, we will have better excuses for not attending these events in person anymore. In many ways, Covid-19 has succeeded in building walls between humans across all countries. All of us live inside our own bubbles of self-dependence: we do not seek human assistance. The 'new normal', with its insistence on machine-bred life that helps in mutual isolation, may soon make our gatherings, parties and *joie-de-vivre* a thing of the past.

What about teachers in this mechanized world? Teachers are not merely knowledge facilitators. They are nurturers of young minds and the creators of responsible human beings. Most of us have had very lovable experiences with a teacher at some point in our lives. They inspired us with their presence, with their personalities and with their scholarship. But most of all they touched us with their feeling minds, they instinctively understood our needs and tailored knowledge according to our capacities and abilities. Where, one may ask, does online teaching allow for such instinctive communication? Teaching, by definition, is a human profession, it gets facilitated by the mutual presence of the learner and the learned. At many crucial points, and in spite of all the state-of-the-art technologies, online teaching falls short of such interaction. From the ancient times to the present, man has looked up to the philosopher, seeking wisdom and solutions to problems. Machines can, perhaps, never be a substitute for human intelligence and resilience.

Coming Together

The Coronavirus pandemic has laid bare many truths about human behavior and human nature across nations all over the world. The virus has neither discriminated between the rich and the poor nor has it shown any racial priority, such that we all felt that we were in the same boat as one species of humanity. While the virus proved to be an equalizer and a leveler on one hand, the socio-political, and socio-economic situation of each country or people, on the other hand, made all the difference in negotiating crises. The pandemic has also revealed that most nations do not concentrate on health resources as much as they do on sectors like defense. The economies of most countries along with the education sector have been affected cruelly. Now, after losing thousands of our fellow humans and having suffered deep psychological and emotional scars, it is only hoped that there are fraternal collaborations between individuals of all countries. Žižek speaks of a 'new' Communism (Žižek 2020, vol. 1, ch. 10) where all humanity, irrespective of caste, creed, and color should come together in a bid to tide over this unprecedented crisis. This could be, and most agreeably so, the only way to combat the diseased world. Other ancillary and possibly contributive factors for this pandemic, namely climate change, and ecological balance should be prioritized by each country. It is only on such shared bonds and communistic ideas that we can think of saving humanity and emerging from this prolonged 'night-time' of disease. This is certainly not the time to isolate oneself from the rest of the world on any narrow sectarian basis.

Notes

1 I myself branched off into some travel writing in my own blog https://anascornernet. wordpress.com/author/anasuyabhar/, apart from indulging in childhood nostalgia and autobiographical musings, some of which were published in the online literary journal *Borderless Journal* https://borderlessjournal.com/. In fact, I am pleased to

admit that Covid interim allowed me to branch off into creative writing in a definitive manner.

2 The history of diseases in India has not only excited historians but also many of our authors like Bankimchandra Chattopadhyay, Rabindranath Tagore, and others, whose works abound in such descriptions.

3 This reference is taken from the first part of Žižek's book on the Pandemic, chapter five, titled 'The Five Stages of Epidemics'.

4 This poem was composed in August 2020 in the middle of the first wave of the Covid-19 outbreak in India. It found brief presence in the online poetry portal 'Ode to a Poetess'.

5 This reference is from a poem by sixteenth century English poet John Donne titled 'The Good Morrow'. The metaphor of self-sufficiency is used in the poem for the surfeit of lovers. The metaphor is here used in an inverse sense of grotesque claustrophobia.

References

"Bodies Pile up as Second Covid -19 Wave Drowns India". 23 April 2021. *News18.com*. https://www.news18.com/photogallery/india/bodies-pile-up-as-second-covid-19-wave-drowns-india-see-gut-wrenching-photos-3671249.html (Accessed on 29th January 2022).

Bhar, Anasuya. 2020a. "The Corridors of the Mind". September. *Borderless Journal*. https://borderlessjournal.com/2020/09/15/the-corridors-of-the-mind/ (Accessed on 30th January 2022).

Bhar, Anasuya. 2020b. "Time and Us". December. *Borderless Journal*. https://borderlessjournal.com/2020/12/14/time-and-us/ (Accessed on 30th January 2022).

Bhar, Anasuya. *Ana's Corner*. https://anascornernet.wordpress.com/ (Accessed on 30th January 2022).

Chatterjee, Tanmay and Thakur, Joydeep. 2021. "All Bengal Rallies Flouting Covid -19 Norms". 15 April. *The Hindustan Times*. https://www.hindustantimes.com/india-news/all-bengal-rallies-flouting-covid-19-norms-101618425712682.html (Accessed on 29th January 2022).

Chauhan, Sukriti, Yachu, Shireen and Butola, Kiran. 2021. "Covid-19 Pandemic: There's a Need to Address Health Challenges Faced by LGBTQ+ Community". 27 June. *The Indian Express*. https://indianexpress.com/article/lifestyle/health/covid-19-pandemic-theres-a-need-to-address-health-challenges-faced-by-lgbtq-community-7378193/ (Accessed on 29th January 2022).

Chowdhury, Subhankar. 2020. "Digital Divide Caution from Jadavpur VC". 2 April. *The Telegraph*. https://www.telegraphindia.com/west-bengal/calcutta/digital-divide-caution-from-jadavpur-vc/cid/1761513 (Accessed on 29th January 2022).

Dawson, Lindsay, Kirzinger, Ashley and Kates, Jennifer. 2021. "The Impact of the COVID-19 Pandemic on LGBT People". 11 March. https://www.kff.org/coronavirus-covid-19/poll-finding/the-impact-of-the-covid-19-pandemic-on-lgbt-people/ (Accessed on 29th January 2022).

"India Devotees Celebrate Holi Festival, Ignore COVID Restrictions". 24 March 2021. *Aljazeera*. https://www.aljazeera.com/gallery/2021/3/24/india-devotees-ignore-restrictions-celebrate-holi (Accessed on 29th January 2022).

Mohanty, Basant Kumar. 2020. "Migrant Deaths Government Won't See". 16 September. *The Telegraph*. https://www.telegraphindia.com/india/coronavirus-lockdown-migrant-deaths-govt-wont-see/cid/1792114 (Accessed on 29th January 2022).

Seshu, Meena Saraswathi, Rai, Aarti and Murthy, Laxmi. 2021. "Locked Down: Sex Workers and Their Livelihoods". *Economic and Political Weekly*, Vol. 56, No. 11, 13 March. https://www.epw.in/engage/article/locked-down-sex-workers-and-their-livelihoods (Accessed on 29th January 2022).

Sontag, Susan. 1977. *Illness as Metaphor*. New York: Farrar, Straus and Giroux.

Vutsinas, Amanda. 2020. "Managing Domestic Violence in a Work at Home World". 10 April. *Security Magazine*. https://www.securitymagazine.com/articles/92085-managing-domestic-violence-in-a-work-at-home-world (Accessed on 29th January 2022).

Žižek, Slavoj. 2020a. *Pandemic! 2 Chronicles of a Time Lost*. New York and London: OR Books.

Žižek, Slavoj. 2020b. *Pandemic! Covid-19 Shakes the World*. New York and London: OR Books.

6 Livelihood of Internal Migrants of India during Covid-19 Pandemic

Concerns and Measures

Debasis Chakraborty

Introduction

India being a multicultural country, overtime has seen human migration of different nature and of different magnitude. Till the first few months of 2020, it was assumed that India has already seen the biggest mass migration in history at the time of partition. But, thanks (!) to this Covid-19 pandemic, India experienced yet another mass migration which was as big as the earlier one to say the least. The main difference is, this time the migration has been inter-state and mostly urban to rural in nature. There were other characteristics of this internal migration flow. One of them was, this time people who migrated along with their families mostly were workers (broadly informal) in nature. These workers earlier migrated from rural part of relatively poorer economic states to the urban areas of wealthier states in search of employment and were largely engaged in urban informal sector jobs like construction, service sector, etc. Some social scientists have rightly pointed out that they are the real 'city-makers' of modern India (Sikdar and Mishra, 2020). These migrants are the most vulnerable class of Indian citizen and most of them are economically (sometime socially) backward. As soon as Covid-19 pandemic started, they became severely susceptible not only to the disease itself but also became threat to the rest of the economy. This pandemic has helped to visualize how the migrant labourers have always been treated as outcasts by the mainstream economy. They were considered neither relevant nor safe for the cities which already had started battling with this Covid-19 pandemic with one and only weapon of 'lockdown'. Earlier these set of migrants, while working in the urban job markets, were exploited in terms of wages, job hour, safety measures etc. But somehow, they became accustomed with all these adverse situations. One of the main reasons was that the job opportunities were higher in these urban centres compared to their rural origin. Therefore, some of them could send money to their family at home state and few others could afford to bring their family to the host state. As soon as lockdown was brought to effect, Indian industries, companies and firms (heavily centred in and around urban spaces) closed their offices and stores, leading to complete shutdown. The first visible blow came in the shape of losing jobs overnight. The impact on the unorganized migrant labourers was multi-faceted, adversely

DOI: 10.4324/9781003300762-7

affecting their life, livelihood and wellness. As they were mainly daily earners, they had little savings. Under the given circumstances, they could only manage a few days of survival in the suburbs of their urban work spaces of host states. After few days, when they exhausted all their savings, they couldn't manage full meal for two main courses of the day (The Hindustan Times, 2020). A considerable section of these migrants couldn't even have access to one course full meal. Coupled with food crisis, they faced problems related to their living condition as well. Most of these labourers rented house or managed to stay in the slums close to work spaces. As soon as they failed to make ends meet, they were forced to vacate rented houses. Without food and shelter, they were forced to stay under the sky for days with their families comprising of children, women and aged people (The Indian Express, 2020a). The employers, the Central government, and the concerned State governments turned a blind eye to the internal migrant labourers' physical and mental crises. To worsen the situation, the labourers were hurled into a state of uncertainty where time and space had lost their meanings. Not knowing when lockdown would end, the homeless and starving labourers became stateless in their own nation.

Exiled in their own workspace, the internal migrants were determined to go back to their homes. As a result, mass migration of a huge group of people started from various parts of the country to reach their homeland. From this point their difficulties increased many folds, apparently unpredicted by any government in India. Since receiving or sending governments didn't arrange for any conveyance whatsoever for the safe (both mental and physical) return journey towards home, a massive stream of hungry, poor, destitute and stranded migrants started their uncertain journey to cross the inter-state boundaries on foot. Later both Central and few State governments arranged some transport facilities (through buses and trains) but that too were visibly short by a significant margin from what was actually required (Bhagat et al., 2020). Not to forget, this transport process was handled inefficiently, triggering the fear of further cross-infection among themselves. Nevertheless, the outcome of this migratory movement was a severe blow to the economy in various aspects as well as specifically to the wellness of the migrants involved. To perform this impossible task (of migrating on foot) many died on streets irrespective of gender, age and caste; many got infected with novel coronavirus who later became carriers of this deadly virus. While some could reach their home state, others couldn't make it. Coming back to the native space, neither their economic problems nor their social issues got eliminated. Indian rural economy had already been facing the problem of surplus labour and low employability. These reverse migrants were addition to the existing agricultural labour (mostly) within the rural economy. Very few got job where most migrant labourers remained unemployed. One of the arguments in favour of them being unemployed could be since they remained in the urban areas for most part of the year (or years) and were involved in non-agriculture sector jobs, they lacked the required skill to be engaged in the agriculture sector. Whatever be the case, a lion's share of them became unemployed and this made adverse effects on their social wellbeing. Soon in their native villages, they started lacking basic livelihoods and was forced to reconsider the risk of re-migrating to the previous host state in search of livelihoods. Hence, when the lockdown was lifted after few months and shops, restaurants and factories started to re-open, and a return migration started from rural to those urban centres in search of a fresh new beginning. The story from the urban side was somewhat different. As soon as those migrants flew from the city, the city came to a stand-still (considering the fact of lockdown). Even when the phase of lockdown was lifted, almost all the developmental projects missed their target dates as the migrants who flew to their rural areas were the main source of supply of labour in those urban projects. Most of the shops, hotels & restaurants, etc. started to work below their potential as there was immense shortfall of labour. The sit-uation of urban households suffered a blow too due to this reverse migration. This is because a considerable share of the migrants (mainly the female family members) was involved in various household works (like maids, cleaning, house-keeping, etc.), involving the 3D jobs – dirty, dangerous and demeaning (Bhagat et al., 2020) which the sophisticated urban dwellers hesitate to perform. As the economy started to move on, factories re-opened. But they were opened only to experience the fact that they were severely understaffed. By then Indian cities became ready to accept the fact that migrants were the lifeline of their daily wellbeing. If Indian cities have to sustain and blossom, it is not possible without the direct and/or indirect involvement of these migrant labourers. So, when these migrants returned to their respective workplaces, urban centres, which once turned their back on those ever-needy migrants, received them with both hands. Even certain shops and factory owners were ready to bear the cost of their migrant workers' return journey from their home state to their respective urban centres (The Hindu, 2020). While some employers waived house rents of their workers until they were able to relocate themselves, few provided cash supports to minimize the loss. Moreover, governmental initiatives (on the part of both Central and State like Delhi, U.P., Haryana, etc.) could be seen as a few trains and busses were run by the inter-state transportations to facilitate the return journey of the migrant workers back to their workspace, unlike the initial unsafe unhygienic uncertain journey on foot. This, in a nutshell, is the story of Indian migrants in both pre- and post-lockdown phases.

The Covid-19 pandemic (unfortunately) was an eye-opener for the Indian policy makers who for the first time considered the significance of the inter-nal migrants in India's economic and social development. Moreover, urban in-migrants from rural areas hitherto were never given importance in the policy framing in urban planning. It's time for the policy-making bodies to consider the developmental potential of these disadvantaged and marginalized groups of people who hadn't been even guaranteed the fundamental rights in their own country. The study therefore focuses on the status of migrant workers during the first wave of Covid-19 pandemic and the role of various policies that have been adopted and prescribed for their wellbeing. After a brief overview of the trend and volume of migrants in India, the study incorporates the status of internal migrants during the Covid-19 pandemic as reported by various government and non-government organizations. In doing so, the next section critically examines various measures adopted by both Central and State governments to improve the wellness of these migrants and analyses some of the key policy issues. The final section offers a conclusion by underscoring the significance of the present findings.

Migration in India: A Broad Overview

Migrants, whether inter-state or intra-state, constitute a determining factor in India's population distribution. In a country like India where there is a lack of opportunity for employment, education and livelihood every 100 kilometres, migration is an inevitable phenomenon. Additionally, this is also triggered by disproportionate allocation of resources between urban and rural. Hence historically, Indian people have moved, sometimes from rural to urban, sometimes from one state to another or even within the state from a relatively deprived region to a well-off province (Table 6.1).

Recent most evidences (Census-2011) show that over the last decade the gross figure of internal migrants has increased by almost 50 per cent, which is a considerable share of population in India. Stream-wise segregation shows that most of them move within the State (due to various reasons like geographical, lingual and economic benefits) as it accounts for almost 400 million in comparison to the inter-state migration accounting for just over 54 million. Though the percentage increase is high for this inter-state migrants (almost 32 per cent) too.

For simplicity, census of India has identified some of the fundamental causes of migration that take place across India. They are classified in terms of economic and non-economic reasons. While reasons like Work/Business/Employment come under economic causes, factors like education, marriage and moving with family or household come under non-economic reasons. 'Others' primarily comprise various natural calamities that have taken place. Table 6.2 suggests that one-third of migration due to economic reason goes for the inter-state movement. This is understandable, as inter-state migration is a long-distance one and someone has to have significant employment opportunities to cross the border of the

Table 6.1 Migrants in India in 2001 and 2011

Streams	2001 (in million)	2011 (in million)	Rate of growth (in percentage)
Inter-State Migrants	41.2	54.3	31.80
Intra-State Migrants	268.2	395.7	47.54
Total Internal Migrants	309.4	449.9	45.41

Source: Census Data (D-Tables), 2001 & 2011.

Table 6.2 Migration according to various reasons for migration (in percentage)

Reasons	Inter-state	Inter-district	Intra-district
Work/Business/Employment	30.3	34.6	35.1
Education	13.8	32.4	53.8
Marriage	8.1	26.5	65.4
Moved with Family	15.9	29.3	54.8
Others	8.3	18.0	73.7

Source: Census Data (D-Tables), 2011.

Table 6.3 Gender-wise distribution of workers by migration stream (in percentage)

Streams	Male	Female	Total
Inter-Country	3.2	1.5	2.6
Inter-State	29.4	12.3	24.0
Inter-District	29.3	25.2	28.0
Intra-District	38.1	61.0	45.4

Source: Khanna (2020).

state. Hence Indian migrants move more within the territory of the country for employment (whether permanent or temporary; circular or seasonal) (Table 6.3).

Gender-wise distribution states that out of total male migrants, almost 30 per cent are migrating across the border of the State, while this figure is 12 per cent for female migrants. This is also logical in the sense that if taking up employment is the fundamental reason for inter-state migration then male migrants have a higher employment probability than their female counterparts. For females, this figure is significantly low as they mostly migrate either with households or after marriage.

Figure 6.1 depicts the changing dynamics of inter-state migration in India over the last three decades. It shows an increasing trend of people migrating across states of origin to move into a new settlement mostly for searching for jobs. It also shows that new cities are becoming hotspots for migrants as India's growth over the years has been city-oriented and urban-biased. The data also reveals that the number of these hotspots is increasing overtime (see Table 6.4). There are several reasons for the changing structures of Indian urbans. Most of these cities provide informal jobs (e.g. contractual, daily wage) in manufacturing and construction sectors which requires almost no specialization on the part of those migrants. Moreover, these migrants provide cheap source of labour as they are huge in number and require very little or no investment in their health, education or similar social sectors from the employer's end. One of the closest examples would be the NRIs who settle abroad (e.g., Silicon Valley) where they are assumed as a cheap source of labour to the native industries, compared to migrants from other countries who are relatively expensive to hire. Hence, in regard to inter-state migration, there is an 'India within India' scenario.

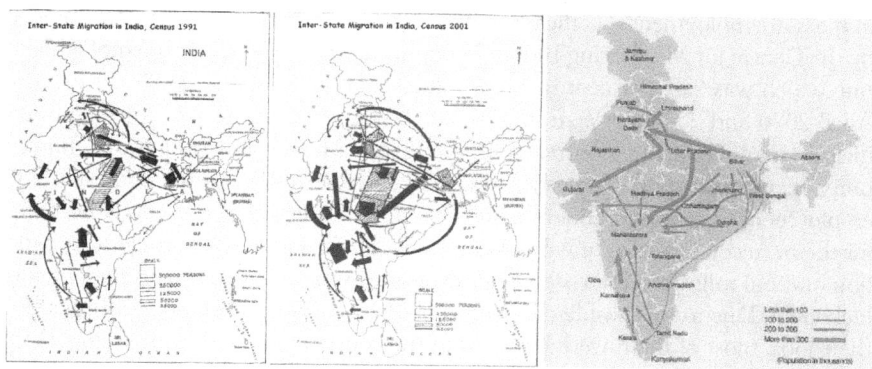

Figure 6.1 Trend of inter-state migration flow in India – 1991, 2001, and 2011.
Source: Das & Saha (2012) and WEF (2017).

Table 6.4 Proportion of migrants and non-migrants in metro cities in India (in percentage)

Cities	2001		2011	
	Migrants	*Non-migrants*	*Migrants*	*Non-migrants*
Bengaluru	36	64	52	48
Chennai	24	76	50	50
Delhi	41	59	42	58
Hyderabad	25	75	64	36
Kolkata	23	77	37	63
Mumbai	43	57	54	46

Source: Census Data (D-Tables), 2001 & 2011.

Migrants during Lockdown: The Indian Experience

With an eye to break the chain of transmission, India went for a nationwide lockdown for a considerable period starting from 25 March and ending on 31 May in a phase-wise manner. The first phase continued for 21 days, while the second phase lasted for 19 days which was a continuation of the first phase. The third and last phases had lasted for 14 days each, and hence, the lockdown ended on 31 May 2020. Immediately after the imposition of the lockdown, the economic activities in India came to a halt and its aftermath directly fell on the urban in-migrants. They soon became helpless amidst other urban odds having lost their jobs and home. Almost 400 million workers of the informal labour force which constitutes nearly 90 per cent of the Indian workforce lost their job during this phase (ILO and ADB, 2020) and were driven into acute poverty. According to some experts, it has been 'the worst economic downturn since the great depression' (Gopinath, 2020). It is the urban centres in India that have been hit most by this lockdown. As these centres were the primary destination of most of the inter-state migrants in

India, they became the worst victim due to the closing of businesses. This resulted in mass unemployment specifically in India's urban metros. According to a report by the Centre for Monitoring Indian Economy (CMIE), the urban unemployment rate which was 9.41 per cent in March 2020 soon increased to 24.95 per cent in April 2020 and 25.79 per cent in May 2020. Few sectors that were affected most include manufacturing, construction, retail trade, hotels and restaurants, hospitality, textile, transport, domestic work, etc. These sectors enjoy the lion's share of employment of migrant labourers and therefore resulted in disastrous conditions for them. According to a study by World Bank (Ratha et al., 2020), roughly 40 million internal migrants (inter-state and intra-state) were affected by this nationwide lockdown. Due to this pandemic, a total of 41 lakh young workforce in India lost their jobs, most of them were involved in the construction and farm sector (ILO and ADB, 2020). There are specific reasons for which domestic migrants all over the world and specifically in a labour-intensive country like India, become more vulnerable in a pandemic situation like this: First of all, in the area of destination they lack proper habitat and are forced to accommodate themselves in already overcrowded slums. In these places, social distancing can hardly be maintained and access to masks and other protective gears simply becomes a luxury to them. This increases their chance of being infected during pandemics or endemics. Additionally, being in the urban informal labour market, they are barely protected by any laws or any legal terms and hence neither get any medical support nor do they receive any financial support specifically for treatment purposes (Ghosh, 2020). Coupled with these there is a lack of unemployment benefits from the government or local authorities (at least at the beginning of the lockdown) and shortages of food, etc. All these factors make the migrant workers most vulnerable in the changing times and bring them along with their family members to the threshold of starvation. This has a direct negative impact on their wellbeing which finally results in a mass exodus from the area to their destination. The pattern of migration that India experienced during the Covid-19 pandemic is basically a 'reverse migration' (Sikdar and Mishra, 2020). According to data provided by the Stranded Workers Action Network (SWAN, 2020a), most of the stranded migrants came from four major states namely, Maharashtra, Karnataka, Delhi and Haryana. The first two cities that contributed the most to this flow of migrants are Mumbai and Bangalore. The report suggests that almost 90 per cent didn't receive any payment from their employer and hence their living standards deteriorated drastically during this span. According to Gaikwad and Nellis (2020) during these testing times also these migrants had to face discrimination from the political leaders. They found in their study that local political leaders tend to support a long-time migrant compared to someone whose duration of migration is relatively shorter. On the contrary, it is evident that short-time migrants do need more support as they are yet to establish themselves in new settlements. Hence there were discriminations on the ground of local support as well. Along with this, there was a delay in government support for these migrant workers who were neither having savings nor food to support their daily life and were left in the hands of destiny only to increase their suffering (Ghosh, 2020). As 'support' delayed means 'support' denied, this actually hit them adversely. Initially, the government didn't allow these inter-state migrants to reverse migrate to their homeland which forced these stranded people to literally travel on foot. This resulted in hundreds of people being killed due to various reasons (e.g. heat, road accidents, and train accidents). As per one report (SWAN, 2020a) as of 4 July 2020, there has been 971 non-Covid death in India during lockdown related to migrant workers out of which 216 were due to starvation and financial distress, while 209 were due to road and train accidents. These are the data which have been reported or collected, but the true figures could be more. Talking about the profile of the workers it has been seen that almost 79 per cent of migrant workers are daily wage factory/construction workers whose average daily wage is merely Rs. 402 (SWAN, 2020b).

There can always be a debate if the lockdown is the best possible way to resort to under a pandemic situation, especially in a diverse country such as India. In the beginning of lockdown (i.e. on March 25, 2020), India had only 320 Covid-19 cases, but by the end of June, it increased exponentially to place India as the third most affected country in the world (Ghosh, 2020). The reason is not only the unprepared imposition of one of the most severe lockdowns in human history, according to the University of Oxford's Covid-19 Government Response Stringency Index (OxCGRT) but also inadequate government relief measures that were necessary to support the most vulnerable class of the people especially the migrants.

Various Government Measures and their Effectiveness

Measures

Untimely and an impromptu lockdown had a severe long-run blow on the Indian economy as it was just trying to recover from the imposition of demonetization and GST. Additionally, it had unique consequences on the life and livelihood of the informal migrant workers which required to be addressed separately by both Central and State governments. It will be unfair to state that none of the governments took any step in this regard but they certainly failed to meet the expectations. Some of the measures were overlapping and it affected the proper implementation of the said scheme as their jurisdictions were not well defined. For this too, in spite of having proper measures, marginalized people and/or migrants had to suffer a lot. As there are numerous strategies that have been advised by different task forces and accordingly adopted by the governments, in this section, we discuss some of the crucial measures taken by them and try to analyse their effectiveness.

Soon after the declaration of a nationwide lockdown, GOI announced a relief package amounting to Rs. 1.70 lakh-crore under the scheme Pradhan Mantri Gareeb Kalyan Yojana (PMGKY). Initially, it was effective till June 2020 which was extended twice till November 2020 and later until 24 April 2021. This particular scheme broadly was distributed in two facets: food security and Direct Benefit Transfer (DBT). These two again were subdivided into various sub-schemes. Direct cash transfer programme was one of them under the name of Prime Minister Jan Dhan Yojana (PMJDY) (mostly for women) where Rs. 500 is transferred to bank accounts held by the poorest of the poor people. Most of the accounts are held in public sector banks and as of August 2020 just over 380 million JDY accounts were in operation (Ray and Subramanian, 2020). The list of beneficiaries of PMGKY includes MNREGA (Mahatma Gandhi National Rural Employment Guarantee Act) workers, farmers, health workers, aged and unorganized sector workers and migrant workers. Rs. 3,000 crores were allotted for widows, senior citizens and differently abled persons. Most coveted Ujjawala Scheme also comes under this umbrella where approx. Rs. 13,000 crores were allotted to provide LPG connections to families who were below the poverty line. Additionally, Rs. 2,500 crores were allocated for Employees' Provident Fund while Rs. 6,000 crores were allocated for the employment of tribals under the scheme named Compensatory Afforestation Management & Planning Authority (CAMPA). The scheme PMGKY included the distribution of an additional 5 kg of wheat or rice and 1 kg of preferred pulses every month to 80 crore beneficiaries for the next three months from the date of its implementation. It was decided that the food would be distributed under the Public Distribution System (PDS). To help the construction workers, a considerable share of which were the stranded migrants, each of the State governments was asked to use Building and Construction Workers Welfare Fund to provide relief to these workers through DBT. The total fund under this scheme was Rs. 52,000 crores. There were provisions for health workers too under this scheme. Medical insurance of the sum assured Rs. 5 million was provided for all the forefront health workers fighting Covid-19. Government expediated the arrangement made by the PM-Kisan Samman Nidhi Yojana scheme for a direct cash transfer of Rs. 6,000 (in three equal instalments) to 87 million farmers during this lockdown. There was a provision for a collateral-free loan for the female SHGs too amounting to Rs. 2 million. As an extension to last year's stimulus, RBI on 5 May 2021 announced a Term Liquidity Facility of Rs. 50,000 crores (The Hindu, 2021). This will specifically be helpful for health workers, medical suppliers and small borrowers under MSMEs.

Some steps were specifically taken to help and facilitate migrant workers who were migrating back to their villages. In June 2020, the Central government launched an employment scheme by the name Garib Kalyan Rozgar Abhiyaan (GKRA), specifically targeting migrant workers, and allocated Rs. 50,000 crores. It was launched initially for 125 days, in 116 districts of six states namely, Bihar, Madhya Pradesh, Uttar Pradesh, Rajasthan, Jharkhand and Odisha which received a considerable number of return migrants. In its brief note published by the GOI, it was claimed that this scheme will broadly help to expedite the implementation of 25 types of public infrastructure works and this in turn will expand livelihood opportunities. The scheme actually aimed to provide at least 125 days of work to migrant workers according to their skills and hence expanding their wellbeing (The Economic Times, 2020). Under the PMGKY scheme Rs. 3,500 crore had been allotted for migrant workers for providing free food to them. Apart from steps taken by the Central government, few State governments took certain measures to comfort these inter-state migrants. Few of them provided free food, shelters, important commodities, etc. to those stranded migrants. States like West Bengal, Bihar, Delhi, Telangana, and Uttar Pradesh arranged facilities like direct fund transfer, cash relief, providing provisional ration cards, etc. Providing employment to the migrants once they came back into their villages has been one of the daunting challenges for both these governments. This is because the rural job market of India which is broadly agri-driven, was already experiencing surplus labour, low growth of employment, etc. due to various bottlenecks of its own. Hence to accommodate these in-migrants the government has to create jobs both temporary and permanent. Thankfully few initiatives were taken in this regard too. There was a direct enhancement of funds by Rs. 40,000 crores, over and above the allocation of Central Budget 2020–2021, that were made for MGNREGA workers. If we go with the claims made by Finance Minister, it would create additionally about 300 crore man days of employment which would specifically be helpful for reverse migrants. As the second phase of relief measures, on 12 May 2020, the Government of India launched a new and unique scheme under the name of Atmanirbhar Bharat Abhiyan (ABA) which was aimed to make India a self-reliant and a manufacturing hub. It focused most valuable five components namely Economy, Infrastructure, Systems, Vibrant Demography and Demand (Government of India, 2020a). It was claimed that this scheme would help integrate the manufacturing sector of India with its predominant agricultural sector. This would not only create sufficient employment opportunities for the whole economy and for reverse migrants in particular but would also create adequate demand in the economy in the long run, much needed to push the cycle of growth ahead once the pandemic is over. This would also help local Micro, Small & Medium Enterprises (MSMEs) to create employment. Under this scheme of ABA, the Centre announced an economic package of Rs. 20 lakh crores which was almost 10 per cent of India's GDP (Ray and Subramanian, 2020). This scheme had a plan for almost every sector of the economy. Out of them few salient features were specifically for migrants and most vulnerable groups of the society. For example, provision for a concessional credit of Rs. 2 trillion for 25 million fishermen, farmers and animal husbandry farmers under PM-Kisan, special credit benefit exclusively for street vendors, additional emergency fund for farmers amounting Rs. 0.3 trillion, promoting affordable housing for migrants, free food grains for 80 million migrants who are not holding any ration card etc. (Government of India, 2020b). As a gesture to extend the helping hands, the Central government had asked each of the states to use money that are left in the State Disaster Relief Fund (SDRF) to provide food, medical facilities and accommodation to migrant workers (Joy and DHNS, 2020). Soon the Ministry of Home Affairs issued a three-way guideline which could be considered a significant step towards the wellbeing of the migrants…

2.1 Migrant workers who are still in the cities of their local residence…

a) Names, local residential and permanent addresses and mobile numbers of the migrant workers shall be recorded. b) District health

administration will depute a team which would include District Surveillance Officer/his representative and public health personnel. Thermal
screening of all such persons shall be done by this team...

2.2 Migrant workers who are on their way and are yet to reach their
destination city/village

2.2.1 Setting/establishment of quarantine center

2.2.2 Health actions at the quarantine facility

2.3 Migrant workers who have reached their destination

a) District health administration will depute a team which would
include District Surveillance Officer/his representative and public
health personnel. b) Such persons shall be contacted by IDSP teams
and interviewed about place of local residence...

(Government of India, 2020c)

Psychological trauma that migrants go through is one of the major concerns at
this point in time as it affects the long-term mental stability and wellness of an
individual. Though of late, the Government of India did make provision for the
mental health of migrants who are always in fear of getting infected by others,
not being able to reach home, having fear of being food-less, etc. So, provisions
were made to make phone calls to their near and dear ones at frequent intervals,
counsellors were appointed for those camps where they were residing temporarily (Government of India, 2020d).

Effectiveness

These measures though gave the much-needed support, they were heavily criticized by various experts as they were far below their requirements. The most
severe critique was that the initial relief plan was even less than 1 per cent of
India's GDP and stands at a very low level compared to the economically well-
off countries (Anderson et al., 2020; Ghosh, 2020) and only 5.6 per cent of the
GOI's planned financial outlay for 2020–2021 (Sengupta and Jha, 2020). Some
experts commented that some of the allocations that have been made under this
relief plan have already been mentioned in the Union Budget (Drèze, 2020).
Even the efficacy of JDY was questioned by the social researchers. People living in rural areas find it difficult to open an account in banks as they mostly
operate in urban centres. Though the number of branches in rural areas has
increased manifold in 2019 compared to 2010 (almost 91 per cent), still 45 per
cent of accounts that have been opened remain inactive due to various reasons
like rising unemployment, low wages, low savings, lack of infrastructures, high
service charges, etc. (Grant Thornton India Report, 2020). Amidst this, the
funds that are to be transferred to those accounts, experts believe, will have
very little impact on the livelihood of those poverty-stricken families. Measures which were migrant-specific were also not spared and experts considered
them to be flawed in various aspects. The free food grain that was allocated
for them through PDS can only reached them if they had ration card. But as

stated earlier, at that point of time most of the migrants were stranded and were on the move from one state to another. Hence, they either didn't have ration card or had ration cards issued from home states which were not valid/applicable in a different host state where they were locked down. They had to wait till they returned to their homes. Therefore, the people for whom this plan was intended didn't get any benefit in times of dire need. Even though some of the food items that were distributed through PDS under the Central government scheme, didn't have that impact as the time taken for distribution was unbearably long (Ray and Subramanian, 2020). The claim of creation of jobs under MGNREGA, through increase in funds, was also highly criticized as experts commented that the initial allotment of Rs. 61,000 crores were already an immense underestimate of fund that was actually required. The additional Rs. 40,000 crores that was allotted under the relief measures, were miniscule in comparison to the actual need of the hour (Bajaj et al., 2020). Additionally, one section of the fund was used for paying past dues which considerably reduced the share for migrant workers making the scheme far below than what was envisioned. Drèze (2020) heavily criticized the effectiveness of PM-Kisan scheme as it was only for those who had certain level of land holdings. But data reveals that most of the migrants were landless and casual workers. Hence the impact of this scheme remains well beyond the reach of those migrants for whom this scheme was actually proposed. One of the major absences that these relief measures had was availability of ransom due to loss of lives that took place due to the reverse migration (Sibal, 2020). Upon getting instructions from the Central government many State governments made shelter for the habitation of the stranded people in their state but the status of those centres was one of the points of criticism by many experts. While some were of the opinions that these centres fast became super spreaders of Covid-19 pandemic due to mismanagement on the part of the local administration (Ghosh, 2020), others pointed out terrible conditions of migrants in those shelters as severe violation of human rights (Libal et al., 2021). Even the famous Atmanirbhar Bharat Abhiyan scheme of GOI was criticized on several grounds. Under this scheme it was decided that the money for the migrants would be distributed through the State and local administration like municipalities, corporations and panchayats. There was a substance of doubt that presence of factors like red-tapism, bureaucratic bottlenecks and overall political biasedness etc. would hamper the motto of this fund transfer as in their presence the amount might not reach the targeted group. Again, though the macro share of this total relief package was almost 10 per cent of India's GDP, micro-segregation revealed that share for migrants and poor households out of this was merely 1.1 per cent of India's total GDP (IMF, 2020). This was because this Rs. 20 lakh crores included measures and financial assistance already taken by RBI and hence the actual additional amount that was spent was considerably less, merely Rs. 12 lakh crores (The Indian Express, 2020b). This shows how less relevant migration status was in the eye of the policy makers which originated from the lack of understanding their real state of being.

Conclusion

Like most of the countries in the world, Covid-19 pandemic has posited an unprecedented situation in India too. Its economy has been shattered like never before, employment scenario dropped an all-time high, and poverty and inequality estimates have risen at a record peak level. Summarily, the welfare of common man or '*AAM -AADMI*' has been affected severely. But amidst this challenging time, there is one ray of hope specifically for the group of people whom we call the '*Internal Migrants*': the Covid-19 pandemic, for the very first time, visibilized the importance of internal migrants as an important sector within the context of mainstream policy making in the Indian economy. These migrants – called the 'city-makers' – were first time guaranteed measures exclusively for their welfare. Though there are debates on the effectiveness and degree of strength of some of these measures that were opted solely for them, they can be enforced by the state through proper monitoring and emphasis, thereby increasing the overall wellbeing of the migrant labourers of India during. This pandemic has been a lesson that these internal migrants indeed need to be 'internalized' in the urban growth process if India really wants to fulfil its dream of sustainable growth.

References

Anderson, J., Bergamini, E., Brekelmans, S., Cameron, A., Darvas, Z., Jiménez, M. D., Lenaerts, K. & Midões, C. 2020. The Fiscal Response to the Economic Fallout from the Coronavirus. Bruegel Datasets. https://www.bruegel.org/publications/datasets/covid-national-dataset/.

Bajaj, A., et al. 2020. Nine Concerns about the Centre's 1.7 Lakh Crore Package. https://thewire.in/government/covid-19-india-government-package.

Bhagat, R. B., et al. 2020. The COVID-19, Migration and Livelihood in India: Challenges and Policy Issues: Challenges and Policy Issues. *Migration Letters*, 17(5), 705–718.

Drèze, J. 2020. View: The Finance Minister's COVID-19 Relief Package Is Helpful, but There Are Gaping Holes in It. *The Economic Times*. https://economictimes.indiatimes.com/news/economy/policy/view-the-finance-ministers-covid-19-reliefpackage-is-helpful but-there-are-gaping-holes-in-it/article show/74853103.cms.

Gaikwad, N., & Nellis, G. 2020. Do Politicians Discriminate Against Internal Migrants? Evidence from Nationwide Field Experiments in India. *American Journal of Political Science*, 1(1). https ://doi.org/10.1111/ajps.12548.

Ghosh, J. 2020. A Critique of the Indian Government's Response to the COVID-19 Pandemic. *Journal of Industrial and Business Economics*, 47, 519–530.

Gopinath, G. (2020). The Great Lockdown: The Worst Economic Downturn since the Great Depression. https://blogs.imf.org/2020/04/14/the-great-lockdown-worst-economic-downturn-since-the-great-depression/.

Government of India. 2020a. AatmaNirbharBharat Abhiyan Portal. https://aatmanirbharbharat.mygov.in/.

Government of India. 2020b. Part-2: Poor, Including Migrants and Farmers. https://cdnbbsr.s3waas.gov.in/s3850af92f8d9903e7a4e0559a98ecc857/uploads/2020/05/2020051751.pdf.

Government of India. 2020c. Advisory for Quarantine of Migrant Workers. https://www.mohfw.gov.in/pdf/Advisoryforquarantineofmigrantworkers.pdf.

Government of India. 2020d. Psychological Issues among Migrants during COVID-19. https://www.mohfw.gov.in/pdf/RevisedPsychosocialissuesofmigrantsCOVID19.pdf.

International Labour Organization and Asian Development Bank. Tackling the COVID-19 Youth Employment Crisis in Asia and the Pacific. Co-publication of the Asian Development Bank and the International Labour Organization, 2020. ISBN: ILO 978–92-2–0326039 (web PDF).

International Monetary Fund (IMF). 2020. Policy Responses to COVID-19 Policy Tracker. https://www.imf.org/en/Topics/imf-and-covid19/Policy-Responses-to- COVID-19.

Joy, S., & DHNS. 2020. Coronavirus: MHA Tells States to Set Up Relief Camps along Highways for Migrant Workers. *Deccan Hearld*, 28 March 2020. https://www.deccan-herald.com/national/national-politics/coronavirus-mha-tellsstates-to-set-up-relief-camps-along-highways-for-migrant-workers-818637.html.

Khanna, A. 2020. Impact of Migration of Labour Force due to Global COVID-19 Pandemic with Reference to India. *Journal of Health Management*, 22(2), 181–191.

Libal, K., et al. 2021. Human Rights of Forced Migrants During the COVID-19 Pandemic: An Opportunity for Mobilization and Solidarity. *Journal of Human Rights and Social Work*. Published online on 19th March. https://link.springer.com/content/pdf/10.1007/s41134-021-00162-4.pdf.

Ratha, D. K., De, S., Kim, E. J., Plaza, S., Seshan, G. K., & Yameogo, N. D. 2020. COVID-19 Crisis through a Migration Lens (No. 147828, pp. 1–50). The World Bank, April.

Ray, D., & Subramaniam, S. 2020. India's Lockdown: An Interim Report. *Indian Economic Review*, 55, 31–79.

Sengupta, S. & Jha, M. K. 2020. Social Policy, COVID-19 and Impoverished Migrants: Challenges and Prospects in Locked Down India. *The International Journal of Community and Social Development*, 2(2), 152–172.

Sibal, K. 2020. On COVID-19, the Centre Has Foisted All Responsibility on the States. https://thewire.in/government/covid-19-modigovernment-states.

Sikdar, S., & Mishra, P. 2020. Reverse Migration during Lockdown: A Snapshot of Public Policies. National Institute of Public Finance and Policy, Working Paper 318.

Stranded Workers Action Network (SWAN). 2020a. 21 Days and Counting: COVID-19 Lockdown, Migrant Workers, and the Inadequacy of Welfare Measures in India. Bengaluru, 15 April. https://www.thehindu.com/news/resources/article31442220.ece/binary/Lockdown-and-Distress_Report-by-Stranded-Workers-Action-Network.pdf.

Stranded Workers Action Network (SWAN). 2020b. 32 Days and Counting: COVID-19 Lockdown, Migrant Workers, and the Inadequacy of Welfare Measures in India. Bengaluru, 1 May. https://covid19 social security.files.wordpress.com/2020/05/32-days-and counting_swan.pdf?fbclid=IwAR0kuFz9pV9drrshn7NLnOUOuVbkv7N-brGzcqMLBMwyel0isEsaoLO-dw0.

The Economic Times. 2020. PM Modi Launches Employment Scheme for Migrant Workers Affected by Coronavirus Lockdown. https://economictimes.indiatimes.com/news/economy/policy/pm-launches-employment-scheme-for-migrant-workers/articleshow/76479291.cms?from=mdr.

The Hindu. 2020. After Turning their Backs during Lockdown, Cities Now Want Migrant Workers Back. https://www.thehindu.com/news/national/after-turning-their-backs-during-lockdown-cities-now-want-migrant-workers-back/article31927237.ece.

The Hindu. 2021. RBI Steps in to Ease COVID-19 Burden. https://www.thehindu.com/business/Economy/rbi-steps-in-to-ease-covid-19-burden-small-businesses-msmes-to-get-relief/article34492630.ece.

The Hindustan Times. 2020. Pandemic Teaches a Tragic Lesson in Migration. https://www.hindustantimes.com/india-news/pandemic-teaches-a-tragic-lesson-in-migration/story-69EIk6MB70zNDX1VsRTx0J.html.

The Indian Express. 2020a. In Goa, Migrant Workers Left with No Money Asked to Leave Rented Houses. https://indianexpress.com/article/coronavirus/in-goa-migrants-workers-left-with-no-money-asked-to-leave-rented-houses-6361545/.

The Indian Express. 2020b. PM Modi's Atmanirbhar Bharat Abhiyan Economic Package: Here Is the Fine Print. https://indianexpress.com/article/explained/narendra-modi-coronavirus-economic-package-india-self-reliance-6406939/.

World Economic Forum (WEF). Migration and Its Impact on Cities – An Insight Report, October 2017.

7 Federalism and Intergovernmental Coordination during a Pandemic

A Special Reference to India

Chitra Roy

Introduction

The Covid-19 Pandemic has caused an unprecedented crisis in human life, posing new challenges to governments all over the world. At the same time, it has forced countries to reconsider the nature of federalism and intergovernmental mechanisms for coping with this global health emergency. In this context, intergovernmental relations have turned out to be an important element in designing an effective measure to respond to the crisis. To put it another way, a strong government response to a Pandemic demands a clear division of roles and responsibilities. Thus, the Covid-19 Pandemic has necessitated intergovernmental cooperation in both the public health and financial sectors since its outbreak, with state and local governments responsible for localized public healthcare and the federal or central government subsidizing the system in order to successfully lead the Pandemic responses.

Federalism, as a political principle, refers to the constitutional distribution of powers among the constituting parties, in which each can enjoy the desired unity and autonomy for some purposes. Many definitions of federalism explain a common feature of the federal system namely the division of power between the two constitutionally established orders of government with some genuine autonomy from each other; each government has a direct electoral relationship with its people; and governments at each level are primarily accountable to their respective electorates. (Anderson 2008, 3–4). A federal system of government also ensures the important elements of divided and shared powers within a decentralized administration to pave the ways to bridge differences in the crisis time and it helps to build the capacity to respond. It expects the federal, state, and local governments to work together to protect public health, while also functioning as separate, autonomous entities to promote and provide for the common good. Downey and Myers writes:

> Generally, within federalism systems, there are enumerated powers given to each branch of government as well as specific policy domains that are under their purview. Under this system of governance, states and the national government are co-sovereign. On one hand, federalism as a form of governance

DOI: 10.4324/9781003300762-8

is notable due to its ability to protect and foster the divergent policy preferences of territorially based groups, thus minimizing coercion by the central government while maximizing policy responsiveness at the subnational level. Federalism in its purest form protects state autonomy, venerates distinct state interests, and ensures separation between state and national interests.

(Downey & Myers 2020, 527)

However, in times of crisis, a federal system of government may face a number of challenges, both horizontally and vertically, in terms of collaboration and coordination with multilevel governance. To be more specific, when a crisis occurs, both cooperation and conflict may exist within the federal paradigm. In this context, recent studies (Benton 2020; Brown & Latulippe 2021; Dagurre & Conlan 2020; Downey & Myers 2020; Kincaid & Leckrone 2020; Lecours et al. 2021) focuses on the various challenges of federalism, intergovernmental relations and policy responses with the outbreak of novel coronavirus in the several federations like the USA, Canada, Australia, etc.

Since the global outbreak of the Covid-19 virus, for example, the United States has experienced serious governance issues, with economic and public health ramifications. In certain areas, the Pandemic has resulted in diverse and contradictory state responses, inadequate federal measures, and ineffective intergovernmental coordination. Downey and Myers make the following observation on the US government's initial response to the Covid-19:

The United States has had an admittedly haphazard response to the COVID-19 pandemic at the national level by all metrics. Inconsistent federal guidance regarding stay-at-home orders, as well as conflicting messages of the use of facemasks for personal protection, and significant problems with coordinating the distribution of personal protection equipment for medical responders has taken up lots of space in national and local newspapers across the country.

(Downey & Myers 2020, 529)

In comparison to the United States, intergovernmental relations in other federations such as Canada and Australia were more collaborative and responsive during the Pandemic. According to Lecours et al. (2021), intergovernmental conflicts were not as evident in these federations because governments avoided denouncing one another's actions and instead focused on improving public health policies and standards, as well as developing several Covid-19 mechanisms to prevent the spread of coronavirus. Lecours et al. also remark:

The acute emergency context triggered by the spread of COVID-19 could be expected to strain intergovernmental relations in federations... Intergovernmental relations in the Canadian and Australian federations were in general harmonious during the first wave of the pandemic. In Canada, where federal–provincial relations are often acrimonious, governments generally refrained from criticizing each other as they managed the pandemic—sometimes even complimenting each other's performance and praising intergovernmental collaboration. In Australia, intergovernmental relations during the pandemic, although not entirely devoid of tensions, were also collaborative. In short, during the first wave of the pandemic, Intergovernmental conflict, understood as public criticism of one government of the federation by another and accompanying actions, was much more significant in the United States than in Canada and Australia.

(Lecours et al. 2021, 514)

However, as Benton (2020, 538-540) points out, despite the enormous challenges posed by the virus, the American federal system has lived up to expectations due to effective interstate and interlocal interactions and greater partnerships among states and local governments. In many regions, the role of state governments in dealing with the Pandemic was commendable. Regional governments have implemented some significant welfare policies, such as 'extending credit to local governments, extending healthcare coverage to those who lost it through unemployment; property tax relief; affordable housing relief, and assistance to colleges and universities, small business, and nursing homes' (Brown & Latulippe 2021, 13–14). Notably, it became possible as a result of the desired cooperation between federal governments. In this case, 'Federal agency responses are, in part, to work closely with allied state agencies such as through coordinating, testing, provisioning equipment, sharing data, and administering various aid programs' (Brown & Latulippe 2021, 14).

The Case of India

The emergence of the Covid-19 Pandemic in India since March 2020 has resurfaced the question of how the Indian multilevel governmental structure functions within the framework of the Constitutional distribution of powers and federal arrangements during a crisis. Does a decentralized federal polity like India has extended its relationships with regional governments and undertaken a variety of strategies to address the issues posed by Covid-19? What is the current state of inter-state relations aimed at preventing virus spread and strengthening intergovernmental coordination? These questions have become relevant in the Indian context, and they deserve serious consideration at the moment. However, before delving into these issues, it is necessary to provide a brief summary of the Indian federal system and its constitutional foundation.

Constitutional Backdrop

A Federal form of government has considered as the most appropriate form of governance in complex, multi-ethnic countries like India. India is a well-known federation not only for the structure of its mere division of powers between the centre and the states but also for retaining or accommodating its internal diversity while maintaining the autonomy of the states. In this regard, Indian federalism has played a significant role. The Indian federal system has aided the country in promoting democracy, strengthening national unity, and achieving a fair level of economic progress (Jain 2017, 17).

The Indian Constitution officially referred to India as a "Union of States" [see Article I (I)]. In India, the Constitution establishes a dual polity with the Union at the top and the states at the bottom, each with their own defined sovereign powers. Dr. B.R. Ambedkar described the Indian Constitution

> federal inasmuch as it's establishes what may be called a dual polity (which)…
> will consist of the Union at the Centre and the States at the periphery each
> endowed with sovereign powers to be exercised in the field assigned to them
> by the Constitution.
>
> (Bhattacharyya 2001, 17)

The framers of the Indian Constitution aimed to create an integrated federal structure. Their main goal was to devise a constitutional arrangement within an organized framework in which the entire subcontinent will be joining together to create a unified, strong India. They attempted to create a federal government that was not as 'tightly moulded' as America's; their objective was to frame a federation with some unitary features. The essence of cooperative federalism, on the other hand, found a place. Members of the Constituent Assembly envisioned a nation built on mutual respect and cooperation between the centre and the states. Sri Brojendra Lal Mittar, a member of the Constituent Assembly, once mentioned, 'We do not believe in isolated independent existence, which can only weaken the Union. We shall join you wholeheartedly in a spirit of co-operation and not in any spirit of securing special privileges at the cost of the Union' (CAD 2014, 367).

The various parts of the Indian Constitution have broadly explained inter-governmental relations. The provisions relating to the distribution of powers between the Union and the Provisional governments have been added in Part XI of the Indian Constitution, titled "Relations between the Union and the States," and have been divided into two chapters in the original Constitution. Union State Legislative Relations (Article 245–255) are defined in Chapter I and Administrative Relations are defined in Chapter II (Article 256–263). Part XII of the Constitution discusses financial provisions separately. The Constitution's Seventh Schedule (Article 246) delineates the functions of all levels of government in three lists: Union List, State List, and Concurrent List, each with its own set of subjects and power distribution. The central government has sole legislative and executive authority over the subject matter of the Union Lists. The States, on the other hand, share the powers specified in the State List. The Constitution empowers both the Union and the state governments to make laws on the Concurrent List; yet, in times of conflict, the Constitution grants Parliament supreme federal powers, and thus the central law prevails (Article 254). The Constitution does, however, guarantee the establishment of an inter-state Council to ensure effective coordination and cooperation between the centre and states, as well as among the states themselves (Article 263). The Council is tasked under the Constitution with investigating and advising on inter-state disputes, as well as coordinating on matters of common interest involving the Union or all of the states. It has also tasked itself with making suggestions on inter-state issues in order to improve policy coordination and implementation (Bakshi 2016, 279).

Despite this, there is no explicit mention of public health emergencies or pandemics in the Indian Constitution. The emergency provisions have not stated any methods associated to this. While the other provisions of the Constitution, such as Article 21, recognize the right to life and personal liberty as fundamental rights of Indian citizens. Public health issues, on the other hand, have been enlisted in Part IV of the Indian Constitution in terms of the Directive Principles of State Policy, which state that it is the "responsibility of the State to provide security to citizens by ensuring the Right to adequate means of livelihood." "provide public assistance in cases of unemployment, old age, sickness, and disablement." "makes provision to protect the health of the infant and mother through maternity benefits." "raising the level of nutrition and the standard of living of people and improving public health" (see Articles 39 (a), 41, 42 & 47). At the onset of the Pandemic in the Indian context, Swenden et al. observe:

> Constitutionally speaking, different authorities may be responsible for handling different aspects of a health crisis such as a pandemic… as per the constitution, the states are largely responsible for health, but the union (centre) controls interstate quarantine and interstate migration. The states occupy the fields of public health and sanitation, hospitals and dispensaries, but social security, social insurance, employment and unemployment as well as 'the prevention of the extension from one state to another of infectious or contagious diseases or pests affecting men [sic], animals or plants' are concurrent subjects. In these concurrent areas both levels can operate, but the centre assumes a dominant role in case of centre–state conflict.
>
> (Swenden et al. 2021, 2)

The Constitution however provides that the Union and the state governments act in collaboration for the common good and ensures adequate means concerning all the matters which have been entrusted to them. Thus, during the Pandemic extensive governmental responses at all levels have become crucial with regard to protecting public health and providing basic healthcare facilities to all the citizens.

The Union-State Relation amidst Covid-19 Pandemic

During the Pandemic, Union-State relations in India became somewhat critical. It has faced a number of challenges since the Covid-19 Pandemic broke out, particularly during the first wave. Lack of trust and disagreements between the governments to take active measures have been observed during this period.

The first confirmed case of Covid-19 infection in India was reported on January 30, 2020, and the World Health Organization (WHO) declared 'COVID-19 as a Public Health Emergency of International Concern (PHEIC)' on the same date (WHO 2020a, 2). Soon after this declaration, the WHO Director-General declared Covid-19 as 'Pandemic' on March 11, 2020, after observing the virus's 'spread' and 'severity,' as well as assessing the number of cases and death rates (WHO 2020b). On March 25, 2020, the Government of India imposed a nationwide lockdown and social distancing policy in order to find an immediate response to prevent the spread of the virus. In this regard, on March 24, 2020, the Ministry of Home Affairs (GOI) issued an order mandating a lockdown in order to contain the Covid-19 epidemic and directed all states and territories to strictly enforce this order.[1]

While the lockdown measures were successful in terms of controlling the spread of infections across the country but on the other side, it raised many questions and generates centre–state conflicts in some areas. Despite the Constitutional provisions of the 'health' and 'sanitation' stated as the state listed subject (List II), the central government had issued the order of the nationwide lockdown under the Disaster Management Act (2005) which according to some state governments (for instance, the state of West Bengal) violates the spirit of federalism. The National Disaster Management Act of 2005 gives the centre exclusive administrative and financial controls that caused myriad issues between the centre and states. Some issues, such as ensuring the right mechanisms for the management of the disease and claiming working policies for the management of the lockdown, as well as demanding adequate financial funds to the state governments to meet the health, social, and economic challenges posed by the virus,[2] sparked disputes in the centre–state relationship in early April 2020.

Other major areas of such clashes include the sealing of inter-state borders, restrictions on the movement of migrant workers, demands by various state governments for the closure of domestic flights[3] and setting up the vaccination policies about procurement and distribution etc. had produced serious tensions and caused number of roadblocks not only between the centre and states but also generated uncertainty and lack of coordination among the states.[4] Apart from these drawbacks, it has been perceived that India's federal response to the Pandemic shifted from its initial stance, i.e. moved from a centralized to a decentralized approach (Tillin 2021), and it has later promulgated some effective policy responses (successful implementation of vaccination drives across the country) in which the various levels of government (national, state, and local) acted cooperatively and responded collaboratively.

India's Response to the Pandemic

It is evident that the Pandemic has had a major impact on people all over the world, causing distress and a large number of deaths. It has instilled fear and dread in the general public, as well as increased uncertainty in all aspects of life. As a result, the role of governments in restoring normalcy through cooperation and solidarity is essential. With the emergence of Covid-19 in early 2020, governments all over the world have responded to arrest the spread of infections by implementing a variety of measures under varying conditions. The virus's nature was largely unknown to the rest of the world at the time. Many countries developed policies in common, such as social distancing and containment strategies, among others. India is not an exceptional case in this regard. Even before the first Covid-19 infection was discovered, the country with a population of nearly 1.3 billion people took some important steps. It has primarily generated surveillance measures, which have been followed by a series of travel advisories and restrictions, as well as a quarantine policy for people arriving from abroad. Following the WHO's official declaration of Pandemic, the first major step taken by the central government was the announcement of a 21-day nationwide lockdown (which was later extended to 75 days), followed by the announcement of 'Do Gaj Ki Doori' (a distance of two yards) by the Indian Prime Minister Narendra Modi. The lockdown certainly hampered the economy and the daily lives of ordinary people however, it initially helped to contain the spread of the virus, lowering the daily number of cases, and it was also perceived as an effective measure for the nationwide preparedness of medical health structures. Jha and Jha (2020) write about India's early lockdown effort to stop the virus's transmission at the beginning of Covid-19:

> India's performance in combating the health crisis has been quite good and certainly much better than that of countries (including USA, UK, Italy, France and Germany) with far more advanced health systems and much lower populations. India's recovery rate is steadily rising (98% on 19 October 2020) and the death rate steadily falling (currently two of all infected cases). This lockdown brought much of economic and social activity to a halt. However, this had a salutary effect on cutting down the mortality from COVID.
>
> (Jha & Jha 2020, 345)

State governments, on the other hand, were prompt to respond to the situation and they 'devised a set of proactive strategies to fight the Pandemic that can truly be considered as 'public actions' in a sense that is closely related to the notion put forward' (Jalan & Sen 2020, 107). At the onset of the crisis, the states enabled themselves on planning, organizing, coordinating, and implementing measures with proper coordination with the centre. Several states issued guidelines on a variety of proactive preventive and mitigating actions under the Epidemic Disease Act (1897), which empowers both the centre and states to take special measures and prescribe regulations during the outbreak of dangerous diseases. As the number of cases has increased, many state governments have been actively investing in the enhancement of their local health infrastructures and have successfully implemented tracing, testing, and containment techniques. Furthermore, in many states, Covid-Care centrer and safe homes have also been established with the help of district administrations and they have also been very proactive in terms of crisis management. Kerala is one of the best examples of this, and its Covid control measures have garnered international recognition from the World Health Organization.[5]

Notably, India's reaction to the crisis would be impossible to achieve without the cooperation of state governments, which are considered to be the most important actors in the Indian federal system. Saxena (2020) also believes that the Indian government's response to the Covid-19 outbreak has been characterised by close collaboration and cooperation between the central and state governments. The Pandemic has highlighted the importance of strengthening cooperative federalism, as no single jurisdiction or level of government is capable of dealing with the crisis alone. The Disaster Management Act (2005) under section 36(f) directs the central government to assist state governments in developing mitigation, preparedness, and response plans, as well as capacity-building, data collection, and identification, and personnel training in disaster management; conducting rescue and relief operations in the affected area; and assessing disaster damage (2005, 18).[6] Keeping this in mind, state governments implemented policies to advise, assist, and coordinate the activities of district authorities, statutory bodies, and other governmental and non-governmental organizations involved in crisis management at the same time.

The catastrophe was much more severe during the second wave, which emerged in mid-May 2021, resulting in a severe oxygen crisis and a greater demand for ICU beds. During this time to ensure a sufficient supply of oxygen to all states, the Government of India took initiatives on adopting collaborative actions to conduct a mapping exercise of the sources of supplies with the demand for medical oxygen in the critically affected states and removed restrictions on the inter-state movement for oxygen carrying vehicles.[7] The central government has also established a green corridor to ensure the timely supply of oxygen cylinders among states. The centre collaborated with the states to keep the inter-state supply chain (including supply of essential drugs) operational. At the time, intergovernmental coordination was much stronger, and the centre delegated responsibility for vaccine procurement and distribution to the states. However, more instances of coordination can be observed when the Prime Minister held several rounds of discussions with the Chief Ministers of the States to address this issue.[8] Hence, ensuring adequate health infrastructure at the district level and maintaining local level best practices for combating the current virus threat will also necessitate intergovernmental coordination in the coming days as well.

Concluding Remarks

Covid-19 Pandemic is a global health crisis with far-reaching consequences for all aspects of life, including health, the economy, and education, for the entire world, including India. Recognizing the severity of the situation, the government across the world has implemented several curative measures, such as lockdown, quarantine, social distancing, and so on. To combat the virus effectively India, as a nation, has been trying to survive the situation, with both government and non-governmental support advancing preventive and healing healthcare facilities, diagnostic and research facilities, and tracking services, in order to reduce the loss of human lives. If vaccination appears to be one of the most important strategies or weapons for preventing further Pandemic spread, as well as providing a sense of security and reassuring people about their health and well-being, then India has successfully driven its immunization process, with nearly 165 billion doses administered to its population till date.[9] In fact, in light of the current situation, the government has announced the need for booster doses for its people. Thus, it has been perceived that the federal response to the Pandemic in India has evolved in numerous ways and the existing federal structures have aided in the efficient control of the virus. Indian federalism is incorporated into the basic structure of the constitution, and India, which stands out in the world for its unity in diversity, is attempting to stand together in the face of this crisis. However, some concerns remain in the current context, especially since the country has yet to fully recover from the deadly virus and its consequences. It is alarming that thousands of people are still suffering from the Pandemic's devastating effects on the economy and health. Thus, rather than blaming and criticizing each other's actions, governments (national and local) must ensure that all cogs in the wheel continue to function properly and that no institution, whether government, private sector, or civil society, operates in isolation within the federal structure, but rather collaborates for the general welfare of the people.

Notes

1 See, Press Information Bureau, Government of India. 'The Government of India Issues Orders Prescribing Lockdown for Containment of COVID19 Epidemic in the Country', New Delhi, March 24, 2020. Accessed December 27, 2021. https://www.mha.gov.in/sites/default/files/PR_NationalLockdown_26032020_0.pdf.

2 See the Article, 'View: Without a Paradigm Shift in Politics, Centre-state Relations Will Only Become More Fractious', *The Economic Times*, April 26, 2020. Accessed November 25, 2021. https://economictimes.indiatimes.com/news/economy/policy/view-without-a-paradigm-shift-in-politics-centre-state-relations-will-only-become-more-fractious/articleshow/75395332.cms.

3 In this case, the states of Delhi and West Bengal are examples. They had asked the Centre to halt domestic and international flights and ensure strict compliance in order to prevent the spread of the virus. *Times of India*, March 23, 2020. Accessed January 20, 2022. https://timesofindia.indiatimes.com/business/india-business/government-suspends-domestic-flight-operations-from-wednesday/articleshow/74775742.cms.

4 For example, when the Karnataka government sealed its border to limit the spread of the virus, the Kerala government objected, claiming that the disruption of vehicle services related to healthcare equipment would be a major problem for the state. In fact, the Kerala High Court issued directions in this regard, instructing the centre to ensure that vehicle services run smoothly while keeping the health emergency in mind.

5 See the story published by the WHO titled 'Responding to Covid-19- Learning from Kerala', July 2, 2020. Accessed November 25, 2021. https://www.who.int/india/news/feature-stories/detail/responding-to-covid-19---learnings-from-kerala. To know more on the Kerala's strategy. see Jalan and Sen (2020), '"Containing a Pandemic with Public Actions and Public Trust: The Kerala Story"'.

6 See The Disaster Management Act, 2005. Accessed from https://ndma.gov.in/sites/default/files/PDF/DM_act2005.pdf

7 See Government of India, Ministry of Home Affairs Order in this regard. Accessed from https://www.mha.gov.in/sites/default/files/MHADMAct_22042021.pdf.

8 See 'PM Narendra Modi Calls for Meeting with CMs on Covid Response', *The Economic Times*, January 10, 2022. Accessed January 24, 2021. https://economictimes.indiatimes.com/news/india/pm-narendra-modi-calls-for-meeting-with-cms-on-covid-response/articleshow/88799342.cms.

9 See the current data on https://www.mygov.in/covid-19.

References

Anderson, George. 2008. *Federalism: An Introduction*. New York: Oxford University Press.

Bakshi, P.M. 2016. *The Constitution of India*, Thirteenth Edition. Noida: Universal Law Publishing.

Benton, J. Edwin. 2020. "Challenges to Federalism and Intergovernmental Relations and Takeaways Amid the COVID-19 Experience." *American Review of Public Administration*, Vol. 50(6–7), 536–542. Accessed August 20, 2021. https://doi.org/10.1177/0275074020941698.

Bhattacharyya, H. 2001, *India as a Multicultural Federation: Asian Values, Democracy and Decentralization (in comparison with Swiss federalism)*. Switzerland: Institut Du Federalisme Fribourg Suisse.

Constituent Assembly Debates. 2014. *Official Report (Vol. III)*. New Delhi: Lok Sabha Secretariat.

Dagurre, Anne, and Tim Conlan. 2020. "Federalism in a Time of Coronavirus: The Trump Administration, Intergovernmental Relations, and the Fraying Social Compact." *State and Local Government Review*, Vol. 52(4), 287–297. Accessed August 20, 2021. https://doi.org/10.1177/0160323X21990881.

Douglous, Brown, and Nic Latulippe. 2021. "Pandemic Federalism: The Covid 19 Response in Canada, Australia and the United States." *Mulroney Papers in Public Policy and Governance*, No. 3. Accessed November 25, 2021. https://www.stfx.ca/sites/default/files/MPPG%20No%203%20March%202021.pdf.

Downey, Davia Cox, and William M. Myers. 2020. "Federalism, Intergovernmental Relationships, and Emergency Response: A Comparison of Australia and United States." *American Review of Public Administration*, Vol. 50(6–7), 526–535. Accessed August 20, 2021. https://doi.org/10.1177/0275074020941696.

Jain, Sumitra Kumar. 2017. *Indian Federalism: Emerging Issues*. Delhi: Kalpaz Publications.

Jalan, Jyotsna, and Arijit Sen. 2020. "Containing a Pandemic with Public Actions and Public Trust: The Kerala Story." *Indian Economic Review*, S105–S124. Accessed November 25, 2021. https://doi.org/10.1007/s41775-020-00087-1.

Jha, Abhay Kumar, and Raghbendra Jha. 2020. "India's Response to COVID-19 Crisis." *The Indian Economic Journal*, Vol. 68(3), 341–351. Accessed November 25, 2021. https://doi.org/10.1177/0019466220976685.

Kincaid, John, and J. Wesley Leckrone. 2020. "Partisan Fractures in U.S. Federalism's COVID-19 Policy Responses." *State and Local Government Review*, Vol. 52(4), 298–308. Accessed August 20, 2021. https://doi.org/10.1177/0160323X20986842.

Lecours, André, Daniel Béland, Alan Fenna, Tracy Beck Fenwick, Mireille Paquet, Philip Rocco, and Alex Waddan. 2021. "Explaining Intergovernmental Conflict in the COVID-19 Crisis: The United States, Canada, and Australia." *Publius: The Journal of*

Federalism, Vol. 51(4), 513–536. Accessed November 25, 2021. https://doi.org/10.1093/publius/pjab010.

Saxena, Rekha, 2020. "Federalism and Covid-19 Crisis: Centre-State Apposite Relations in Pandemic Federalism-India." *Forum of Federations*, April 22, 2020. http://forumfed.org/2020/04/rekha-saxena-federalism-and-covid-19/.

Swenden, Wilfried, Rekha Saxena, and Chanchal Kumar Sharma. 2021. "Understanding Multilevel Dynamics in India: Constituent Power and Multilevel Governance." *Territory Politics, Governance*, 1–11. Accessed November 25, 2021. https://doi.org/10.1080/21622671.2021.1972830.

Tillin, Louise. 2021. "Center and States Need to Coordinate, Not Compete." *Centre for Advanced Study of India*, May 24, 2021. https://casi.sas.upenn.edu/iit/louisetillin.

World Health Organization. 2020a. "COVID-19 Public Health Emergency of International Concern (PHEIC) Global Research and Innovation Forum." Accessed January 17, 2022. https://www.who.int/publications/m/item/covid-19-public-health-emergency-of-international-concern-(pheic)-global-research-and-innovation-forum#:~:text=On%2030%20January%202020%20following, of%20International%20Concern%20(PHEIC).

World Health Organization. 2020b. "WHO Director-General's Opening Remarks at the Media Briefing on Covid-19-11 March 2020." https://www.who.int/director-general/speeches/detail/who-director-general-s-opening-remarks-at-the-media-briefing-on-covid-19---11-march-2020.

8 Hate in the Times of Covid-19

Can We Blame the Print Media in India?

Rumela Sen and Nusrat Farooq

Introduction

In late 2019, a small cluster of pneumonia of unknown cause began in one part of the world and spread rapidly across several continents, to emerge as the deadliest pandemic the world has ever faced, surpassing the 1918 flu pandemic.[1] Alongside the severe havoc that Coronavirus (also known as SARS-CoV-2) wreaked in the global economy, the worst since World War II, it also unleashed a worldwide pandemic of hate and stigmatization of various marginalized groups. The Muslims and the East Asian diaspora in various countries were among the worst victims worldwide (Xu et al. 2021). How do we explain the correlation between the outbreak of an infectious disease and ensuing prejudice against certain religious or racial groups? In India, for example, anxieties over coronavirus (or Covid-19) became grounds for violence, discrimination, and misinformation campaigns against the Muslims, who constitute 14.2 per cent of the population. This chapter traces the trajectory of anti-Muslim hate and fear as it unfolded in India alongside the Covid-19 outbreak, and specifically highlights the role of misinformation and rumors circulated by the print media in this process. It analyzes how a biological contagion was used by the print media in India to amplify notions of ethnic purity and magnify the pre-existing architecture of hate in India.

It is worth mentioning that this spike in Islamophobia and Covid-19 deaths in India is hardly an exception. For example, during the outbreak of syphilis in Europe and Asia as far back as the 1500s, each affected country blamed their adversarial and neighboring countries for the spread (Tampa et al. 2014). There is a long history of stigmatization and violence against victims of smallpox outbreaks in slave ships. Jewish populations in Europe were targeted and murdered during plague outbreaks, and systematic discrimination against Italian and German immigrants in America during the yellow fever and influenza epidemics are well documented (Finley et al. 2018). More recently, the Chinese community was scapegoated as a source of the foot-and-mouth outbreak in the United Kingdom in 2001.[2] More recently, Chinese students reportedly expressed their fear of racism being worse than their fear of the coronavirus itself.[3] The immigrant African community in Guangzhou China also expressed similar fears when they were identified as a source of contamination in China and were subjected to

DOI: 10.4324/9781003300762-9

repeated and excessive tests and quarantine.[4] These examples illustrate the prevalent and well-documented correlation between pandemic and hate.

The primary contribution of this chapter is in presenting both quantitative and qualitative evidence on how the top five newspapers in India vilified a Muslim seminary group (Tablighi Jamaat) that organized an event at the onset of the Covid-19 pandemic in India, and by extension, the entire Muslim community. To be sure, press coverage of the pandemic did not create Islamophobia, it merely acted as a catalyst accelerating the process. It also highlights how the same press did not condemn a Hindu congregation at Kumbh, an event of much larger scale and attendance, organized a year later, with similar or worse ramifications for the pandemic. Specifically, we conduct machine learning-based textual analysis using the Latent Dirichlet Allocation (LDA) model to analyze 1,539 newspaper stories (1307 for Tablighi event and 232 for Kumbh) published by five major Indian newspapers across the left-right ideological spectrum. The disproportionately smaller number of articles on Kumbh is due to reduced reporting on the Kumbh compared to the coverage of the Tablighi event in the Indian press. As shown in Table 8.1, the top five English newspapers reduced the reporting frequency on Kumbh by 82.2 per cent when compared to the Muslim event. For example, Economic Times reduced its reportage by 93.5 per cent; The Hindu, The Statesman, and Hindustan Times reduced their reporting by 92.8 per cent, 86.9 per cent, and 78 per cent, respectively, with The Telegraph recording the lowest reduction rate of 64.9 per cent.

Second, based on the widely divergent media coverage of the two events, we investigate the underlying mechanisms of the correlation between the outbreak of an infectious disease and the intensification of prejudice against marginalized communities.[5] Third, this chapter also raises bigger questions of what the specific ramifications of such misinformation campaigns against

Muslims could be for minority rights in an electoral democracy like India. To that end, we theorize three mechanisms of otherization of minorities through the language of viral contagion in media viz. coordination channel, persuasion channel, and social norm channel. Vilification of minorities changes the costs

Table 8.1 Frequency of articles on the Tablighi Jamaat event (March 15 - April 30, 2020) and the Kumbh Mela (March 15 - April 30, 2021)

Newspaper (Tablighi Jamaat)	Frequency (Tablighi Jamaat)	Newspaper (Kumbh Mela)	Frequency (Kumbh Mela)	Percentage reduction
Hindustan Times	749	Hindustan Times	158	78
The Hindu	320	The Hindu	23	92.8
The Telegraph	114	The Telegraph	40	64.9
The Economic Times	78	The Economic Times	5	93.5
The Statesman	46	The Statesman	6	86.9
TOTAL	1307	TOTAL	232	82.2

of coordinating hate crimes between potential perpetrators (*a coordination channel*), changes people's beliefs (*a persuasion channel*), and changes perceived societal acceptance of xenophobic beliefs or actions (*a social norms channel*). This chapter is organized as follows: Section 8.1 provides the background and timeline of the outbreak of Covid-19 in India and situates the two cases in this timeline. Section 8.2 introduces our research methodology, specifically how we collected and analyzed the data on print media coverage. Section 8.3 presents our main findings. Section 8.4 theorizes the ramifications of this dynamic of hate perpetrated by the print media on the larger issues of minority rights in a democracy like India.

Section 1: Background and Timeline

The first Covid-19 case in India was detected on January 31, 2020, almost one and a half months before the government of India put its first one-day Covid-19 restriction (janta-curfew) in place on March 22, 2020.[6] On March 13, 2020, the Delhi government banned "all sports gathering (including IPL)/conferences/ seminars beyond 200 people".[7] The first case examined in this chapter is the gathering by Tablighi Jamaat between March 13 and 15. Tablighi Jamaat is a century-old Islamic missionary movement that has its global spiritual center or markaz in the Indian capital city of Delhi. On March 16, three days after the Jamaat event began, the Delhi government issued a new notification clarifying that the ban included religious gatherings as well.[7] On April 1, 2021, the Delhi government took legal action, filing a First Information Report, against the leader of the Tablighi Jamaat and seven other Jamaat officials before the nationwide lockdown on March 24.[7] Tablighi members were blamed for the uptick in India's Covid-19 cases and were accused of carrying a 'coronajihad' in a deliberate attempt to spread disease and death to the population of India.[8] In India, "jihad" is a blanket term for 'holy war' terrorism carried out in the name of Islam, and "love jihad" and "population jihad" have also been routinely employed against Muslims.[9] The media identified Tablighi mosques as top coronavirus hotspots and vilified the entire Muslim community for spreading the virus, instigating nationwide social boycott and attacks against Muslims.[10] The subsequent images of Tablighi leaders, charged under India's National Security Act for violating quarantine, handcuffed, and surrounded by police, reinforced the public perception of them as law breaking criminals. After Tablighi members were arrested and jailed, widespread surveillance and contact tracing was meted out to Muslim communities across India.

The second case examined in this chapter is a majority/Hindu event known as the Kumbh Mela, which occurred between April 1 and 30, 2021 in the Indian state of Uttarakhand. It is worth noting that India saw its cases drop by nearly 90 per cent between September 2020 and February 2021, with many heralding the country's apparent success in controlling infections.[11] But when hundreds of thousands of devotees started assembling for Kumbh Mela, India saw cases rise rapidly, raising the alarm of a second wave, starting in March

2021.[12] On March 21, 2021, however, a full-page newspaper advert featuring the Prime Minister of India, invited devotees to the festival, assuring them it was "clean" and "safe". By April 15, more than 2,000 Kumbh attendees had already tested positive for Covid-19. On April 17, the Prime Minister called for the Kumbh Mela to be "symbolic".[13] By the time the festival ended, on 28 April, it was estimated that more than 9.1 million people had attended.[14] The true toll of the Kumbh Mela will never be known, and thousands of pilgrims returned home without having been tested or quarantined and without any track of them kept by the government. However, a few days later, the horror of floating corpses in Ganga first came to light on 10 May, and over 2,000 dead bodies were retrieved from Ganga by various district administrations in Uttar Pradesh and Bihar.[15]

Although much larger in scale and attendance than the Tablighi event, Kumbh did not receive comparable media scrutiny. The Tablighi attendees were pilloried as purveyors of disease, the Kumbh attendees were not. The choice of comparative method in this chapter, highlighting the difference in media portrayal of a minority and a majority religious event during a pandemic, is not only a preference but a requirement, particularly because there is no possible recourse to experimental techniques and statistical techniques in this case (Table 8.2).

The contrast between the media attack against the Muslim/Tablighi event and the Hindu/Kumbh event needs to be understood in the context of a groundswell of protests in India in the preceding months against the new controversial citizenship laws enacted by the Indian government on 12 December 2019. Although a full discussion of the events leading to the Covid outbreak in India is outside the scope of this chapter, it is worth noting that citizenship laws promised to fast-track asylum claims of all irregular immigrants from neighboring countries of Afghanistan, Bangladesh, and Pakistan, except the Muslims.[20] These laws made religion the basis of Indian citizenship for the first time. Together with a planned nationwide citizenship verification process, through a National Population Register and a National Register of Citizens (NRC) aimed at screening "illegal migrants", these laws threatened the citizenship rights of millions of Indian Muslims.[16] While work on the population register was deferred to prevent the spread of a pandemic, Indian Muslims living in India for generations feared

Table 8.2 Dates, Attendees, and Location of the Muslim and the Hindu Events

	Muslim Event	*Hindu Event*
Dates	– March 13, 2020 to March 15, 2020[16]	– April 1, 2021 to April 30, 2021
		– The first shahi snan took place on March 11, 2021[17]
Attendees	– Between 3,000 and 4,500[18]	– 9.1 million[19]
Location	– Delhi, India	– Uttrakhand, India

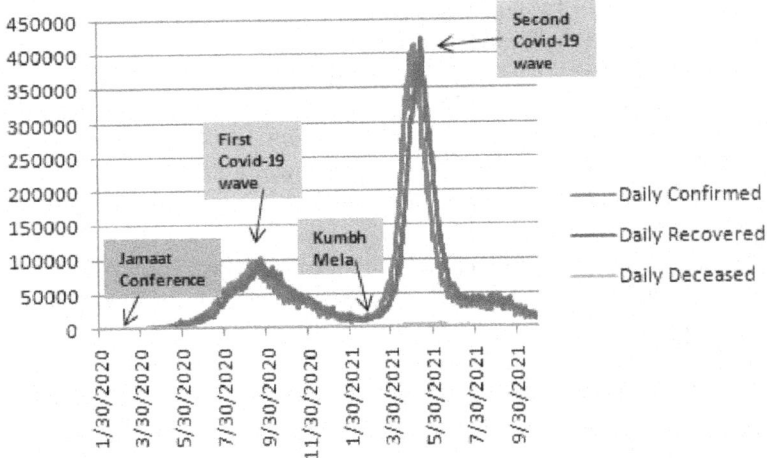

Figure 8.1 First and second Covid-19 wave in India.
Source: data.covid19.bharat

stripping of citizenship rights and disenfranchisement. In this contextual back-drop, it is not too farfetched to argue that citizenship legislations and the result-ant public reaction provided a fertile ground for intensification of anti-Muslim xenophobia, with the virus acting as the catalyst. Subsequent reports of Muslim vendors being stopped from selling in the streets in the National Capital Region (NCR), reports of some gated communities convening residents' meetings to keep Muslims out of their compounds, and the proliferation of hateful hashtags against Muslims on the social media must be understood in this context. The following diagram shows the timeline of the Tablighi and Kumbh gatherings in the context of the two peaks of the first and the second wave of Covid in India (Figure 8.1).[21]

Section 2: Research Method

This chapter uses machine learning-based textual analysis techniques to build datasets on media coverage of the two above-mentioned events, viz. the Tablighi gathering in 2020 and the Kumbh gathering in 2021. Using text as data is one of the most fruitful areas of machine learning applications in political science. It has a long tradition in political science. Computerized text analysis allows exploration of massive amounts of politically relevant text, in this case, media reports, using increasingly sophisticated tools. The first step was to identify the top five English newspapers in India.[22] Next, we extracted stories from all five of these newspapers on Factiva and created two datasets: one on their coverage of the Muslim event and another on their coverage of the Hindu gathering. A screenshot of one of our Factiva searches is provided below (Figure 8.2).

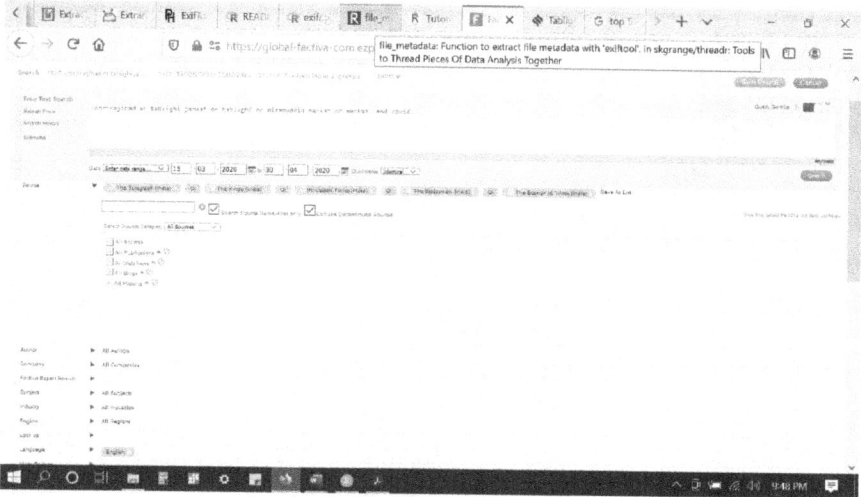

Figure 8.2 Example of Factiva Boolean keyword search screenshot for Muslim/Tablighi Event: (coronajihad or tablighi jamaat or tablighi or nizamuddin markaz or markaz) and Covid.

For stories related to the Muslim/Tablighi event, we selected the date range of March 15, 2020, to April 30, 2020.[23] For stories related to Hindu gatherings, we selected the date range from March 15, 2021 to April 30, 2021.[24] We used separate keyword combinations on Factiva to access the newspaper articles in above-mentioned date ranges for the two events in the top five newspapers in India.[25] Following collection and subsequent pre-processing of data on Tablighi and Kumbh events, the next step in the analysis, which includes both supervised and unsupervised methods, was cleaning the data for both the cases removing numbers, infrequent terms, stop words such as 'a', punctuation marks and URLs. Once the data was clean, we performed machine learning-based analysis, including topic analysis (quantitative) and thought analysis (qualitative). A detailed five-step explanation of this data processing is provided below (Figure 8.3).

The statistical topic models, which allow for rich latent topics to be automatically inferred from the text, were used to discover the abstract "topics" and hidden semantic structures that occur in the collection of many newspaper articles. Topic models, as used in this chapter, are often referred to as "unsupervised" methods because they *infer* rather than *assume* the content of the topics under study, and they have been used across a variety of fields (Blei et al. 2003; Wang et al. 2011). More than supervised learning, unsupervised methods used in this chapter allow for the discovery of patterns and classification of topics without the extensive prior labeling efforts often required for supervised learning methods. In other words, unsupervised topic modeling, as employed in this chapter,

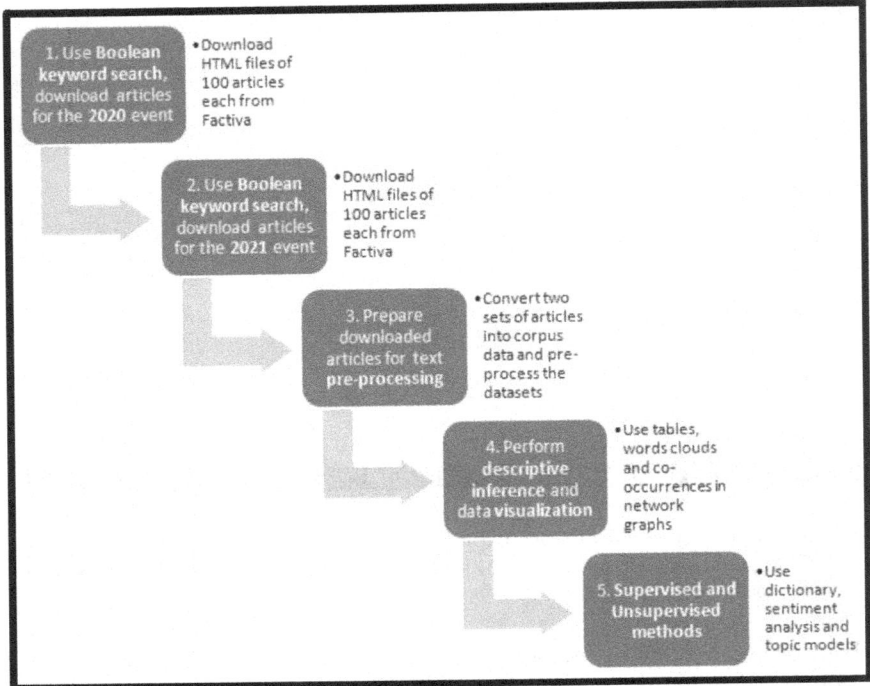

Figure 8.3 Five steps in data processing.

looked for themes (or topics) that lie within the two cleaned sets of text data that we created on the two events.[26]

Section 3: Analysis and Findings

This section of the chapter showcases the central findings of the chapter based on topic models that cluster the most frequent words in media coverage of the two cases (Tablighi and Kumbh), followed by qualitative thought analysis which situates these frequently used words in the context of news stories they occur in. The topic models should be understood as exploratory analyses that include counting words and allowing the algorithm to identify and group similar word patterns to infer topics within the unstructured data. The diagram below depicts the top flex words in the coverage of the Muslim/Tablighi event clustered into ten top topics. Once topic models identify word clusters, we use deep case knowledge of India to infer and label what meaning and framing each word cluster conveys. We call this thought analysis, a qualitative inference method based on the analysis of the most representative documents for a particular topic identified using FindThoughts function in R, as depicted in Figure 8.4. This allows us to get a better sense of the content of actual documents with a high topical

Top Topics

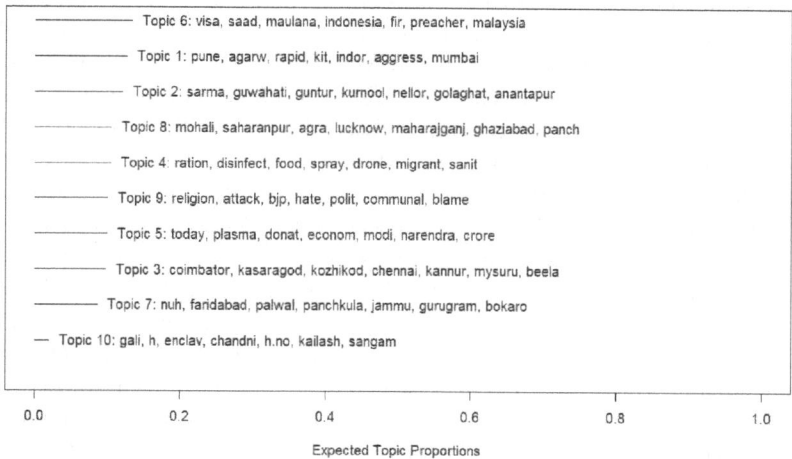

Figure 8.4 High-frequency words in coverage of Muslim/Tablighi event in top five newspapers.

content. Together the topic models and subsequent thought analysis provide additional evidence for our central contention that the media associated the Tablighi event with words and meanings that implicated them in three mutually reinforcing frames of reference.

Based on the topic model above, the predominant theme in the way the newspapers framed the Tablighi episode was as a law & order issue, portraying attendees as criminals and terrorists unleashing a biological war on India. The highest frequency words clustered as Topic 6 include *FIR, visa, maulana, preacher, names of places like Malaysia and Indonesia* (where the Jamaat attendees came from), and reference to Jamaat leader Maulana Saad Kandhalwi. The most reported aspect of the Tablighi/Muslim event was the First Information Report lodged against the leader of the Jamaat conference, Mr. Saad Kandhalwi—a maulana (Islamic Scholar), and six other organizers, under Section 3 of the Epidemic Disease Act for holding a Muslim religious congregation which spread Covid-19 "across the country". In addition, the newspapers harped on transnational networks of the Tablighis, particularly highlighting that their members came from Malaysia (60 per cent Muslim) and Indonesia (99 per cent Muslim). This illustrates framing of the Tablighi conference as a law and order issue, a framing further bolstered by images of Tablighi members handcuffed and surrounded by law enforcement.

The second frequent word clusters are Topics 1, 2 and 3, which refer to *government policy of aggressive testing of jamaat attendees, contact tracing of attendees and their close contacts*. Together these three high-frequency topics include flex words like the last name (*Agarwal*) of an Indian Joint Secretary who made media statements on the mass testing requirements of Tablighi attendees, as well as names of places across India where the Tablighi attendees were accused of spreading the disease too. It is clear from this analysis that words like *rapid, kit* and *aggressive* testing, and contact tracing were repeatedly used alongside the names of places across India where the attendees returned, which conveyed the extent and intensity of harm done by one conference on the health and wellbeing of ordinary people. Not only were Tablighi attendees depicted as purveyors of disease, but the newspapers also reported frequently how Delhi's Nizamuddin area where the event took place was the "biggest hotspot of the disease in the country". Identification of Muslims and their living quarters as the fountainhead of the disease makes them vulnerable to concerted attacks and creates legitimation for violating privacy and other rights of the minority community, all in the name of health and wellbeing. In other words, public perception of the Muslim/Tablighi event had two main elements: first, it was illegal (Topic 6), and second, it's cavalier handling of a contagious disease exposed many others to its dangers, increasing casualties from Uttar Pradesh and NCR to Haryana (Topics 8, 7, 10), which necessitated testing as well as contact tracing. For example, deaths and containment of Covid-19 cases in Uttar Pradesh (Topic 8), Haryana (Topic 7) and in the National Capital Region (Topic 10) were blamed on the Tablighis. The birth of the hashtag coronajihad (Topic 9) needs to be understood in this context.

The third theme that emerges from the topic model and subsequent thought analysis is that the pandemic created an opportunity for politicians, administrators, and media personnel to completely violate the privacy and security of ordinary Muslim citizens of India. Reports on contact tracing of attendees of the Tablighi conference publicly named Muslims who tested positive after coming in contact with Jamaat attendees. The plight of sanitation workers in India, who complained about the lack of effective protective Covid-19 gear for first responders, was blamed on the Tablighis as well. The South Delhi Municipal Corporation (SDMC) started a drive to sanitize areas near the Nizamuddin area where the Tablighi event had taken place. It also used drones to spray disinfectants in Nizamuddin East, Nizamuddin Basti, and surrounding areas. Topic 10 (Containment Zones in National Capital Region) also shows that reports on containment zones in Delhi began with reference to "House no-152 to 162 in Block D of Shaheen Bagh", which captured newspaper headlines as the symbolic site of Muslim-led peaceful resistance. The following table sums up our labeling of the top ten prevalent topics in the media coverage of the Muslim/Tablighi event (Figure 8.5).

In sharp contrast to the Tablighi event, the top topics picked by the algorithm in the coverage of Kumbh Mela in Indian print media do not exhibit negative stereotyping of the Hindu religious leaders or ordinary people who attended the event. This mass gathering was not implicated in breaking the law and endangering the rest of the population. While the government response to Tablighis ranged from aggressive testing to keep the rest of the population safe to FIR against Tablighi leaders, the Kumbh gathering was almost immune to public or policy censureFor example, the most frequent topic (Topic 1) includes words like *akhada,*

Top Topics

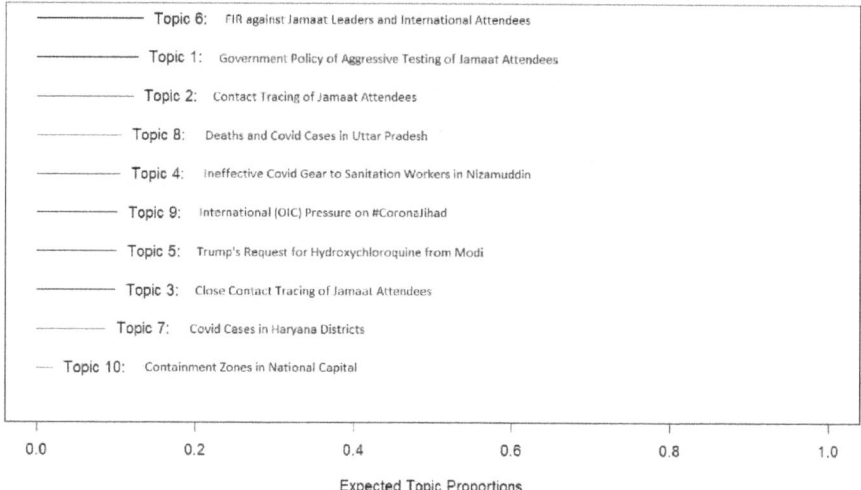

Figure 8.5 Most prevalent topics in coverage of Mulsim/Tablighi event in top five newspapers.

seer, parishad, ganda, ghat, mahant, which are the sites, actors, and main ritual of the holy dip in river Ganga (Shahi Snan) associated with Kumbh Mela. In other words, the print media reported most extensively and descriptively (as seen in the highest frequency topic, Topic 1) on the rites and rituals of Kumbh Mela, without reference to implications of this gathering, either legally given ongoing restrictions on mass gatherings or socially in terms flouting social distancing guidelines. In fact, the second most frequent topic identified by the algorithm in this corpus is that negative Covid-19 tests were not required to attend Kumbh. The Indian state of Uttarakhand scrapped the requirement for a negative test inviting devotees from across the world for Kumbh Mela, with the then Chief Minister, Tirath Singh, saying, "nobody will be stopped in the name of Covid-19 as the faith in God will overcome the fear of the Coronavirus"[27] (Figure 8.6).

We argue that this kind of neutral to positive reporting on Kumbh gives readers an impression of legitimacy of the Kumbh gathering, recommended as safe by authority figures, which is in sharp contrast to depiction of the Tablighi event as irresponsible, illegal and dangerous. A point of clarification here: the argument in this chapter is not about whether or not the Tablighi leaders acted responsibly by continuing their gathering amidst tightening government control. Instead, we highlight that the media scrutiny was disproportionately harsh for the Tablighi event compared to the Kumbh. There were reports on experts criticizing the Kumbh gathering as "superspreader" and others blaming the Prime Minister (PM) of India, Narendra Modi, for listening to astrologers instead of epidemiologists, for holding the Kumbh Mela in the 11th year of the usual 12-year cycle.

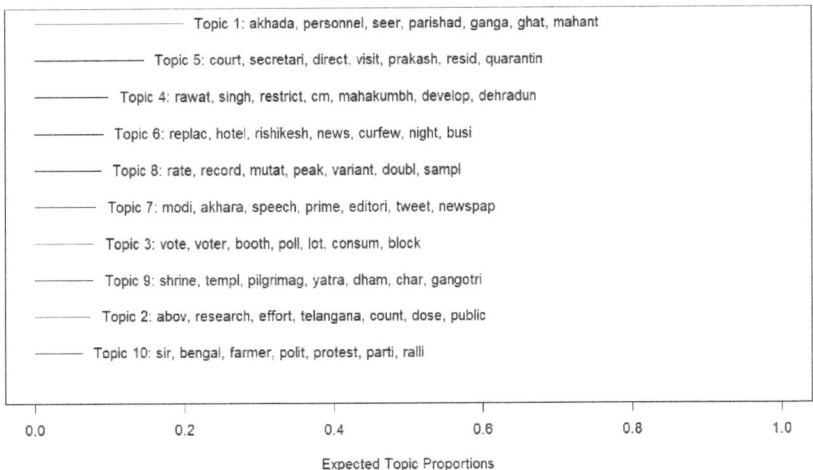

Figure 8.6 High-frequency words in coverage of Kumbh Mela in top five newspapers.

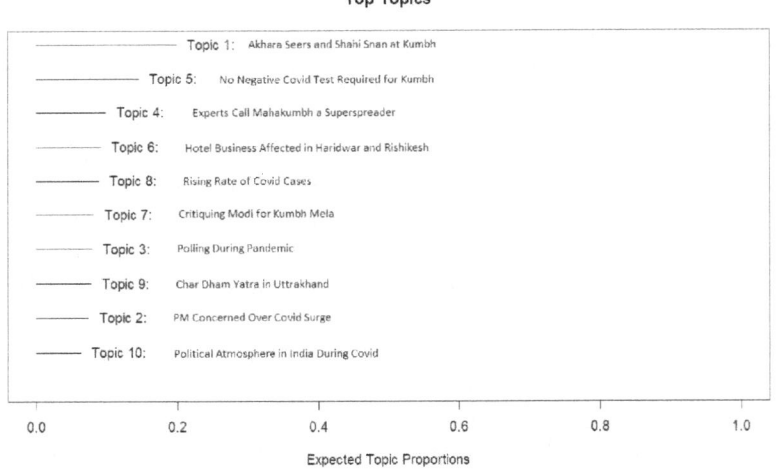

Figure 8.7 Most prevalent topics in coverage of Kumbh Mela in top five.

However, these stories were reported alongside the PM's concern on the growing number of cases (Topic 2) and many other events that assembled large numbers of people such as polling, another pilgrimage (Char Dham Yatra) in the state of Uttarakhand (Topic 9) and the Indian Cricket Premier League (Topic 10). The following table shows the most prevalent topics in the coverage of Kumbh by the print media (Figure 8.7).

Newspapers Section 4: Mechanisms of Otherization

This section analyzes what the specific ramifications of the divergent approach of Indian print media do to two religious events during a pandemic, one organized by the majority/Hindu and the other by the minority/Muslim community could be on otherization of minorities in an electoral democracy like India. This inquiry is contingent on two assumptions: first, we assume that electoral democracies combine majority rule with minority rights and protections. A democratic regime cannot allow unrestricted power of the majority to tyrannize the minority (De Tocqueville 2015). Second, we assume that the media does not merely relay what it sees as the government line, in which case, we might have dismissed the marked divergence in reporting on two events depicted above as inconsequential. However, if we are to assume that the media plays a vital role in generating a democratic culture by supplying information that not only influences how voters make their decisions but also builds deeply ingrained perception in the public consciousness over time, our findings are highly significant. Even if the lack of negative stereotyping of the Kumbh attendees in the media merely indicates the absence of censorship and sanctions against Kumbh in government policies and announcements, this chapter assumes that the role of the media, often referred to as the fourth estate, is not to simply follow the government line. This discussion contributes to ongoing research on the relationship between traditional media consumption and violence against marginalized groups attacked in the media (Adena et al. 2015; DellaVigna et al. 2014; Yanagizawa-Drott 2014). For example, traditional media is known to increase ethnic hatred and sometimes, instigate short-lived spikes in violence (Card et al. 2011) and increase in sex crimes (Bhuller et al. 2013). This section shows how the language of viral contagion that villainized the Tablighis and, by extension, the entire Muslim community, engendered three mechanisms of otherization of the Muslim minorities in India (Müller et al. 2021).

First, we argue that the vilification of Muslims and implicating them in the deliberate spread of an infectious disease reduces the costs of coordinating hate crimes among potential perpetrators. We call this mechanism of otherization of Muslims *coordination channel* based on the game theoretic assumption that a player's best option is to do what they think others would do. In other words, widespread propagation, and acceptance of negative stereotyping of Muslims makes it easier and less costly for individuals, who are predisposed to hate the "other" to participate in hate crimes because they expect others, primed by similar negative stereotyping of the target group, to join and support them (Manekin et al. 2022). For example, media reports mentioned close contact tracing of four Jamaat attendees from Kerala long after they returned from the Tablighi event in Delhi Nizamuddin. Reports disclosed personal details about the attendees, such as the railway station they traveled to, the mosque they prayed at on their journey back home, the airport they went to, whether they took a cab from the airport, which hospital four attendees were admitted to for observation and so on.[28] In addition, the Indian government has also blacklisted more than 2,500 foreign nationals, all Muslims, associated with the Tablighi Jamaat and barred their entry into the country for ten years. In his daily media briefing on Saturday, Lav Agarwal, joint secretary of the Ministry of Health and Family Welfare (MoHFW), chose to highlight the role of Tablighi Jamaat repeatedly, saying that of the 14,378 positive Covid-19 cases countrywide, 4,291 of them were linked to its congregation in Delhi's Nizamuddin area.[29]

About 45 days after the Tablighi event, there were reports of a young Muslim man being beaten for attending the event. This episode in the village of Harewali, near Delhi was filmed, and the mob was heard demanding if this Muslim man planned to spread the virus to the rest of the village.[30] In 2020, a Public Interest Litigation asked the Central Government of India to stop the dissemination of fake news and to take strict action against the sections of the media spreading bigotry and communal hatred concerning the Tablighi (Nizamuddin Markaz) issue.[31] After the health ministry repeatedly blamed Tablighi Jamaat for spreading the coronavirus, with the ruling party officials referring to them as "human bombs" and "corona jihad", a spree of anti-Muslim attacks broke out across the country.[32] Young Muslim men organizing a food drive for the poor were assaulted with cricket bats; many were nearly lynched, run out of their neighborhoods or attacked in mosques, branded as virus spreaders. In Punjab, loudspeakers reportedly broadcast messages advising people not to buy milk from Muslim dairy farmers because the milk was infected with the coronavirus. Videos falsely claiming to show members of the missionary group spitting on police and others quickly went viral on social media.[33] Only when incidents of backlash against Muslims were reported, the health ministry issued a statement (April 2020) on the need to counter such prejudices.

In addition, consistent media vilification of a particular community also changes in people's beliefs (a persuasion channel) and increases the likelihood of societal acceptance of xenophobic beliefs or actions (a social norms channel). The attack against Tablighis in the media, we argue, can make already radicalized individuals more willing to commit violent acts against Muslims in real life. According to a report by the human-rights group Equality Labs, #CoronaJihad was used in nearly 300,000 tweets, with a potential reach of 170 million users, between March 31and April 6.[34] Existing research on the subject shows that the effects of the media on the uptick of hate crimes are largely driven by areas that are more likely to harbor pre-existing hatred of minorities, which is explained by the media persuading people that certain actions toward minorities, otherwise impermissible, are now socially acceptable (Müller et al. 2021).

When a handful of visible individuals, in this case, the ruling party politicians and mainstream media aggregate discourse on important issues, they influence what is socially acceptable and make people more susceptible to extreme viewpoints. This re-enforcement process has often been called "echo chambers" which instigate a small set of potential perpetrators to take hateful actions online or offline (Bessi et al. 2015; Del Vicario et al. 2016; Schmidt et al. 2017; Sunstein 2017). In other words, reports of authority figures, such as bureaucrats and politicians, attacking Muslims as purveyors of the disease may enable those with extreme viewpoints to find sources of social legitimacy. It signals to potential perpetrators of hate crimes that their actions are more widely accepted than they really are. Here are a few examples. Mukhtar Abbas Naqvi, the minority-affairs minister, called the Jamaat's actions a "Talibani Crime" in a March 31, 2020 tweet.[35] Shobha Karandlaje, a Bharatiya Janata Party MP from Udupi Chikmagalur, used the phrase "corona jihad" during a speech in her constituency, on April 4, 2020, as did many others.[36] Karnataka Bharatiya Janata Party legislator MP Renukacharya on Wednesday attacked the members of Tablighi Jamaat, suggesting they were "traitors" and should be shot dead for evading tests and spreading Covid-19 in the country.[37] Haryana Home Minister Anil Vij maintained that a sharp spike in the total number of Covid-19 cases in Haryana was due to the sizable chunk of positive cases belonging to the Jamaat members. Vij said that so far, nearly 1,550 of the Jamaat members, including 107 foreigners, had been tracked down in the state.

The World Health Organization (WHO) warned that harmful stereotypes would "drive people to hide the illness to avoid discrimination, prevent people from seeking health care immediately, and discourage them from adopting healthy behaviours", thus compounding the public health problem. The consequences of this stereotyping are already evident in many parts of India, where Hindu vigilantes have begun boycotts of Muslim vendors and even resorted to violence. In some Muslim localities, the stereotyping has fueled paranoia about the intention of government health workers and led to tension and violence.

Conclusion

The primary contribution of this chapter is in presenting comprehensive quantitative and qualitative evidence on how the top five newspapers in India vilified a Muslim seminary group (Tablighi Jamaat) and by extension, the entire Muslim community, for organizing a mass event at the onset of Covid-19 pandemic in India. It also highlights how the same press failed to condemn a Hindu congregation at Kumbh, an event of much larger scale and attendance, organized a year later, with similar or worse ramifications for the pandemic. Topic analyses of the two events clearly demonstrate that the Indian press associated very different sets of words and meanings with the two events, effectively portraying only the Muslim event as illegal, socially pernicious, and a threat to national security as well as health and wellbeing of the people.

We also theorize three mechanisms of otherization of minorities through the language of viral contagion in media viz. coordination channel, persuasion channel, and social norm channel. Vilification of minorities changes the costs of coordinating hate crimes between potential perpetrators (*a coordination channel*), changes people's beliefs (*a persuasion channel*), and changes perceived societal acceptance of xenophobic beliefs or actions (*a social norms channel*). The larger question here is about what the specific ramifications of such misinformation campaigns against Muslims could be for minority rights in an electoral democracy like India. Moreover, from the perspective of the Muslim minority in India, the crucial question is if their negative stereotyping amounts to dehumanization of a people that can eventually cause sharp polarization in society and extreme violence including genocide.

Future research on negative stereotyping of minorities, pandemic-induced or not, needs to explore how such "othering" of minority groups by the networked media has long-term effects on the political preferences and electoral outcomes as well. Researchers are now interested in exploring how conspiracy-like narratives aimed at explaining reality provide an unprecedented opportunity to study the dynamics of narratives' emergence, production, and popularity in the media. The more users are exposed to unsubstantiated rumors, the more they are likely to jump the credulity barrier. Most of this research focuses on social media. However, newspapers also hold an influential place in disseminating information, forming attitudes, and motivating behavior, more so in India because it has defied the global trend of declining readership of newspapers.[38] In general, the findings on the role of print media in the process of exacerbation of Islamophobic hate, and the three mechanisms of otherization of minorities through the language of viral contagion in the media can resonate with other cases of pandemic-induced hate outside India as well.

Notes

1 COVID-19 is now the deadliest disease in American history, surpassing the death toll of the devastating 1918 flu pandemic. More than 676,000 people in the United States have lost their lives to the disease in the last year and a half since the World Health Organization first declared a pandemic on March 11, 2020. https://www.nationalgeographic.com/history/article/covid-19-is-now-the-deadliest-pandemic-in-us-history

2 Kandil CY. CNBC. Asian Americans Report over 650 Racist Acts over Last Week, New Data Says. https://www.nbcnews.com/news/asian-america/asian-americans-report-nearly-500- racist-acts-over-last-week-n1169821.

3 Rajagopalan M. BuzzFeed News. Men Yelling "Chinese" Tried to Punch Her off Her Bike. She's the Latest Victim of Racist Attacks Linked to Coronavirus. 2020. https://www.buzzfeednews.com/article/meghara/coronavirus-racism-europe-covid-19.

4 Marsh J, Deng S, Gan N. CNN. Africans in Guangzhou Are on Edge, After Many are Left Homeless Amid Rising Xenophobia as China Fights a Second Wave of Coronavirus. https://www.cnn.com/2020/04/10/china/africans-guangzhou-china-coronavirus-hnk-intl/index.html

5 The argument in this paper is not about Tablighi Jamaat's conservativeness, value systems or their response or lack of it to an unfolding global pandemic. The central argument in this paper is how the media in India depicted it's mass event versus a much larger Hindu event.

6 Chandna H, Basu M. The Print. Modi Announces 'Janata Curfew' on 22 March, Urges For resolve, Restraint to Fight Coronavirus. 2020. https://theprint.in/india/modi-announces-janata-curfew-on-22-march-urges-for-resolve-restraint-to-fight-coronavirus/384138/.

7 Chisti S. Caravan Magazine. The Nightmare: The Modi Government's Persecution of the Tablighi Jamaat. 2021. https://caravanmagazine.in/politics/nightmare-persecution-tablighi- jamaat.

8 Social media was rife with hashtags like #CoronaJihad or #NizamuddinIdiots and #BanJahilJamat, often accompanied by fake photos and videos of Muslims engaged in the act of spreading corona virus by licking plates. For example, see https://twitter.com/BJYMinWB/status/1244917375339835394.

9 This is an example of narrative building in India around a negative connotation of the term "jihad". See, for example, https://time.com/5815264/coronavirus-india-islamophobia-coronajihad/

10 Zaffar H, Abdulla S. Aljazeera. Tablighi Jamaat Men India Held for 'Spreading COVID' Share Ordeal. 2021. https://www.aljazeera.com/news/2021/3/25/tablighi-jamaat-members-held- for-spreading-covid-stuck-in-india.

11 Addressing the World Economic Forum's (WEF) Davos Agenda on Monday via videoconference, Prime Minister Narendra Modi said India has showcased its strength by fighting the COVID-19 pandemic. https://www.firstpost.com/india/india-gifted-world-bouquet-of-hope-pm- modi-at-wefs-online-davos-2022-summit-10294651.html.

12 Although there were election rallies in West Bengal, Indian Premier League (IPL) in Maharashtra and other mass events going on simultaneously, the cases were rising because of them as well before the second wave. However, (1) those events did not have as large a gathering as Kumbh (9.1 million), (2) those events were not religious gathering, and most importantly (3) if elections and IPL had shown cases were increasing in various states, the government should have immediately canceled the Kumbh mela gathering.

13 Sharma A, Bhasin S. NDTV. "Strengthen Covid Fight": PM. 2021. https://www.ndtv.com/india-news/pm-modi-urges-people-to-focus-on-fighting-covid-by-taking-all-precautions-2407943

14 Rawat S. Hindustan Times. 9.1 Million Thronged Mahakumbh Despite Covid-19 Surge: Govt data. 2021. https://www.hindustantimes.com/cities/dehradun-news/91-million-thronged-mahakumbh-despite-covid-19-surge-govt-data-101619729096750.html.

15 See https://www.bbc.com/news/world-asia-india-57154564.

16 Zaffar H, Abdulla S. Aljazeera. Tablighi Jamaat Men India Held for 'Spreading COVID' Share Ordeal. 2021. https://www.aljazeera.com/news/2021/3/25/tablighi-jamaat-members-held-for-spreading-covid-stuck-in-india

17 eUttranchal. Haridwar Kumbh Mela. 2021. https://www.euttaranchal.com/tourism/kumbh-mela-haridwar.php

18 Kidwai R, Sahar N. Let's Talk about How Tablighi Jamaat Turned Covid Hate against Muslims Around. 2020. https://theprint.in/opinion/lets-talk-about-how-tablighi-jamaat-turned- covid-hate-against-muslims-around/458728/.

19 Rawat S. Hindustan Times. 9.1 million Thronged Mahakumbh Despite Covid-19 Surge: Govt data https://www.hindustantimes.com/cities/dehradun-news/91-million-thronged-mahakumbh- despite-covid-19-surge-govt-data-101619729096750.html.

20 Hausman G. Columbia University Blogs. Citizenship Amendment Act (CAA) and National Register of Citizens (NRC). 2020.https://blogs.cul.columbia.edu/global-studies/2020/12/10/citizenship-amendment-act-caa-and-national-register-of-citizens-nrc/.

21 We downloaded the case_time_series dataset from data.covid19.bharat. This graph is based on daily confirmed, daily recovered and daily deceased cases in India, from January 30, 2020 to October 31, 2021.

22 The Hindu, Hindustan Times, The Economic Times, The New Indian Express, The Statesman were identified as the top five English language newspapers. However, Factiva did not show any results for The New Indian Express, even when we entered the word 'covid' in its keyword search. So, we used the sixth top newspaper, The Telegraph, instead of The New Indian Express. Since Telegraph is known as more left leaning than The New Indian Express, we can reasonably expect that inclusion of

The New Indian Express would generate more (and not less) evidence of anti-Muslim bias. Secondly, use of English language versus vernacular newspapers does not lead to any systematic bias in our findings. Covid, and the two cases of Tablighi and Kumbh gathering were very much national news. In addition, The Hindu is most circulated in the South, and the Statesman and The Telegraph are most widely circulated in the East, which makes the sample representative of regional variations as well.

23 We chose the start date as March 15, 2020 because the Muslim event concluded on March 15, 2020 and the Tablighi Jamaat and the Indian Muslims, on the whole, started facing backlash in the coming weeks. We decided the end date as April 30, 2020 because it matches the end date of the Hindu event. We could choose 1.5 months or more for both events. But, we chose the exact same data collection period for both events in their respective years. In the 1.5 month during which Kumbh Mela took place, there were only 232 articles. This is way less than the number of articles for a three- to four-day Jamaat event for which 1,307 articles were published in 1.5 months. The vilification of Jamaat by television and social media, and the Delhi government started after the event ended. The legal action, the societal boycott also happened after the event ended. Hence, the 1.5 months data collection for the Jamaat event.

24 On March 11, 2021, the first shahi snan (royal dip in the river Ganga) was performed following which Covid cases rose. So, we decided to choose March 15, 2021 as the start date for Kumbh data colelction to match the start date of the Muslim event in their respective years. The Hindu event ended on April 30, 2021.

25 The Boolean keyword search for the Muslim event was: (coronajihad OR tablighi jamaat OR tablighi OR nizamuddin markaz OR markaz) AND covid. The Boolean keyword search for the Hindu event was: (kumbhmela OR kumbh mela OR maha kumbh OR mahakumbh OR shahi snan) AND covid.

26 It is important to conceptually differentiate "unsupervised" from "supervised" methods where the analyst defines the topics ex ante, usually by hand-coding a set of documents into pre- established categories (Laver et al. 2003).

27 CM Tirath Singh of Uttarakhand Later Tested Covid Positive Himself. https://www.tribuneindia.com/news/nation/uttarakhand-cm-tirath-singh-rawat-tests-positive-for- coronavirus-228880.

28 We found this through thought analysis after doing qualitative analysis of top ten topics.

29 The Wire Staff. The Wire. Despite Its Guidelines against 'Stigmatisation', Govt Hypes Jamaat Role in COVID-19 Spread. 2020. https://thewire.in/government/health-ministry-covid-19-tablighi-jamaat.

30 Gettleman J, Schultz K, Raj S. New York Times. In India, Coronavirus Fans Religious Hatred. 2020. https://www.nytimes.com/2020/04/12/world/asia/india-coronavirus-muslims-bigotry.html.

31 PTI. Muslim Body Moves SC, Seeks Hearing of 2020 PIL on Fake News Regarding Tablighi Congregation. 2022. https://economictimes.indiatimes.com/news/india/muslim-body-moves-sc- seeks-hearing-of-2020-pil-on-fake-news-regarding-tablighi-congregation/articleshow/89098551.cms.

32 Ellis-Petersen H, Rahman SA. Coronavirus Conspiracy Theories Targeting Muslims Spread in India. 2020. https://www.theguardian.com/world/2020/apr/13/coronavirus-conspiracy-theories- targeting-muslims-spread-in-india.

33 For more information on this, please see https://time.com/5815264/coronavirus-india-islamophobia-coronajihad/

34 Equality Labs. Coronajihad. 2020. https://www.equalitylabs.org/coronajihad.

35 "This is not negligence, it's a 'serious criminal act,'" he wrote. "When the entire country is fighting united against Corona, such a 'sin' is unpardonable." At an event organized by Aaj Tak in May, he claimed that the third phase of the nationwide lockdown would not have been necessary if the Jamaat had not acted as a "super spreader." https://twitter.com/naqvimukhtar/status/1244968702157586432.

36 Special Correspondent. Tablighi event: Shobha Smells 'Corona Jihad.' 2020. https://
www.thehindu.com/news/national/karnataka/tablighi-event-shobha-smells-
corona-jihad/article31259288.ece
37 ANI on Twitter. 2020. https://twitter.com/ANI/status/1247738113503277058.
38 Newspaper circulation in India has grown from 39.1 million copies in 2006 to 62.8
million in 2016, recording a 60 per cent increase during the decade. The Indian
Readership Survey (IRS) data released for 2019 reveals that the overall readership
of newspapers has grown from 407 million readers in 2017 to 425 million readers at
the end of the first quarter of 2019. In fact, English newspapers saw a 10.7 per cent
growth, compared to Hindi and regional dailies that grew at 3.9 per cent and 5.7 per
cent, respectively. English newspaper readership went up from 28 million to 31 million
between the 2017 and Q1 2019 surveys. https://www.business- standard.com/article/
current-affairs/print-readership-in-india-jumps-4-4-to-425-million-in-two-
years-report-119042700079_1.html.

References

Adena M, Enikolopov R, Petrova M, Santarosa V, Zhuravskaya E. Radio and the rise of
the Nazis in Prewar Germany. *The Quarterly Journal of Economics*, 2015;130(4), 1885–1939.
Bessi A, Coletto M, Davidescu GA, Scala A, Caldarelli G, Quattrociocchi W. Science
vs conspiracy: Collective narratives in the age of misinformation. *PloS One*, 2015;10(2),
e0118093.
Bhuller M, Havnes T, Leuven E, Mogstad M. Broadband internet: An information super-
highway to sex crime?. *Review of Economic Studies*, 2013;80(4), 1237–1266.
Blei DM, Ng AY, Jordan MI. Latent dirichlet allocation. *Journal of Machine Learning
Research*, 2003;3, 993–1022.
Card D, Dahl GB. Family violence and football: The effect of unexpected emotional cues
on violent behavior. *The Quarterly Journal of Economics*, 2011;126(1), 103–143.
DellaVigna S, Enikolopov R, Mironova V, Petrova M, Zhuravskaya E. Cross-border
media and nationalism: Evidence from Serbian radio in Croatia. *American Economic
Journal: Applied Economics*, 2014;6(3), 103–132.
Del Vicario, M., Vivaldo, G., Bessi, A., Zollo, F., Scala, A., Caldarelli, G., & Quattro-
ciocchi, W. (2016). Echo chambers: Emotional contagion and group polarization on
facebook. *Scientific reports*, 6(1), 1–12.
Del Vicario, M., Bessi, A., Zollo, F., Petroni, F., Scala, A., Caldarelli, G., ... & Quattro-
ciocchi, W. (2016). The spreading of misinformation online. *Proceedings of the National
Academy of Sciences*, 113(3), 554–559.
De Tocqueville, A. *Democracy in America-Vol. I. and II*. 2015. Read Books Ltd.
Farrell, J. (2016). Network structure and influence of the climate change counter-move-
ment. *Nature Climate Change*, 6(4), 370–374.
Finley, A. (2018). OK Google, You've Been Served. *The Wall Street Journal*.
Finley T, Koyama M. Plague, politics, and pogroms: The Black Death, the rule of law,
and the persecution of Jews in the Holy Roman Empire. *The Journal of Law and Eco-
nomics*, 2018;61(2), 253–277.
Laver M, Benoit K, Garry J. Extracting policy positions from political texts using words
as data. *American Political Science Review*, 2003;97(2), 311–331.
Manekin D, Mitts T. Effective for Whom? Ethnic identity and nonviolent resistance. *American Political Science Review*, 2022;116(1), 161–180. doi:10.1017/S0003055421000940.
Müller K, Schwarz, C. Fanning the flames of hate: Social media and hate crime. *Journal
of the European Economic Association*, 2021;19(4), 2131–2167.

Schmidt AL, Zollo F, Del Vicario M, Bessi A, Scala A, Caldarelli G, Quattrociocchi W. Anatomy of news consumption on Facebook. *Proceedings of the National Academy of Sciences*, 2017;114(12), 3035–3039.

Sunstein CR. A prison of our own design: divided democracy in the age of social media. *Democratic Audit UK*, 2017.

Tampa M, Sarbu I, Matei C, Benea V, Georgescu SR. Brief history of syphilis. *Journal of Medicine and Life*, 2014;7, 4–10.

Wang C, Blei DM. Collaborative topic modeling for recommending scientific articles. In *Proceedings of the 17th ACM SIGKDD international conference on Knowledge discovery and data mining*, 2011; pp. 448–456.

Xu J, Sun G, Cao W, et al. Stigma, discrimination, and hate crimes in Chinese-speaking world amid Covid-19 pandemic. *Asian Journal of Criminology*, 2021;16(1), 51–74. doi:10.1007/s11417-020-09339-8.

Yanagizawa-Drott D. Propaganda and conflict: Evidence from the Rwandan genocide. *The Quarterly Journal of Economics*, 2014;129(4), 1947–1994.

9 Neoliberal Turn in the Domain of Health Care

The Emergence of Corporate Health Care Sector in India

Amrita Bagchi

Introduction

Indian hospitals were mostly run by government or private charities and Trusts till the 1970s. In the early 1980s, the state encouraged private nursing homes and small and medium hospitals to supplement government health care and facilities to meet the growing needs of the sick poor. But soon a significant shift in government policy led to the recognition of hospitals as an industry. The present chapter looks into the neoliberal turn in health care delivery services in India from the early 1980s and describes the systematic failures in the Indian health system. The eighth five-year plan in keeping with the selective health care approach adopted a new slogan. This chapter examines how the neoliberal turn shaped the health care policies and plans of the consecutive Indian governments. Instead of 'Health for All by 2000 AD,' it chose to emphasize Health for the Underprivileged. Simultaneously it continued the support for privatization[1] and subsequently towards corporatization. The chapter is divided into two segments: Neoliberal Turn: Reflections in Health Sector and Reflections of Neoliberal Turn in formulating Health Care Policies: A Brief Overview.

Neoliberal Turn: Reflections in Health Sector

The advent of the wave of liberalism in India in the post-1991 era had three characteristics that questioned the state's ability to provide an alternative mode of service delivery: the marginalization of the state, primacy to markets, and ceding space to NGOs. As a result, the gap between rich and poor did not exhibit a positive picture and poverty did not decline. Nehru's brand of socialism had indeed become passe.[2] Systematic failures in India's health infrastructure and the retreating nature of welfare state were further accelerated due to the shift towards a neoliberal economy from the late 1980s. Neo-colonialism in thought and practice, with the World Bank and other bilateral and multilateral agencies and donors with a particular source of ideological and financial support, has encouraged those who have pushed for liberalization of the Indian economy. These neoliberal policies have transformed India's health care system.[3] These policies found their echo in the attitude of the political class and large sections of bureaucracy whose trust in

DOI: 10.4324/9781003300762-10

the public sector was eroding. Both the Congress governments of Indira Gandhi and Rajiv Gandhi played a significant role in effecting several policy changes for hospitals to be recognized as an industry. Large government investments made in medical education not only allowed the private sectors to access subsidized and affordable treatments, but also provided good quality doctors. Stoppage in government recruitments left little choice for the medical graduates but to join the private sector or fly overseas. These public subsidies were meant to boost FDI and attract professionals back to India. The liberalization of the health sector is reflected in the Health Policy 1982, which actively sought to engage both the for-profit and non-profit sectors.[4] Moreover, a crisis in global capitalism has required a shift to 'surplus extraction without welfare'. The privatization of health care since the late 1980s must be seen in this wider context of structural changes in capitalism. Welfare sector expansion played an important role in rejuvenating the economy. The emergence of institutions like the IMF, World Bank, and GATT no doubt helped to concentrate power in the hands of the western block over the 1930s to the 1960s, where most of the transnational corporations were located. The search for new markets created inter-imperialist conflicts within capitalist economies. The hegemony of the US control over this search was threatened and the oil crisis added to the woes of the western countries which intensified the business of loans and aid and fresh wars in West Asia.[5]

From 1991 onwards, there was a drastic reduction in the central government budgetary allocation for health care which favored the establishment of private hospitals in India. Successive governments stimulated the growth of private sector, in various ways, such as releasing the prime building land at low rates, providing exemption from taxes and duties for importing drugs, high-tech medical equipment, and so forth.[6] The liberalization policy and health sector reforms provided opportunities in the health care markets for local and international corporations. State facilitated the growth of corporate health sector to establish tertiary level super specialty hospitals to achieve 'high quality' care and this continued through the 1990s and 2000s. The government opened up in 2000 the FDI route in hospitals and mobilization of capital stimulating the growth of corporate hospitals. Thus, there was a slow paradigmatic shift in the domain of health care services where health care itself was commodified. Hospitals became lucrative commercial enterprises; medical education became investment destinations and patients became clients. Moreover, the shift from the family doctor to a professionally managed health machine was also inevitable. In the face of technological innovation in medical devices, discovery of new drugs, and rapid changes in disease profile towards non-communicable diseases that required better diagnostic tools, more sophisticated laboratory facilities, and institutionalized treatment, health care became specialist dependent, organizationally structured, and resource-intensive. By 1990, private players accounted for 58 per cent of hospitals and 29 per cent of beds.[7] Meager government spending on health care led to the abandoning of the vision of Comprehensive Primary Health Care (Health for All by 2000 AD). With the transformation in the health policies and programs and in the patterns of allocation, the exogenous factors started playing a dominat role. With international and bilateral funding of some of the programs, there is a gross distortion of priorities in health development and disease control[8]. According to Rural Health Statistics Bulletin (2017–2018),[9] there were 1.39 health centers (either of SCs or PHCs) per 10,000 people nationally with a shortage of 32,900 Sub Centers & 6,430 Primary Health Centers (PHC). Besides the existing 46 per cent shortfall of doctors in PHCs, 74 per cent of the current graduate doctors reside in urban India leaving a large chunk of the rural population underserved. The vacancy rate of doctors is 24.9 per cent across rural PHCs.

India's ability to expand universal access to primary health care is seriously hampered by the persistent gaps in infrastructure required to deliver a basket of services. There is still a normative gap of 3,469 Community Health Centers (CHC) for a population of 0.1 million, 5,887 Primary Health Centers (PHC) for every 30,000 people, and 27,430 subcentres for every 5,000 people. Seventy per cent of the gap is in the poorly performing states that also have the disease burden. Besides, the existing facilities are not equipped and have an inadequate infrastructure with 10 per cent of the PHCs and 35 per cent of the subcentres housed in thatched huts located more than 3 kilometers away from the village, seriously impacting access.[10] Studies on the private sector in several developing countries show that the world recession of the late 1970s hindered the financing of the public services and resulted in the growth of markets in the welfare sector.[11] This is evident from the fact that in 1973 the percentage of beds in public hospitals was 71.2 while that in private hospitals was 28.8. In 1993, the percentage of beds in public hospitals got reduced to 42.3. On the contrary, the percentage of private hospital beds increased to 57.7. In the next phase, the private health sector, including the hospital sector, expanded rapidly on the one hand, and on the other the public health system was being reformed to fit the market model through the introduction of user charges and contracting out of services. The figure changed in 1996, when the percentage of hospital beds in the public sector decreased to 39 and as against the private sector which increased to 61.[12] In 2010–2011, the share of allopathic facilities was around 76 per cent, consisting of hospitals (7.8 per cent), medical (55.6 per cent), dental (4.1 per cent), nursing (4.1 per cent) and diagnostic (4.4 per cent) labs/centers, whereas the shares of service providers of homeopathy and ayurveda medicines were recorded to be around 11.2 per cent and 7.4 per cent, respectively. It is interesting to note that after Independence, roughly 1,352 private health enterprises were recorded in 1950, which cumulatively increased to 10.4 lakh in 2010–2011.[13] Approximately, an estimated 54.3 per cent of the medical institutions, 75 per cent of the hospitals, 51 per cent of the hospital beds, 75 per cent of the dispensaries and 80 per cent of all qualified doctors are in the private sector.[14] The share of government health enterprises in 2016 was found to be only 20 per cent.[15] During the 1980s, public health spending peaked and this was reflected in major health infrastructure expansion in rural India via the Minimum Needs Program. In fact, the entitlements mentioned above were achieved during this decade in most states. However, in the 1990s, the public health sector was woefully neglected with new public investments being virtually stopped and expenditures declining.

The expenditure on health as a percentage of total government expenditure was 5.5 in 1977; it declined to 3.2 in 1981, rose to 5.5, and peaked to 6.5 in 1989. During the 1990s, it declined from 5 per cent to 4.1 per cent.[16] The government health spending on medical care and public health, as a proportion to the total government expenditure, declined in real terms from 3.2 per cent to 2.7 per cent. Worse, the reduced spending had a higher proportion of salaries that increased from 39.93 per cent to 58.97 per cent and a corrosponding decline in capital expenditures from 4.37 per cent to 2.58 per cent. In terms of GDP, public spending increased from 0.98 per cent in 1975 to 1,36 per cent in 1986, only to fall to 1.28 per cent by 1991—this contracted even further to 0.09 per cent by 2000, resulting in the marginalization of the state as the primary player in the health service.[17] This poor investment pattern in health care retarded the expansion of public health services and this was the phase when 'welfare state' driven growth of private health sector started flourishing.

The Asian countries, despite their relative economic resilience, started getting trapped in the debt burden. Information technology became the instrument of this growing phenomenon of finance capital. The North, especially the US, protected its own agriculture and labor to the extent possible and attempted to practice austerity, the ex-socialist states were forced to face the consequences of the economic shock and the developing periphery of the capitalist system was offered Structural Adjustment Programs (SAP). The strategy was to deepen the links between public and private sectors, shift state subsidies to the private sector, focus on technology-based services (with the promotion of hi-tech) and commoditize them, and create low-cost alternatives for the poor to contain social unrest. Thus, balancing corporate interests, elite demands for personalized hi-tech services, and needs of the majority were attempted. The nature of technological inventions in sectors such as medicine (antibiotics, vaccines, chemicals for vector control, nutritional supplements), drinking water supply (filtration plants and piped water supply) and sanitation (sanitary pits and waste disposal technologies), and transport (roads, railways, bus systems), made extensive population coverage possible and economically feasible, thereby scaling up these services. The second crisis of the 1970s preceded by the electronics-based communication revolution, was tackled partially by this very technology for faster movement of financial capital.[18] It increased wealth without actually increasing production. The invention of the chip revolutionized the invasive power of medical technology, and made it more individualized, costly, and restrictive of employment within the sector.[19] India's official acceptance of SAP not only further integrated the country into the periphery of the capitalist system but also set the stage for a major transformation of its welfare sector including health sector challenging to expand and transform the scope of the medical market.

In line with the neoliberal priority of opening up investment opportunities for the private sector, India threw open the health insurance sector to private players in 1999, setting the foreign direct investment (FDI) cap in health insurance at 26 per cent. Generally, the private insurance funds access to hospitalization services from private providers.[20] Health insurance schemes are likely to be merely a further means of allowing the private sector to 'facilitate further consolidation of capital at the expense of people's money'. The Government of India policy documents, particularly the Tenth and Eleventh Plans, also recognized the growing inequalities in access to health care and the rising out-of-pocket expenditure as a serious concern. The National Health Policy Draft (2015) indicates that inequalities in access need to be addressed through policies that would ensure inclusion of the poor and other vulnerable sections of the population. This in fact pushed the government to develop a stronger contractual arrangement with private sector providers in both the non-profit and for-profit sectors.[21] The consolidation and transformation of markets in the Indian health service system present the features of a medical-industrial complex. Drawing on the analogy of the military-industrial complex, Arnold Relman, the former editor of *The New England Journal of Medicine,* characterized the rise of diverse business interests in medicine as a medical-industrial complex in the US during the 1980s. He along with several others who were critical of private interests in medical care wrote extensively on the entrenched network of power relations, the rise of business lobbies, and their influence on policy. Capital consolidated itself in medical services through pharmaceutical, medical devices, insurance, and provisioning corporations in the US. Public health reforms were diluted during the Clinton and Obama regimes and the interests of corporate American medical care remained largely protected.[22] This similar pattern is also reflected in the development of health care service in the post-reform phase.

President and CEO of GE Health Care India has observed that India is the first country to have a large number of multinational health care providers. There are seven to eight very active MNCs. It opens a whole host of opportunities.[23] Increasingly over the past decade, there is strong advocacy and promotion by the industry of the idea that 'Health care infrastructure should not just be viewed as a social good but also as a viable economic venture with productivity'.[24] The Confederation of Indian Industry (CII) projects health care sector as one with immense importance for the national economy, due to its rising contribution to GDP and the potential to be an engine of growth for the nation as it can create '70 to 80 million jobs in the next 10 years….' The CII National Health Care Division, comprising hospitals, diagnostic centers, and medical equipment companies, regularly organizes the India Health Summit since 2002 to promote private investment in the health care sector and lobby for concessions and favorable policies.[25] One of the demands of the Federation of Indian Chambers of Commerce and Industry (FICCI) Health Services Division is that the government should attract private health care investment to supplement the public funding deficit in health care allocations, by giving various fiscal and non-fiscal incentives.

'Corporatization of healthcare in India: The liberalization effect'[26] gave an excellent overview of the health care situation in the post-liberalization era. One of the most significant trends emerging in the wake of liberalization is the new vigor of the entry of corporate hospitals and multinationals into the health care scenario. The reason for this new tempo is the potential that India offers to

NRIs and multinationals. Since the early 1990s, when health care was seen as a "sunrise industry", several big corporate houses, Fortis Health Care (promoted by Ranbaxy Labs), Wockhardt Hospitals (promoted by the pharma company Wockhardt), and Max Health Care announced plans to set up hospital chains across the country. In addition to these big hospital chains, including the oldest one Apollo, other private hospitals and specialized health care facilities have been created for specialized services such as cardiac care, renal care, eye care, orthodontics, and laparoscopic surgery.[27] Mention should be made that International Finance Corporation (IFC), a private sector lending arm of the World Bank, has granted loans to several hospital projects that include Max Health Care, Rockland, Artemis, Apollo, and Duncan Gleneagles. Since 2002, IFC has extended loans to Apollo twice. In June 2009, IFC provided loans amounting to $50 million to Apollo Hospitals Enterprises Limited (AHEL) to expand its Apollo Reach network, specifically to set up smaller hospitals in the next three years in semi-urban and rural areas, in Tier II cities, to provide 'affordable health care' to low-income populations in these areas, using cross-subsidization between 'high-income and low-income consumers'. IFC is promoting this activity of AHEL as an 'innovative and inclusive business model'. More recently international private equity firms like AIG, J P Morgan Stanley, Carlyle, Blackstone Group, Quantum, and Blue Ridge have been investing in hospital projects. In a further sign of international involvement in financing commercial health care in India, smaller groups such as Portea (Healthvista India) and Regency (based in Kanpur) have also recently accessed loans.[28] In a recent study by the Centre for Disease Economics and Policies (India) and Princeton University,[29] it has been shown that India has approximately 1.9 million hospital beds, 95,000 ICU beds, and 48,000 ventilators. Nationally, hospital beds are concentrated in the private sector (hospital beds: 1,185,242 private vs 713,986 public). ICU beds and ventilators follow a similar trend (ICU beds: 59,262 private vs 35,699 public; ventilators: 29,631 private: 17,850 public).

Reflections of Neoliberal Turn in formulating Health Care Policies: A Brief Overview

With the coming of the World Bank on the stage in 1993, three key features had been clearly discerned[30]:

* The concept of an essential health service package as opposed to the grand vision of comprehensive primary care articulated at Alma Ata.
* Confining the role of government in implementing selective disease control programs justified on principles of Disability Adjusted Life Years (DALY's).
* Allowing markets to provide hospital and medical care with government engagement on the basis of public–private partnerships.

This vertical intervention program of the World Bank has to be seen within the Structural Adjustment Program (SAP), where the investment in social sectors is viewed as important for cushioning the vulnerable sections from the impact of the SAP. World Bank emphasized building health infrastructure and preventing and controlling communicable diseases. Thus the World Bank has emerged as the single largest fund loaning agency during the early nineties.[31] From 1990 to 2000 the influence of the World Bank, the WHO, and donor agencies on policy formulation was strong, though the share of their funding was less than 2 per cent of the total health spending. Complex health problems were simplified into single-lined technical solutions—DOTS for TB, immunization for infant mortality, early diagnosis and distribution of chloroquine tablets for malaria, and cataract surgeries for blindness. Health problems of India are being addressed through technological solutions while ignoring the social dimension of disease causation and neglecting the importance of social determinants.[32] Another crucial development of neoliberal health policies in India was the introduction of user fees. In 1987, the World Bank, in its report 'Financing Health Services in Developing Countries: An Agenda for Reform', recommended the introduction of user fees in government health care services, steering the debate towards the financial efficiency of these institutions rather than addressing the financial crisis of the poor households and critically analyzing the financial schemes of the government health care system. Several policy documents of the World Bank also recommended the introduction of user charges in the public hospitals of India.

In the context of making the public sector hospitals autonomous, proponents of user fees see it as a revenue mobilizing avenue. However, revenue generated from a user fee has not been very encouraging. In a district hospital of West Bengal, from 2002–2003 to 2005–2006, the share of user charges to the total expenditure showed a decline from 2.1 per cent to 1.8 per cent and the major share of revenue was generated from diagnostic services.[33] World Bank pushed the private sector agenda, introducing the concept of Public–Private Partnership (PPP). Justified on the grounds of organizational efficiencies, the concepts of 'outsourcing' and contracting services such as sanitation, laundry, diet, and the delivery of allied services took root, gradually expanding to co-opt NGOs and private sector care providers as partners. There was a clear shift towards the growth of curative (tertiary)services with a strong commercial focus on the neglect of primary health services. Attempts were initiated to take over hospital land for other purposes, non-renewal of land leases to charity hospitals, attempts to hand over primary health centers to private organizations, and so on were some major reforms that occurred in the last two decades. These measures have been justified by the state as being reform measures to increase the viability of health care services.[34] In 1993, World Bank published a report on "Investing in Health",[35] which acknowledged the role of government efforts in improving health outcomes and argued that the public health care system in developing nations was confronted with several challenges in the areas of efficiency and equity. It insisted that government involvement in the health care and health insurance sectors had only a limited role to play and that the government should restrict its role in these areas. The report rejected the idea of health care as a public good and proposed that health care provisions were a matter of individuals and families, with their strikingly different health needs, and they should be able to choose freely.[36]

On the eve of the Tenth Plan, the Draft National Health Policy 2001 was announced and for the first time feedback was invited from the public. 'Universal, comprehensive, primary health care services', the NHP 1983 goal, was not even mentioned in the NHP 2001 but the latter bravely acknowledged that the public health care system was grossly short of defined requirements, functioning was far from satisfactory, that morbidity and mortality due to easily curable diseases continued to be unacceptably high, and resource allocations were generally insufficient.[37] The second National Health Policy was called realistic and equitable. The BJP-led National Democratic Alliance (NDA), which came to power in 1999, condemned the policies of the previous government. Though there were some people-oriented promises, those were not implemented. World Bank-IMF-generated policies on health care failed to bring about any positive outcome by 2004. The post-liberalization rhetoric, namely, 'New Public Health' (NPH), has replaced the primary health care approach. The NPH is in harmony with the World Bank's essential package of services. It has eliminated the concept of planning for the population as a national agenda and talks of healthy 'cities' and 'communities' thereby shifting responsibility to the local organizations.[38] The NRHM (2005–2007) was launched on 12 April 2005 by the Prime Minister to improve the status of health services in India. It is based on the understanding that under the prevailing circumstances States required additional funds and technical and institutional support from the Center to improve the health status of their population. The stated aim of the NRHM was to provide accessible, affordable, and accountable quality services to the rural population.[39] The NRHM failed to achieve its stated objectives. The most important lesson that ought to be learnt is that 'the health of the people is not a standalone phenomenon that can be improved through health care alone. It requires a comprehensive action plan encompassing food security, employment and poverty alleviation as well'.[40] Another significant development in health care was the introduction of Rashtryia Swasthya Bima Yojana.

In recent years, several developing countries have introduced tax-financed health insurance coverage for their poor populations. India too, joined this effort in 2008, with the Indian Ministry of Labour and Employment (MoL&E) launching the '*Rashtriya Swasthya Bima Yojana*' (RSBY) to protect poor Indian households from financial risks associated with hospitalization expenses.[41] Several studies[42] have been undertaken on the impact of RSBY on Indian population. However, it has been inferred that overall our analysis shows that RSBY has not provided any significant financial protection for poor households. Government of India drafted the National Health Bill[43] in 2009, by advising the legal framework to recognize the 'right to health' and 'right to healthcare' with a stated recognition to address the underlying social determinants of health. Imrana Qadeer has pointed out the government's real intention behind this Bill. Explicit definitions of terms were neglected by the Bill making multiple legal interpretations possible.[44] The Bill was more concerned with the private providers and did not specify the responsibility of the public sector except for its role in public health services for the marginalized. The issue of universalization therefore remained vague and devoid of a time plan. The World Health Assembly adopted the term 'Universal Health Coverage' in 2005 and it has become the most widely used phrase in the global discourse on access and affordability of health services. The WHO defines UHC as a 'state of health system performance, when all people receive the quality health services they need without suffering fiancial hardship'.[45]

In India, UHC entered policy dialogue through the Public Health Foundation of India (PHFI), an initiative of the McKinsey consulting company. PHFI, chaired by a corporate honcho, was set up with a corpus of Rs 65 billion from the Indian government, Rs 65 billion from the Bill and Melinda Gates Foundation, and about Rs 4 billion of contributions promised by other corporate leaders.[46] It was a partnership between the government and the private sector and emerged as a think-tank and became a one-stop solution for all donor and foreign-funded research, including multinational pharmaceutical companies in the country. Contracted to come up with a plan to advocate UHC, the PHFI was provided handsome grants from the Rockefeller Foundation in 2009 and flagged UHC as a global priority.[47] The High Level Expert Group (HLEG) recommendations were drawn from global best practices and lessons provided by Indian experience. The HLEG upheld the principle of universality, equity, and higher investments in the health sector. It was clear that the state must be 'primarily and principally responsible for universal health care which is an entitlement to comprehensive health security'. Hence public sector services must be strengthened, improved, and brought to the center stage to ensure 'access and services' to all sections of the people. It recommended that user fees in public institutions should be discontinued and participation of citizens must go beyond existing forms of community involvement in preconceived programs of provisioning and monitoring health care.[48] The Twelfth Plan based on the HLEG report made a reasonable effort to assess the current health scenario and suggested a strategy that would entail a substantial increase in public health spending from 1.04 per cent of GDP at the end of the Eleventh Plan to 1.87 per cent by the end of the Twelfth Plan, the expansion of RSBY, expansion of medical education, access to free medicines in public facilities, regulation of the private health care sector, contracting in private services where public facilities were deficient, and so on.[49] There was no clarity on the nature of health financing with regard to creation of a single-payer system from the welter of government-funded social insurance schemes. The role of private sector was emphasized without caveats on the nature of contracting, accountability and regulation. While integrated care was mentioned, no pathway was indicated for the continuum of care across primary, secondary, and tertiary services across the maze of India's mixed health system.[50] Instead of an integrated health service with primary health care getting support from the secondary and tertiary, the thrust of the planning process had been to fragment health service into independent components—UHC, tertiary care and NRHM—in the name of providing rural and urban health services. In each of these strategies, public–private partnerships, commercialization and appropriation of the public resources were the dominant trends. UHC thus no more remained the state-led integrated and inclusive service but became a "Trojan horse of the neoliberal strategy".[51]

A new draft National Health Policy 2015 was introduced for comments by the government in January 2015 and new hope for UHC arose. The draft NHP 2015 gave emphasis on equity, universality, inclusive partnerships, affordability, pluralism, and accountability among its key principles. The political drive to ensure universal access to inexpensive health care services in an assured mode–the promise of Health Assurance—is an important catalyst for the framing of a new Health Policy.[52] NHP 2017 assures a comprehensive primary care to one and all. Both the quantifiable and measurable goals have been laid down. It has been proposed to set up health and wellness centers which would provide a full range of preventive and promotive services to prevent diseases and enhance well-being. To make this a reality, every family would have a health card that links them to a primary care facility and be eligible for a defined package of services anywhere in the country. Though the NHP 2017 provided a road map for future development in the health care sector, there were certain challenges and contradictions. Considering the budget allocation made by the Government of India for the health sector, the targets mentioned in the NHP seem over-ambitious. The expenditure on health in India is one of the lowest in the world at 1.4 per cent of the GDP. The NHP 2017 aims to increase this to about 2.5 per cent, which again is much less than the required 5–6 per cent. The money allocated for health in the Union Budget 2017 was nowhere near to achieving the target of even 2.5 per cent. The next concern is the weak commitment made to building the required infrastructure in urban and rural areas for delivering primary health care services. NHP 2017 affirms the desire to achieve the Indian Public Health Standards (IPHS), but fails to assess its fiscal implications.[53]

Following on the NHP 2017, the Government of India announced the Ayushman Bharat Program (ABP) in February 2018 to achieve the vision of Universal Health Coverage with two components:

a   Health and Wellness Centers (HWCs) to strengthen and deliver comprehensive Primary Health Care (CPHC) services for the entire population and

b   Pradhan Mantri Jan Arogya Yojana.

This initiative has been designed to meet the Sustainable Development Goals and their underlining commitment, which is to 'leave no one behind'.[54]

The second component under Ayushman Bharat is the Pradhan Mantri Jan Arogya Yojana or PM-JAY as it is popularly known. PM-JAY is the largest health assurance scheme in the world which aims at providing a health cover of Rs 5 lakh per family per year for secondary and tertiary care hospitalization to over 10.74 crore poor and vulnerable families (approximately 50 crore beneficiaries) that form the bottom 40 per cent of the Indian population. The government is "steadily but surely progressing towards the goal of Universal Health Coverage." This mega health care project, named 'Modicare' or 'Namocare' (by Union Home Minister Amit Shah) indeed promises to provide secondary and tertiary care hospitalization and covers both prevention and health promotion. Four in ten Indians can avail of secondary and tertiary care in government and private hospitals, within the insurance cap earmarked per family. A new national health agency will be instituted under the scheme to oversee its implementation at the state level.[55] Modicare, as it stands now, is geared more towards taking care of the corporate health care industry's interests in the name of the poor. It is (actually) insurance of insurance companies. Health insurance schemes are likely to be merely a further means of allowing the private sector to 'facilitate further consolidation of capital at the expense of people's money'. The Government of India policy documents, particularly the Tenth and Eleventh Plans, also recognized the growing inequalities in access to health care and the rising out-of-pocket expenditure as a serious concern. The vision of the neoliberal state proposes that gains from the improved management could be obtained within a contracting framework. Hence, the Indian state adopted contract-based models within a publicly set framework and expanded contractual relationships between the public and private health sectors. In pursuit of this model, public health budgets have been re-directed to subsidize social insurance for those sections of the population (BPL) that have been judged to be unable to pay. Health insurance became one of the viable strategies of the state which skillfully tried to address both the growing cost of medical care and accessibility concerns.[56] Between 2000–2001 and 2006–2007, more than 40,000 new establishments have come up, largely in the urban areas. At the same time, small enterprises have almost gone down. These clearly point out that a rapid transformation toward organized forms of production is taking place in urban areas of the country. Parallely there was also the disappearance of general practitioners who are being included in the medico industrial complex. Given the assurance from the government about cashless services, a lot of people would tend to enroll them with the better looking secondary and tertiary care institutions wherever they are available. In order to incentivize the growth process further, the government of India has included the health sector in the Viability Gap Funding scheme under which 20 per cent of expenses would be borne by the government if hospitals and medical colleges are set up in non-metros. This, coupled with the market guarantee mechanisms provided under the 'managed care' model can create conditions for further expansion of the private vis a vis corporate sector.[57]

Conclusion

The global pressure of investing more in private health care and reforming the degenerating public health care services brought about far-reaching consequences in the entire health care culture. The dependence upon the market forces and the technocentric approach to health strengthened the significance and the expansion of corporate health care. The allocation for health care had always been meager compared to the demand of the vast population in India. Since this inadequate infrastructure failed to come up with positive outcomes, it collapsed within three decades of Independence, providing the space for the private health sector to flourish as the alternative for health care delivery services. Further decay was brought about with the shrinking of the welfare state towards the provisioning of funds for the health care sector. This process received a boom in the post-liberalization era with the coming of the international donor agencies with a new package of reforms for public health care and the thrust toward converting the private health care sector to corporate one. The impact of neoliberalism on health care policies, plans and program reveals that none of the governments at the Center has given serious attention to the health issues of this vastly populated nation. It was not the inability that stood as the hindrance, but the will to restructure the health care services. Proposals were made in several policies, but the issue of implementing them to reduce inequity was not seriously addressed. The primary health care sector which needed more attention for addressing health problems of the rural masses was ignored. On the contrary, policies of health care tried to strengthen the tertiary and secondary level health care sectors. State-sponsored health insurances promoted not only the large-scale utilization of hospital beds in private sector for public purposes, but also result in channelizing public funds to the private sector, contracting out the existing public health care sector and deepening of the crisis of getting proper treatment from the giant health sector corporates.

Notes

1 Planning Commission, Government of India, Eighth Five Year Plan Highlights. New Delhi: Directorate of Advertising and Visual Publicity, Government of India, 1992.
2 Rao, Do We Care, 17.
3 Roger Jeffery, "Commercialisation in Health Service," in *Global Health Governance and Commercialisation of Public Health in India: Actors, Institutions and Dialectics of Global and Local,* eds. Anuj Kapilashrami and Rama V. Baru (London and New York: Routledge, 2019), 80–81 (Hereafter cited as Jeffery, Commercialisation in Health Service). Also see Indranil Mukhopadhyay, "Universal Health Coverage: The New Face of Neoliberalism," *Social Change* 43(2013), 177.
4 Rama V. Baru, "Medical-Industrial Complex," in *Equity and Access: Health Care Studies in India,* eds. Purendra Prasad and Amar Jessani (New Delhi: OUP, 2018), 81.
5 Qadeer, Universal Health Care: The Trojan Horse of Neoliberal Policies, 149–164.
6 Purendra Prasad, "Health Care Reforms: Do They Ensure Social Protection for the Labouring Poor?" in *Equity and Access: Health Care Studies in India,* eds. Purendra Prasad and Amar Jessani (New Delhi: OUP, 2018) (Hereafter cited as Prasad, Health Care Reforms).
7 Rao, Do We Care, 16. Also see Sunil Nandaraj, "Unregulated and Unaccountable: Private Health Providers," *Economic and Political Weekly* 42, No. 4 (January 2012), 12–17.
8 *Report of the Independent Commission on Health in India.* New Delhi: Voluntary Health Association of India, 2000, 40.
9 Rao, Do We Care? 53.
10 Rural Health Statistics Bulletin, Government of India Ministry of Health and Family Welfare Statistics Division (2017–2018).
11 Rama V. Baru, *Private Health Care in India: Social Characteristics and Trends* (New Delhi: Sage Publications, 1998) and M. Price, "Explaining Trends in the Privatisation of Health Services in South Africa," *Health Policy and Planning,* 4, No. 2 (1989), 50–62. Baru, "Health Sector Reform", 268. See also Gertler and Jacques, *Willingness to Pay,* 2.

12 GoI, Min of Health and Family Welfare, Health Information of India, Central Bureau of Health Intelligence (New Delhi: Govt of India, 2000–2005).

13 Shailender Kumar Hooda, "Private Sector in Healthcare Delivery Market in India: Structure, Growth and Implications", Working Paper 185 (New Delhi: Institute for Studies in Industrial Development, 2015), 7 (Hereafter cited as Hooda, Private Sector in Health Care Delivery).

14 Shailender Kumar, Private Sector in Health Care Delivery Market in India: Structure, Growth and Implications. New Delhi: Intern report, Institute for Studies in Industrial Development (ISID), 2015 .

15 GOI (Government of India). "Report of Sixth Economic Census." *Ministry of Statistics and Programme Implementation*, Central Statistical Office, Government of India (2016).

16 Baru, Privatisation of Health Services, 4434.

17 Rao, Do We Care? 17

18 Carlota Perez, *Technological Revolution and Financial Capital: The Dynamics of Bubbles and Golden Ages* (Cheltenham: Edward Elgar, 2002), cited in Qadeer, Universal Health Care: The Trojan Horse of Neoliberal Policies, 149–164.

19 Qadeer, Universal Health Care: The Trojan Horse of Neoliberal Policies, 149–164.

20 Sathia Suthanthiraveeran, The Five Year Plans in India: Overview of Public Health Policies (researchgate.net). Accessed on 19 October 2021.

21 *Public Health and Private Wealth: Stem Cells, Surrogates and Other Strategic Bodies*, eds. Sarah Hodges and Mohan Rao (New Delhi: Oxford University Press, 2016) cited in Purendra Prasad, Health Care Reforms: Do they Ensure Social Protection for the Labouring Poor?

22 A.S. Relman "The New Medical Industrial Complex," *The New England Journal of Medicine* 303, No. 17, 963–970 and P. Starr, *The Social Transformation of American* Medicine (New York: Basic Books, 1982), cited in Baru, Medical Industrial Complex, 75–76, in *Equity and Access: Health Care Studies in India*, eds. Purendra Prasad and Amar Jessani (New Delhi: OUP, 2018).

23 P. Bose, India Presents Challenging Paradigms, Opportunities: Terri Bresenham. Interview with President and CEO, GE Healthcare India, *Business Standard*, 26 March 2012, cited in Indira Chakravarthi, "The Emerging 'Health Care Industry' in India: A Public Health Perspective", *Social Change* 43, No. 2 (2013), 165–176 (Hereafter cited as Chakravarthi, Healthcare Industry).

24 FICCI (2008). Fostering Quality Healthcare for all. FICCI HEAL 2008, Federation of Indian Chambers of Commerce and Industry Health Services Division, New Delhi, cited in Chakravarthi, Healthcare Industry.

25 Confederation of Indian Industry (CII) (2011). Addressing the Unfinished Agenda: Universal Healthcare, cited in Chakravarthi, Healthcare Industry.

26 http://www.article alley.com_882070_15.html. Accessed on 14 June 2010.

27 Indira Chakravarthi, "Corporate presence in the Health Care Sector in India," *Social Medicine* Vol. 5, No. 4 (December 2010), www.socialmedicine.info. Accessed on 7 February 2021 (Hereafter cited as Chakravarthy, Corporate presence in Health care Sector).

28 B. Levebre, "The Hospital Chains in India: The Coming of Age?" Published by Centre Asie Ifri (2010) cited in Baru, Medical Industrial Complex 83, Jeffery, Commercialisation in Health Service, 89. Also see Chakravarthi, Healthcare Industry.

29 https://doi.org/10.1101/2020.06.16.20132787. Accessed on 14 September 2020.

30 Rao, Do We Care? 17.

31 Mukhopadhyay, Report of the Independent Commission, 41.

32 Rao, Do We Care? 21–22. Also see Mukhopadhyay, Report of the Independent Commission.

33 For details on user fees, see World Bank Documents (See 1985, 1987,1993,1997). Bijoya Roy, Siddharta Gupta, "Public-Private Partnership and User Fees in Healthcare: Evidence from West Bengal," *Economic and Political Weekly* xlvi, No. 38 (September 2011).

Mylene Lagardea and Natasha Palmer, "The Impact of User Fees on Health Service Utilization in Low- and Middle-Income Countries: How Strong Is the Evidence," *Bulletin of the World Health Organization* 86 (April 2008), 839–848; West Bengal Health Policy Note, *World Bank South Asia Region*, June 2004; Oommen C. Kurian, Suchitra Wagle, and Prashant Raymus, Mapping the Flow of User Fees in a Public Hospital (Bombay: Centre for Enquiry into Health and Allied Themes, 2011), Amrita Bagchi, "Reforms or Dictates: The Role of the Donor Agencies on Health Care in West Bengal," *Global South –Sephis E-magazine* 7, No. 3 (July 2011). ISSN 2347-8594.

34 Rao, Do We Care? 18. Also see Rama Baru, "Commercialisation and the Poverty of Public Health Services in India," in *Public Health and Private Wealth: Stem Cells, Surrogates and Other Strategic Bodies*, eds. Sarah Hodges and Mohan Rao (New Delhi: Oxford University Press, 2016).

35 World Bank, *World Development Report 1993: Investing in Health* (New York: Oxford University Press, 1993).

36 M. Fisk "Neoliberalism and the Slow Death of Public Healthcare in Mexico," *Journal of Socialism and Democracy* 14, No. 1 (2000), 63–84, cited in Shailendra Hooda, "Health System in Transition in India: Journey from State Provisioning to Privatization," *World Review of Political Economy* 11, No. 4 (Winter 2020), 506–532.

37 Duggal, Historical Review of Health Policy Making, 38.

38 See Imrana Qadeer, Kasturi Sen, and K.R. Nayar, eds. *Public Health and Poverty of Reforms* (New Delhi: Sage Publications, 2001).

39 National Rural Health Mission, *Meeting People's Health Needs in Rural Areas: Framework for Implementation 2005–2012* (New Delhi: Ministry of Health and Family Welfare, Government of India).

40 Vikas Bajpai and Anoop Saraya, "NRHM — The Panacea for Rural Health in India: A Critique," *Indian Journal of Public Health Research and Development* 1, No. 3 (January 2013), 24–30.

41 A. Wagstaff, M. Lindelow, G. Jun, X. Ling and Q. Juncheng, "Extending Health Insurance to the Rural Population: An Impact Evaluation of China's New Cooperative Medical Scheme," *Journal of Health Economics* 28, No. 1 (2009), 1–19 and U. Giedion, E.A. Alfonso, and Y. Diaz, *The Impact of Universal Coverage Schemes in the Developing World: A Review of the Existing Evidence*, Universal Health Coverage (UNICO) Studies Series, Vol. 25 (Washington DC: The World Bank, 2013) cited in Anup Karan, Winnie Yip, and Ajay Mahal, "Extending Health Insurance to the Poor in India: An Impact Evaluation of Rashtriya Swasthya Bima Yojana on Out of Pocket Spending for Healthcare (nih.gov)," *Social Science & Medicine* 181 (May 2017), 83–92. doi:10.1016/j.socscimed.2017.03.053. Accessed on 28 November 2022 (Hereafter cited as Karan, Yip, Mahal, Extending health insurance to the poor in India).

42 Sonalini Khetrapal and Arnab Acharya, "Expanding Healthcare Coverage: An Experience from RashtriyaSwasthya BimaYojna," PubMed (nih.gov). Accessed on 28 November 2021. Madhurima Nundy, Rajib Dasgupta, Kanica Kanungo, Sulakshana Nandi, and Ganapathy Murugan, The Rashtriya Swasthya Bima Yojana (RSBY) Experience in Chhattisgarh: What Does It Mean for Health for All?, A paper published by SAMA: A Resource Group for Women and Health (New Delhi, 2013); R.A. Palacios, "New Approach to Providing Health Insurance to Poor in India: The Early Experience of Rshtriya Swasthya Bima Yojna," in *India's Health Insurance Scheme for the Poor: Evidence from the Early Experience of the Rashtrita Swasthya Bima Yojana*, eds., Robert Palacios, Jishnu Das, and Changqing Sun (New Delhi: Centre for Policy Research, 2011); Sakthivel Selvaraj and Anup K. Karan, "Why Publicly-Financed Health Insurance Schemes Are Ineffective in Providing Financial Risk Protection?" *Economic & Political Weekly* 47, No. 11 (2012), 460–468.

43 http://mohfw.nic.in/nrhm/Draft_Health_Bill/General/Draft_National_Bill.pdf. Accessed on 28 November 2021.

44 Imrana Qadeer, "Universal Health Care: The Trojan Horse of Neoliberal Policies," *Social Change* 43, No. 2 (2013), 154–155 (Hereafter cited as Qadeer, Universal Health Care: The Trojan Horse).

45 https://www.worldbank.org/en/topic/universalhealthcoverage#1. Accessed on 2 December 2021.

46 For more details on PHFI see Rao, Do We Care, 25.

47 Rao, Do We Care, 58.

48 High Level Expert Group Report on Universal Health Coverage for India (New Delhi: Instituted by the Planning Commission of India, November 2011). Also see Imrana Qadeer, "Universal Health Care: The Trojan Horse of Neoliberal Policies," *Social Change* 43 (June 2013), 149–164.

49 Planning Commission, *Social Sectors; Twelfth Five Year Plan (2012–2017)* (New Delhi: Planning Commission of India, 2013).

50 Reddy and Mathur, "Universal Health Coverage," in *Equity and Access: Health Care Studies in India*, eds. Purendra Prasad and Amar Jessani (New Delhi: OUP, 2018), 313.

51 See Imrana Qadeer, "Universal Health Care: The Trojan Horse of Neoliberal Policies," 149–164. Also see Imrana Qadeer, "Universal Health Care in India: Panacea for Whom?" http://www.ijph.in. Accessed on 22 November 2021.Also see Indranil Mukhopadhyay, "Universal Health Coverage: The New Face of Neoliberalism," *Social Change* 43 (2013), 177.

52 National Health Policy 2015 Draft, Ministry of Health & Family Welfare December (New Delhi, 2014).

53 For Critique of the NHP 2017, see Vikas Bajpai, "National Health Policy, 2017: Revealing Public Health Chicanery," *Economic and Political Weekly* LIII, No.28 (July 2014); Rajiv Kumar Gupta and Rashmi Kumari, "National Health Policy 2017: An Overview," *JK Science* 19, No. 3 (July to September 2017); S. Sharma et al., National Health Policy 2017: Can It Lead to Achievement of Sustainable Development Goals?, https://www.researchgate.net/publication/322287585. Accessed on 10 December 2021.

54 Nirupam Bajpai and Manisha Wadhwa, Health and Wellness Centres: Expanding Access to Comprehensive Primary Health Care in India, *ICT India Working Paper #13*, Centre of Sustainable Development, Earth Institute, Columbia University (July 2019).

55 www.thehindu.com. Accessed on 23 September 2018.

56 Purendra Prasad, Health Care Reforms: Do they Ensure Social Protection for the Labouring Poor? and Rama V. Baru, *Medical Industrial Complex: Trends in Corporatization of Health Services in Equity and Access: Health Care Studies in India*, eds. Purendra Prasad and Amar Jessani (New Delhi: OUP, 2018), 34. Also see Jeffery, Commercialisation in Health Service; Indranil Mukhopadhyay, "Universal Health Coverage: The New Face of Neoliberalism," *Social Change* 43 (2013), 177.

57 Indranil Mukhopadhyay, "Universal Health Coverage: The New Face of Neoliberalism," *Social Change* 43 (2013), 177–190. Also see Hooda, Health System in Transition in India, 509–510.

References

Bagchi Amrita, "Reforms or Dictates: The Role of the Donor Agencies on Health Care in West Bengal," *Global South –Sephis e-magazine*, Vol. 7, No. 3, July 2011. ISSN 2347-8594.

Bajpai Nirupam and Wadhwa Manisha, Health and Wellness Centres: Expanding Access to Comprehensive Primary Health Care in India, ICT India Working Paper #13, Centre of Sustainable Development, Earth Institute, Columbia University, July 2019.

Bajpai Vikas, "National Health Policy, 2017: Revealing Public Health Chicanery," *Economic and Political Weekly*, Vol. LIII, No. 28, pp. 31–35, July 2014.

Bajpai Vikas and Saraya Anoop, "NRHM — The Panacea for Rural Health in India: A Critique," *Indian Journal of Public Health Research and Development*, Vol. 1, No. 3, January 2013. Doi:10.1016/j.socscimed.2017.03.053. Accessed on 28 November 2022.

Chakravarthi Indira, "Corporate Presence in the Health Care Sector in India," *Social Medicine*, Vol. 5, No. 4, pp. 192–204, December 2010.

Chakravarthi Indira, "The Emerging 'Health Care Industry' in India: A Public Health Perspective," *Social Change*, Vol. 43, No. 2, pp. 165–176, 2013.

GOI (Government of India), *Report of Sixth Economic Census*. Ministry of Statistics and Programme Implementation, Central Statistical Office, Government of India, 2016.

GOI, *Ministry of Health and Family Welfare, Health Information of India, Central Bureau of Health Intelligence*, New Delhi: Govt of India, 2000–2005.

Gupta Rajiv Kumar and Kumari Rashmi, "National Health Policy 2017: An Overview," *JK Science*, Vol. 19, No. 3, pp. 135–136, July to September 2017.

High Level Expert Group Report on Universal Health Coverage for India, Instituted by the Planning Commission of India, New Delhi, November, 2011.

Hodges Sarah and Rao Mohan, Ed., *Public Health and Private Wealth: Stem Cells, Surrogates and Other Strategic Bodies*. New Delhi: Oxford University Press, 2016.

Hooda Shailender Kumar, "Health System in Transition in India: Journey from State Provisioning to Privatization," *World Review of Political Economy*, Vol. 11, No. 4, pp. 506–532, Winter 2020.

Hooda Shailender Kumar, *Private Sector in Healthcare Delivery Market in India: Structure, Growth and Implications*, Working Paper 185, New Delhi: Institute for Studies in Industrial Development, 2015.

http://mohfw.nic.in/nrhm/Draft_Health_Bill/General/Draft_National_Bill.pdf   .
Accessed on 28 November 2021.

http://www.article alley.com_882070_15.html.

https://doi.org/10.1101/2020.06.16.20132787.

https://www.researchgate.net/publication/322287585. Accessed on 10 December 2021.

https://www.worldbank.org/en/topic/universalhealthcoverage#1. Accessed on 2 December 2021.

Imrana Qadeer, "Universal Health Care in India: Panacea for Whom?" http://www.ijph.in. Accessed on 22 November 2021.

Imrana Qadeer, "Universal Health Care: The Trojan Horse of Neoliberal Policies," *Social Change*, Vol. 43, pp. 149–164, June 2013.

Imrana Qadeer, Kasturi Sen, and K.R. Nayar, *Public Health and Poverty of Reforms*. New Delhi: Sage Publications, 2001.

Kapilashrami Anuj and Rama V. Baru, Ed., *Global Health Governance and Commercialisation of Public Health in India: Actors, Institutions and Dialectics of Global and Local*. London and New York: Routledge, 2019.

Kurian Oommen C., Wagle Suchitra, and Raymus Prashant, *Mapping the Flow of User Fees in a Public Hospital*. Bombay: Centre for Enquiry into Health and Allied Themes, 2011.

Lagardea Mylene and Palmer Natasha, "The Impact of User Fees on Health Service Utilization in Low- and Middle-income Countries: How Strong Is the Evidence," *Bulletin of the World Health Organization*, Vol. 86, pp. 839–848, April 2008.

Madhurima Nundy, Rajib Dasgupta, Kanica Kanungo, Sulakshana Nandi, and Ganapathy Murugan, The Rashtriya Swasthya Bima Yojana (RSBY) Experience in Chhattisgarh: What Does It Mean for Health for All?, A paper published by *SAMA: A Resource Group for Women and Health*. New Delhi, 2013.

Mukhopadhyay Indranil, "Universal Health Coverage: The New Face of Neoliberalism," *Social Change*, Vol. 43, pp. 177–190, 2013.

Nandaraj Sunil, "Unregulated and Unaccountable: Private Health Providers," *Economic and Political Weekly*, Vol. 42, No. 4, January 2012.

National Health Policy 2015 Draft, Ministry of Health & Family Welfare December, 2014, New Delhi.

National Rural Health Mission, *Meeting People's Health Needs in Rural Areas: Framework for Implementation 2005–2012*, New Delhi: Ministry of Health and Family Welfare, Government of India, 2012.

Paul Gertler and Van der Jacques Gaag, *Willingness to Pay: Evidence from Two Developing Countries*. Washington D.C: World Bank Publication, 1990.

Planning Commission, *Social Sectors; Twelfth Five Year Plan (2012–2017)*. New Delhi: Planning Commission of India, 2013.

Planning Commission, *Government of India, Eighth Five Year Plan Highlights*. New Delhi: Directorate of Advertising and Visual Publicity, Government of India, 1992.

Prasad Purendra and Jessani Amar, Ed., *Equity and Access: Health Care Studies in India*. New Delhi: OUP, 2018.

Rama V. Baru, *Private Health Care in India. Social Characteristics and Trends*. New Delhi: Sage Publications, 1998.

Rao K. Sujatha, *Do We Care? India's Health System*. New Delhi: OUP, 2020.

Report of the Independent Commission on Health in India. New Delhi: Voluntary Health Association of India, 2000.

Robert Palacios, Jishnu Das, and Changqing Sun, Ed., *India's Health Insurance Scheme for the Poor: Evidence from the Early Experience of the Rashtrita Swasthya Bima Yojana*. New Delhi: Centre for Policy Research, 2011.

Rural Health Statistics Bulletin, Government of India Ministry of Health and Family Welfare Statistics Division, 2017–2018.

Sakthivel Selvaraj and Anup K. Karan, "Why Publicly-Financed Health Insurance Schemes Are Ineffective in Providing Financial Risk Protection?" *Economic & Political Weekly*, Vol. 47, No. 11, 2012.

Sathia Suthanthiraveeran, "The Five Year Plans in India: Overview of Public Health Policies." https://www.researchgate.net/publication/327238255_The_five_year_plans_in_India_Overview_of_Public_Health_Policies?enrichId=rgreq-75427869e04335eeaf 36aa5fbc749671-XXX&enrichSource=Y292ZXJQYWdlOzMyNzIzODI1NTtBU zo2NjQxNjY4ODA3ODAyODhAMTUzNTM2MTEzMjM4MA%3D% 3D&el=1_x_2&_esc=publicationCoverPdf

Shailender Kumar, *Private Sector in Health Care Delivery Market in India: Structure, Growth and Implications*. New Delhi: Intern report, Institute for Studies in Industrial Development (ISID), 2015.

World Bank, *West Bengal : Health Policy Note*. Washington, DC. © World Bank, 2004.

World Bank, *World Development Report 1993: Investing in Health*. New York: Oxford University Press, 1993.

www.thehindu.com. Accessed on 23 September 2018.

Zakir Hussain, Saswata Ghosh, and Bijoya Roy, "Socio Economic Profile of Patients in Kolkata: A Case Study of RG Kar and AMRI," Kolkata: Institute of Development Studies, Occasional Paper. July 2008.

Section II

Cultural Perspective

10 Disease and the Desire for Health in Shakespeare's *Macbeth*

Subhajit Sen Gupta

I

In a famous letter to Pope Clement VI, the Italian Renaissance humanist Petrarch, while acknowledging that the presence of physicians was comforting, wrote:

> … find yourself a single one of their band who is worthy, not on account of the grace of his expressions, but because of his knowledge and his integrity. For in the act of forgetting their profession, they are eager to step out of their sphere; they set their feet upon the blooming acres of poesy and the wide fields of rhetoric, as though it were not their province to heal but to convince.
> (Castiglioni 1947, 400)

Guy de Chauliac, the Pope's physician, happened to read the letter, and this started his famous quarrel with Petrarch, prompting the latter to write satires against physicians. In the same letter, which appears to exaggerate some of the commonly felt misgivings against physicians, Petrarch writes, "Oh, Most Gentle Father, look upon their band as an army of enemies" (399). The general attitude of the age towards physicians was ambivalent. Their presence in society was necessary, and by the close of the fifteenth century, the medical profession in Renaissance Italy was fairly well organized. Laws were framed to regulate the practice of physicians. Castiglione informs us that they needed to consult with colleagues, were forbidden to dig graves, and were fined if they spoke ill of any other physician (1947, 401). And yet, people never seemed to tire of deriding them. Will Durant refuses to see this ambivalence as an exclusively Renaissance attitude, and his statement that "In all civilized lands and times physicians have rivalled women for the distinction of being the most desirable and satirized of mankind" (1953, 531) offers a holistic view of the situation. That said, one must be very myopic to miss the irony, intended or otherwise, in Durant's use of "civilized" to describe such denigration. Medicine, for all this ambivalence, progressed in Renaissance Italy, and the study of anatomy proved to be particularly popular. The Bolognese professor Mondino de' Luzzi's *Anatomia* (1316), described by the Vesalian scholar C. D. O'Malley as "the first modern book on anatomy" (Infusino, Win and

DOI: 10.4324/9781003300762-12

O'Neill 1995, 71), retained its influence into the seventeenth century. Mondino's scarcity of practical experience was compensated for by his reliance on translations of Arabic and Greek texts on the subject which had been made between the eleventh and thirteenth centuries.[1] Durant's assessment of medical knowledge in Italy during the Renaissance is a reminder that even the best anatomists and physicians of the age were inferior in terms of possession of medical knowledge to Hippocrates, Galen, and Soranus of classical antiquity, and that the regulation of medical practice by law did little to curb the dubious operations of quacks (1953, 532). Durant eventually redeems the prestige of Renaissance Italian physicians by speaking of Fracastoro's achievement in the field of medical knowledge (1953, 536), and by his assertion that, after 1500,

> it was because of … high qualifications, devotion, and practical success, that the better class of physicians was … recognized as belonging to the untitled aristocracy of Italy. Having completely secularized their profession, they made it more respected than the clergy.
>
> (1953, 537)

Hieronymi Fracastorii, also called Girolamo Fracastoro (1483–1553), is a name that must feature even in any brief glance at the evolution of medical knowledge in the period. He was a man of literary as well as scientific interests and was the author of a poem called *Syphils, sive de morbo gallico* (1521). Fracastoro's poem is important in the history of medicine because it not only speaks about the early appearance of syphilis but also establishes "the use of the term 'syphilis' for this terrible and inexplicably transmitted disease, often referred to as 'French disease' by the people of the time and by Fracastoro himself" (Pesapane, Marcelli and Nazzaro 2015, 684). The importance of medicine, of course, had been emphasized centuries earlier by Titus Lucretius Carus, the Roman classical poet, in his philosophical poem *De rarum natura*, frequently translated into English as *The Nature of Things*:

> And since we realize that medicine affects and heals
> The mind as well as ailing flesh, this evidence reveals
> The living mind is mortal …
>
> (Stallings 2007, 87. 510–512)

Medical practitioners of the European Renaissance were not aware of germs and viruses. Classical physicians such as Hippocrates and Galen had considered a disease as a problem *within* the body caused by a lack of balance of the humors.[2] Although epidemics were common and highly infectious diseases such as the bubonic plague and syphilis caused severe devastation, physicians were unable to detect germs and viruses. Therefore, to say that the early modern understanding of contagion was inadequate will be an understatement. Nevertheless, concern for the transmission of diseases was common and was not restricted to practitioners of medicine. Early modern writers deliberated much on the subject and expressed awareness of the possibility of infection from touch, or even from the mere presence of others around an individual. Transmission could also occur, as Chalk and Floyd-Wilson tell us, "through various kinds of exchange, or if [someone were] exposed to certain ideas, practices, or environmental conditions" (2019, 1).

Speaking of contagion, no time and place could probably have matched William Shakespeare's late sixteenth-century and early seventeenth-century London for filth, disregard for health, hygiene, and safety, appalling standards of cleanliness, and nauseating odors. This inevitably led to regular deaths from infectious and, sometimes, mysterious, diseases.[3] The city was rat-infested, unclean sewage flowed in the Thames, and sexual promiscuity was rampant. It is hardly a matter of surprise, then, that the London of the time should have become home to some of the most dreadful and most infectious diseases known to mankind. Among these were plague, smallpox, syphilis, typhus, and malaria. The public theatres, in an age so obviously less concerned about hygiene than ours, were possible sites for the manifestation and spread of bodily diseases, and antitheatrical writing in early modern England repeatedly identifies the theatre with contagion. Several plays of the period, including those by Shakespeare, refer to a "physician" or a "doctor", or mention or suggest specific diseases, or use the rhetoric of disease and contagion to construct metaphors for the ill-health of individuals' bodies and minds and of the state. Doran, citing examples from plays such as *Richard II* and *Cymbeline*, points out that "in Shakespeare's England 'physician' and 'doctor' were already understood, as now, to be almost synonymous" (1916, 413).

II

This chapter focuses on Shakespeare's *Macbeth*, and critically examines not only the representations of sickness in the play but also the play's articulation of the desire for good health. The decades preceding Shakespeare's *Macbeth*—the years between 1596 and 1606—saw the publication in London of at least two major works of medical science. The earlier of these, Philip Barrough's *The Method of Physic*, moved into its third edition in 1596. The second, *A Brief Discourse of a Disease Called the Suffocation of the Mother*, was published in 1603.[4] Editors annotating Shakespeare's *King Lear* almost invariably draw upon the latter to gloss Lear's "Histerica passio down, thou climbing sorrow" (*King Lear*, II.ii.232).[5] Nick Moschovakis's discussion of dualistic readings of *Macbeth*[6]—such as dualistic receptions of the play's moral language, explications of the play's dualistic symbols, and dualistic critical perceptions of the Macbeth couple (2008, 41–42)—inspires a similar approach to the discourse on sickness in the play. Dualistic critics, seizing upon the strong moral positions adopted by the characters in the play, posit a world wrought by the oppositionality of the good and the bad, of heaven and hell, of darkness and light, of faith and treachery, of reality and appearance. The last mentioned, ironically, encourages an attack upon the very dualism that it appears to represent: characters and incidents, attitudes and speeches in the play are not always what they *seem* to be, Dualistic readings fail to address the inherent contradictions in the characters, or, for that matter, the moral and ideological ambiguities that destabilize the world of the play. Moschovakis illustrates the point by saying that irrespective of the extent to which

> the characters seem to insist on the viciousness of Duncan's murder (for instance), one need not believe everything that a given individual says — even one whom others valorize, or who attains power at the play's conclusion.
>
> (2008, 46)

Dualistic readings, their limitations notwithstanding, facilitate an initial response to the concepts of "good" and "bad" in *Macbeth* before that easy distinction is problematized and criticism begins to allow ambivalence to replace easy binaries. The witches' mention of the fog in the play's opening scene, suggesting obscurity of vision, offers an early hint of this resistance to dualistic criticism. *Macbeth* holds up dualistic criticism that recognizes binary moral distinctions, but it also interrogates such distinctions by exposing ambiguities, inherent contradictions, and uncertainties. Moschovakis, in this context, refers to an essay by Richard C. McCoy where the latter walks a tightrope and argues that *Macbeth*, though dualistic, is ethically and morally ambiguous (2008, 40).[7] Dualistic criticism stretches to the play's response to and discourse on sickness. Images of sickness pervade the play: sickness of the body, sickness of the mind, a prayer to the "spirits/That tend on mortal thoughts" (I.v.39–40) to reverse the natural "run" of the body, sickness of the state (Scotland, in this case), but these are set against appeals for restoration of health of both individuals and state and against images of healing. If the dualists cite Renaissance texts such as the *Homily against disobedience and willful rebellion* (1570) to foreground connections between "Christian morality and conservative ideology" and the sanctification of the monarch and condemnation of resistance (2008, 42), such citations may also explain the confrontationality of the morally "correct" and "conservative" desire for health and the "rebellious" images of sickness that prove to be impediments to that desire in *Macbeth*. Early in the First Part, the *Homily* attributes diseases, sickness, death, and "other miseries wherewith mankind is now infinitely and most miserably afflicted and oppressed" to man's original act of disobedience to God, and proceeds to declare:

> Thus do you see, that neither heaven nor paradise could suffer any rebellion in them, neither be places for any rebels to remain in. Thus became rebellion, as you see, both the first and the greatest, and the very foot of all other sins, and the first and principal cause, both of all worldly and bodily miseries, sorrows, diseases, sickness, and deaths, and which is infinitely worse than all these, as is said, the very cause of death and damnation eternal also.
>
> (Jewel 2019)

The application of the polemic against rebellion to the discourse on sickness and good health in *Macbeth* allows us to presume that the desire for good health invoked in the play is a desire for an ideal, paradisiacal state of being whose survival depends on its disallowance of sickness. Such an application of the *Homily's* assertion to *Macbeth* intensifies the logic that ascribes miseries, diseases, sickness, and deaths to rebellion against God by identifying sickness itself with the inglorious rebel. Rebellion becomes metaphorical as the several images of misery, sickness and disorder in *Macbeth* consistently resist the possibility of good health till, finally, the protagonist's near madness and gruesome death at the hands of his adversary, the avenging Macduff, bring in some semblance of health and order. Even that is unstable and insecure; the witches, the prime architects of sickness in the play, survive beyond the play's closure and the threat of disease and sickness looms large even as Malcolm prepares to be crowned the new king.

While the representation of disease and ill-health in *Macbeth* has invited extensive critical attention, the play's articulation of the desire for good health has been frequently ignored. *Macbeth* has the highest concentration of doctors in the Shakespearean canon: there are two doctors in this play (if one does not take into account the healing powers of the English king, Edward the Confessor, whom the English doctor refers to in IV.iii 142–146 and IV.iii 147–160), one of whom is English and the other Scottish. Tomaszewski's observation that these unnamed doctors "are both present at key moments of the play and provide spiritual and moral commentary that appears to exceed their professional boundaries" (2008, 182) points to the play's appropriation of sickness and good health to address larger ethical and moral questions.

Witches in Shakespeare's time, like the pile of the city's refuse, dwelt on the margins of the city, and human miseries and calamities were attributed to their supposedly nefarious powers. They were considered major sources of infection, both of humans and of the air, and early modern writers on witchcraft frequently associated them with contamination and disease. The tone is set early in *Macbeth*, and the short opening scene exemplifies the association of witches with an inversion of moral values and with disease when the three weird sisters exclaim, "Fair is foul, and foul is fair, / Hover through the fog and filthy air" (I.i.10–11). Lucinda Cole's statement that "witches, rats, and plague became associated in the early modern imagination as part of a developing theory of contagion" (2010, 66) foregrounds the miasmic atmosphere of the early modern period but needs to be read with our present-day understanding of witches, superstitions, misplaced beliefs, and medical science. Images of sickness pervade the text of *Macbeth*, and in I. iii, soon after the witches mysteriously disappear, Banquo asks:

> Were such things here as we do speak about,
> Or have we eaten on the insane root
> That takes the reason prisoner?

> (I.iii.81–83)

Banquo is alluding here to the qualities of hemlock which ancient wisdom recognized as poisonous and capable of causing insanity. Though Banquo and Macbeth have really encountered the witches (as also has the audience), Banquo's question seems to anticipate Macbeth's subsequent sacrifice of reason at the metaphorical altar of unbridled and destructive ambition. Late in the play, Macbeth's tyranny compels Caithness to remark on the former's inability to restrain his madness:

> Some say he's mad, others that lesser hate him
> Do call it valiant fury; but for certain
> He cannot buckle his distempered cause
> Within the belt of rule.

> (V.ii.12–16)

The "distempered cause" here is not merely Macbeth's diseased mind over which he is fast losing grip; it is also the disorganized Scotland that is beginning to rebel against him. In an archaic sense, "distemper" could mean political disorder.[8] But the disorder of the mind, too, is significant: after all, as so often in early modern writing, the disorder of the mind is a microcosmic version of larger and more wide-ranging disorders in the macrocosm. Brutus drives the point home with his comparison of the vexed human mind with a troubled kingdom:

> and the state of man,
> Like to a little kingdom, suffers then
> The nature of an insurrection.

> (*Julius Caesar*, II.i.67–69)

Macbeth's disease of the mind, therefore, translates into a telling metaphor for the ill-health of a Scotland ravaged by the supernatural utterances of witches and by treachery and killing.

When Macbeth sees a dagger, resembling his own, leading him towards Duncan's bedchamber which he must shortly enter to assassinate the king, he questions the floating dagger. But no sooner has he done this than he begins to consider the possibility that this dagger is unreal and is a construct of his oppressed mind:

> Or art thou but
> A dagger of the mind, a false creation
> Proceeding from the heat-oppressed brain?

> (II.i.37–39)

When, on becoming king, he secretly plans the killing of Banquo, all that he lets his wife in on is the anguish in his mind: "O, full of scorpions is my mind, dear wife! / Thou know'st that Banquo and his Fleance lives" (III.ii.37–38).

The ambiguities and confusion that are central to the play and its characters reflect an uncertainty about ethics and morality, and this uncertainty, or lack of knowledge, spills over into other domains. While the furious storm and other strange events on the night of Duncan's murder—"Lamentings heard i'th' air, strange screams of death, / And prophesying with accents terrible" (II.iii.55–56)— are typical of the kind of premonition of catastrophe that we find in Shakespeare,[9] the occurrences of the following morning beg the question of how such unnatural phenomena may be explained. Ross speaks to the unnamed old man, an embodiment of wisdom that has been perplexed by the strangeness of the most recent events, about divine admonition of Duncan's murder. This foregrounds the binary of good and evil spoken about earlier, but this binary is tempered by the confusion wrought by the unexplainable:

> Ha, good father,
> Thou seest the heavens, as troubled with man's act,
> Threatens his bloody stage, By th' clock 'tis day,
> And yet dark night strangles the travelling lamp.
> Is't night's predominance or the day's shame
> That darkness does the face of earth entomb
> When living light should kiss it?
>
> (II.iv.4–10)

Empson's somewhat unconvincing argument that Ross, at this point, is feeding the old man's credulity and is lying about the unnatural happenings follows from an attempt to see the play too much in terms of the real and the credible:

> Surely even a very superstitious audience would realise that he has waited to see how much Old Man will swallow; he is "spreading alarm and despondency". But this isn't meant to reduce the magic of the play to farce; the idea is that a fog of evil really has got abroad, and as likely as not did produce prodigies; the fact that Ross is telling lies about them only makes it all worse.
>
> (1986, 144)

The conversation between Ross and the old man is best seen as reflecting beliefs of Shakespeare's age and as representing, through the symbolic aberration in the cosmos, the sickening unnaturalness of the human act of murder. The cosmic manifestations give way later in the play to a disorder concentrated in Scotland as the country becomes a wounded and bleeding mass of land, assaulting the Scottish conscience with the disturbing image of a helpless "mother" (IV.iii.167) wronged and left to fend for herself. Macduff's anguished apostrophe evokes once more the binary of good and evil which dualist critics fall back on:

> Bleed, bleed, poor country!
> Great tyranny, lay thou thy basis sure,
> For goodness dare not check thee. Wear thou thy wrongs;
>
> (IV.iii.32–33)

Malcolm's professions "of every sin/ That has a name" (IV.iii.60–61), designed to test Macduff's integrity, hardly come in the way of his immediate attestation of Macduff's words:

> I think our country sinks beneath the yoke,
> It weeps, it bleeds, and each new day a gash
> Is added to her wounds
>
> (IV.iii.40–42)

The discourse on the sickness of the state is extended when Ross's vivid images of pain and death and the infected air strengthen our imagination of a grievously ailing Scotland. Ross's rhetoric of disease and contagion reconstruct around 1606 when *Macbeth* was presumably written and first performed,[10] the monstrosity of the bubonic plague:

> Alas, poor country,
> Almost afraid to know itself. It cannot
> Be called our mother, but our grave, where nothing
> But who knows nothing is once seen to smile;
> Where sighs and groans and shrieks that rend the air
> Are made, not marked; where violent sorrow seems
> A modern ecstasy. The dead man's knell
> Is there scarce asked for who, and good men's lives
> Expire before the flowers in their caps,
> Dying or ere they sicken.
>
> (IV.iii.165–74)

The plague was the most dreaded of all diseases in Shakespeare's England. No one knew at that time what caused it; it was only much later that rat fleas were discovered to be the conveyors of the plague germ. The outbreaks in 1563, 1582 and 1603 were the most devastating, and each killed more than a quarter of London's population. Symptoms would include red, inflamed, and swollen lymph nodes called buboes (hence the name bubonic). This would be accompanied by high fever, delirium, and convulsions. Sometimes, the infection could spread to the lungs and cause pneumonic plague, or to the bloodstream and cause septicemic plague. In most cases, death would be certain, horrific, and quick, usually within hours of the arrival of the symptoms.[11] The word 'plague', which occurs as many as eight times in *King Lear*, is heard only once in *Macbeth*:

> But in these cases
> We still have judgement here, that we but teach
> Bloody instructions which, being taught, return
> To plague th'inventor.
>
> (I.vii.7–10)

This is surprising, since references to the plague, probably the most dreaded of all diseases in late sixteenth and early seventeenth-century England, are not uncommon in Shakespeare.[12] This scarcity in Macbeth notwithstanding, the play is preoccupied with the idea of disease. Jaecheol Kim's recent description of the play as "A Narrative of Medicine" (2020, 69) is an exaggeration, but it pays attention to the subjects of disease, diagnosis, and the desire for healing and good health that characterize the play. Less convincing is his over-tidy division of the play into two halves:

> Shakespeare's *Macbeth*, as a diptych, is a two-fold narrative where the first half of the play is a narrative of disease and the second half is a narrative of healing.
>
> (2020, 69)

The entire texture of the play, to me, is an intricate interweaving of images of ill-health, disease, and the restoration of good health, though, admittedly, the second half underscores the narrative of healing as it brings in the two doctors — one English and the other, Scottish — and the audience hears of the miraculous healing powers of Edward the Confessor. The wounded sergeant, gasping for breath as he speaks of his "knowledge of the broil" (I.ii.6), offers the first visual spectacle of physical suffering in the play; although he has been wounded in battle and has not been afflicted with disease, he still needs medical assistance and Duncan asks his attendants to "get him surgeons" (I.ii.44). It is worth mentioning at this point that despite the several references to surgeons and surgery in Shakespeare, no surgeon appears as a character on the stage in any of his plays.[13]

Duncan and Banquo's description of the gentleness of the air at the entrance to the castle of Inverness where the martins build their nests is ironical because the king's murder has already been planned.[14] Nevertheless, the unsuspecting Duncan is charmed as he reaches the threshold of the castle and waxes eloquent about the hospitable air:

> The air
> Nimbly and sweetly recommends itself
> Unto our gentle senses.
>
> (I.vi.1–3)

Banquo very nearly echoes Duncan, adding that he has always observed the air to be "delicate" (I.vi.10)[15] where the martins build nests and breed in summer. This beginning to the scene, in emphasizing good health and positive energy, cuts almost pitifully into the tragic web that is being spun. The irony is heightened, for the audience knows what lies in wait for Duncan. The images of sickness will soon take over. Duncan and Banquo's reference to the air recalls Andrew Boorde's thoughts on the subject. Boorde, an English traveler, writer, and physician who lived between 1490 and 1549, lays out the contrasting effects of clean air and impure air in *The Boke for to Lerne a man to be wyse in the building of his howsw for the health of body* (1540). Ian Mortimer quotes the relevant passage in *The Time Traveller's Guide to Elizabethan England*:

> If the air be fresh, pure and clean about the mansion house it doth conserve the life of man, it doth comfort the brain and the powers natural, engendering and making good blood, in which consisteth the life of man. And contrarily evil and corrupt airs doth infect the blood and doth engender many corrupt humours and doth putrefy the brain and doth corrupt the heart, and therefore it doth breed many diseases and infirmities through which man's life is abbreviated or shortened.
>
> (2013, 265)

In Shakespeare's play, the "delicate" air is deceptive: it does not help conserve human life, for Duncan dies, and other deaths follow. A castle is hardly a place where the brain may be comforted. Not long after the audience sees Duncan and his train enter the castle, Macbeth, puzzled by the illusory dagger, asks it in a passage quoted above whether it is produced by a disease of the brain. Shakespeare may or may not have read Boorde, but he appears to be using the very tropes that Boorde does — for Boorde speaks, as we have seen, of clean air conserving human life and comforting the brain — only to foreground the deceptive quality of the air that greets Duncan and Banquo. This is firmly in keeping with the theme of deceit and treachery and the play: things are not what they appear to be, and what seems fair may be foul. Contrary to the suggestions offered by the "delicate" air, the human characters and Scotland in *Macbeth* experience the suffering that Boorde says is caused by "evil and corrupt airs".

The figurative uses of disease and healing make *Macbeth* a remarkable play: equally remarkable is the way it blends its essentially political discourse with its medical discourse.[16] The suggestions and images of sickness and good health grow denser as the play moves through Act IV into Act V. The conversation between Malcom and Macduff in IV.iii compresses the sickness-healing discourse. Malcolm's initial suspicion that Macduff might be Malcolm's agent is indicative of how Shakespeare conflates the political issues at stake in the play with the subject of disease and puts the latter to figurative use. The diseased air that envelops Scotland under Macbeth's rule has created this air of suspicion owing to which Malcolm, fearing for his safety, tells Macduff with disturbing candidness:

> This tyrant, whose sole name blisters our tongues,
> Was once thought honest. You have loved him well.
> He hath not touched you yet. I am young, but something
> You may discern of him through me:
>
> (IV.iii.12–15)

Such suspicion, simultaneously a disease of the mind and a defense against what might be a nefarious political strategy, is hardly surprising since Macbeth's despicable treachery has reduced Scotland to a veritable hell, a thoroughly disquieting site of agony and anguish where

> Each new morn
> New widows howl, new orphans cry, new sorrows
> Strike heaven in the face that it resounds
> As if it felt with Scotland and yelled out
> Like syllable of dolour.
>
> (IV.iii.4–8)

The scene compresses the sickness-healing discourse in two ways. First, Shakespeare allows the description of a grievously ailing Scotland and Malcolm's suspicion of Macduff to be tempered by Malcolm's eventual dismissal of "the black scruples" (IV.iii.117) that had made him wary of Macduff. Figurative sickness or disease gives way to figurative healing, and Malcolm conveys news that may easily be described as political: Old Siward,[17] "with ten thousand warlike men" (IV.iii.135) is on his way to Scotland to launch an assault on Macbeth. Malcolm and Macduff will join forces with him so that the "warranted quarrel" (IV.iii.138) may reintroduce good times in Scotland. The suggestions of figurative healing thrown up here are extended by the English doctor's reassuring words about King Edward's powers of healing disease by touch. The disease that the English doctor speaks about is scrofula, also called the "King's Evil". We are told that James I had mixed thoughts about healing by touch and did not want to admit the idea of a miracle that Malcolm mentions while explaining the "malady" (IV.iii.143) which Edward cures: "A most miraculous work in this good King" (IV.iii.148).[18] Malcolm's description of the symptoms and bodily manifestations of the disease would have reminded Shakespeare's earliest audiences of the series of plagues they had lived through:

> but strangely visited people,
> All swoll'n and ulcerous, pitiful to the eye,
> The mere despair of surgery
>
> (IV.iii.151–53)

In *Macbeth*, we hardly have diseases of the body if we leave aside the wounds of the sergeant in I.ii. But even they "smack of honour" (I.ii.44) rather than of disease. The images of diseases of the mind, on the other hand, are many and vivid. These are inextricably connected with the ill-health of the state, and IV.iii brings together images of suffering body and suffering state. Ross arrives shortly and paints a grim picture of Scotland which echoes Macduff's description of Scotland in IV.iii.4–8 quoted above:

> Alas, poor country,
> Almost afraid to know itself. It cannot
> Be called our mother, but our grave, where nothing
> But who knows nothing is once seen to smile;

> Where sighs and groans and shrieks that rend the air
> Are made, not marked; where violent sorrow seems
> A modern ecstasy. The dead man's knell
> Is there scarce asked for who, and good men's lives
> Expire before the flowers in their caps,
> Dying or ere they sicken.
>
> (IV.iii.165–74)

This ailing state seems as much the "despair of surgery" as the people afflicted with scrofula that Malcolm describes. There is, however, the English king's healing, miraculous touch that cures his subjects: in Scotland, by contrast, Macbeth has to ask the Scottish doctor to find a remedy for the state's sickness:

> If thou couldst, doctor, cast
> The water of my land, find her disease,
> And purge it to a sound and pristine health,
> I would applaud thee to the very echo,
> That should applaud again.
>
> (V.iii.52–56)

This invites us back to the question of binaries in the play: the good English king, with his powers of healing the sick, is set against the bad Scottish king who has brought the state to this miserable pass and now, ironically, appeals to the doctor for help. The doctor, however, cures bodily ailments. He is a physician, as physicians were understood in Shakespeare's England. It is hardly a surprise, then, that he has no cure, no medicine, no drugs, to recover Lady Macbeth from her tormented sleepwalking. Her disease, like Macbeth's, is of the mind; only, she surrenders to it more easily, and with hardly a question. Pettigrew, writing of medical practices in Shakespeare's age, speaks of mental conditions such as those of the Macbeths as proceeding from a guilt-ridden conscience:

> Mental anguish could also be caused by moral impairment when the afflicted confronted the guilt arising from his or her sins, and practitioners were employed to carefully distinguish between physical melancholy and spiritual affliction.
>
> (2016 Vol. I, 814)

Lady Macbeth's crime has been against nature itself, and her disease transcends earthly, physical maladies to whose cure the doctor's expertise is limited. "Unnatural deeds/ Do breed unnatural troubles" (V.i.68–69), and so, given the unnaturalness of the ailment, the doctor recommends divine intervention: "More needs she the divine than the physician" (V.i.71). B. H. Traister argues along the same lines:

> Macbeth desires a chemical cure for his wife and purgatives for his country, neither of which the doctor can supply. Present in part to testify to the ill

health of Macbeth's wife and country, the doctor also testifies to the limits of his profession and its inability to deal with moral illness.

(46)

The Scottish doctor and his English counterpart merely articulate the limits of their profession. The former, having no chemical cure for Lady Macbeth's *moral* disease, tells the Gentlewoman: "This disease is beyond my practice" (V.i.56). The English doctor, on the other hand, confesses that it requires King Edward's heavenly touch to cure the disease of the English since the best attempts of physicians have failed:

> Their malady convinces
> The great assay of art, but at his touch,
> Such sanctity hath Heaven given his hand,
> They presently amend.

(IV.iii.143–46)

Shakespeare is creating here a triangle of three categories of diseases: bodily diseases, as those of King Edward's English subjects; diseases of the mind caused by immoral conduct, as those pushing Macbeth and his wife to the brink of life itself; and diseases of the state, such as those holding sway over Scotland. While the English king is foregrounded as a healer of the sick, Macbeth is the source of a dreadful contagion; indeed, he is the disease itself that he so ironically asks the Scottish doctor to "find".[19]

III

The discourse on disease and healing in *Macbeth* would have been very relevant in the early seventeenth century. Not only was England still recovering from a series of devastating plagues, but the general state of hygiene too was also poor. The Elizabethans and Jacobeans did not conceptualize and understand contagion the way we do today. They did not understand germs and were unaware of what precisely had caused deadly diseases such as the bubonic plague and syphilis. This ignorance notwithstanding, people were fully aware of the possibility of transmission of diseases. There was the prevailing notion that a person could be infected if he were in the presence of others or, particularly, if he were exposed to a large gathering of people or to certain kinds of environment.[20] The plague of 1603, which "broke out during April" (Chambers Vol. IV 1923, 349) took a heavy toll. Chambers speculates that stage performances of plays, restrained in March on account of Elizabeth's illness, may not have resumed. The Elizabethan pamphleteer Thomas Dekker's *The Wonderful Yeare*, published that year, gives a very horrifying account of the despair wrought by the plague, Addressing the sufferers apostrophically, Dekker writes:

> you desolate hand-wringing widowes, that beate your bosomes ouer your
> departing husbands: you wofully distracted mothers that with disheueld

haire falne into swounds, whilst you lye kissing the insensible cold lips of your breathlesse Infants: you out-cast and downe-troden Orphanes, that shall many a yeare hence remember more freshlly to mourne, when your mourning garments shall looke olde and be for gotten.

(1603, pages unnumbered)

And then, in terms that anticipate Macduff and Ross's descriptions of Scotland (*Macbeth*, IV.iii) quoted above, Dekker graphically chronicles the despair:

In euery house griefe striking vp an Allarum: Seruants crying out for maisters: wiues for husbands, parents for children, children for their mothers: here he should haue met some frantickly running to knock vp Sextons; there, others fearlfully sweating with Coffins, to steale forth dead bodies, least the fatall hand-writing of death should seale vp their doores. And to make this dismall consort more full, round about him Bells healuily folling in one place, and ringing out in another: The dreadlfulnesse of such an houre, is in vtterable: let vs goe further.

Antitheatrical writing in early modern England repeatedly identifies the theatre with contagion. The public theatres, in an age less concerned about hygiene than ours, were possible sites for the manifestation and spread of bodily diseases. Authors such as Stephen Gosson, William Prynne, and William Rankins expressed antitheatrical prejudices, seeing performance on the early modern stage, and the player's art, as capable of viciously contaminating the audience by assaulting their senses and bodies alike. Stephen Gosson's *The School of Abuse, containing a pleasant invective against Poets, Pipers, Plaiers, Jesters and such like Caterpillars of the Commonwealth* (1579) is an antitheatrical pamphlet that developed some extremely compelling arguments against plays, players, and the theatre, including one that posited the Devil as the essential inspiration behind plays. There were strong reactions to Gosson's arguments, and Thomas Lodge refuted them in a counterargument titled *Honest Excuses* (1579). In 1580, having read Lodge, Gosson developed a longer and even more violent invective against the theatre called *Plays Confuted in Five Actions* (1582) where he defended his own earlier indulgence in playwriting and, ironically, imitated the five-act structure of a play. The Puritan attack on the theatre rested largely on their displeasure over the dramatic appropriation of scriptural themes, but their resentment was hardly less even when the theatre was secular. They argued that tragedies provided corrupting examples of murders, treacheries, and other gross crimes while comedies celebrated wantonness. Besides, they strongly disapproved of the constant presence of prostitutes in the public theatres and were obsessed with the connections they discerned between the public stage and sexual immorality.[21]

Renaissance theatre, as a means of entertainment, was popular and powerful. Equally powerful were the Puritan attacks upon the theatre. It was, for the most part, an exciting, eventful, and even contest, until the theatres were closed down in 1642. Interestingly, those who advocated the cause of the theatre as well as those who attacked it recognized the great hold that theatre had over audiences. For the former, this hold was positive, and for the latter, contaminating. For the former, the influence of the theatre was benevolent; for the latter, its influence was malevolent. Leah Marcus argues that the misgivings against the theatre were grounded "in a vitalist materialist belief in the ability of elements of a community to influence other elements through the power of emotional contagion" (2017, 184), and that the theatrical audience was "a particularly well-defined and vulnerable group" exposed to morally contaminating acts within the enclosed and, therefore, secret space of the public playhouse. Like Gosson, William Prynne also structured his antitheatrical work *Histrio-Mastix* (1633) in the form of a play, with Acts and scenes, and made it bear the subtitle *the Players Scourge, or, Actors Tragaedie.* Prynne's attack on the theatre was unequivocally violent and Marcus reminds us that he was tried for sedition when he "indirectly cast aspersions on Queen Henrietta Maria (who took speaking parts in pastoral drama performed at Court) by calling women actors 'notorious whores'" (2017, 186). Other well-known antitheatricalists were Anthony Munday, William Rankins, John Rainolds and Philip Stubbs. Munday wrote *A second and third blast of retrait from plaies and Theaters* (1580), and both he and Rankins, author of *Mirrour of Monsters: Wherein is plainely described the manifold vices, & spotted enormities, that are caused by the infectious sight of Playes* (1587) where he described two of London's public playhouses as the Chapel of Adultery, proceeded to write plays themselves.[22] Rankins writes that players infect with poison those that visit the playhouses which, for him, resonate with the deadly virulence of the plague. John Rainolds goes beyond suggestions of resonance in his *Th'overthrow of Stage-Playes* (1599), and argues, convincingly for his age, that, given the transformative power of imitation, acting or playing a diseased person may lead to contracting infectious diseases in real life.[23] Philip Stubbes, in *Anatomie of Abuses* (1583), criticizes elements of popular Elizabethan culture through an imagined dialogue between Philoponus, a wise and educated traveller, and Spudeus, a country bumpkin. Stubbes attributes the invention of the theatre to the Devil, and, like his contemporary antitheatricalists, sees the stage as a site for corruption.

The images of healing in *Macbeth* that counterpoise those of sickness and disease represent the play's, and, more significantly, the period's articulation of the desire for good health. The essential vitality of this articulation in *Macbeth* questions and destabilizes the prejudices expressed by Shakespeare's antitheatrical peers who see performance on the early modern stage, the player's art, and theatre itself, as capable of vicious contamination of body and mind. It is possible that the desire for health and wellness in *Macbeth* is Shakespeare's deliberate and ingeniously devised ploy to repudiate misgivings against the theatre. *Macbeth* abounds in images of healing: Duncan's command that the wounded sergeant be treated by surgeons; the Scottish doctor's close observation of Lady Macbeth's sleepwalking and his brief prescription for her well-being; Macbeth's tormented pleas to that same doctor to cure both his wife and the land that he rules; Malcolm and the English doctor's report of the miraculous healing conducted by King Edward; and the final cleansing of Scotland through

Macbeth's death in single combat with Macduff. These pave the way for the
"newer comfort" (V.xi.19) that Macduff brings when he emerges on the stage
with Macbeth's severed head. The head, cut off from his body, becomes, in a
sense, a gruesome and distorted image of surgery. It is, after all, "The'usurp-
er's cursèd head" (V.xi.21), the disease, and its severing with Macduff's sword
is akin to the removal of an infectious sore with a surgeon's knife. Macduff
becomes the metaphorical surgeon, and yet his beheading of Macbeth and dis-
playing of his head bear a fundamental resemblance to the "physical" elements
of a surgical act. Macduff's announcement that "The time is free" reverberates
in the playhouse with all the delight and contentment of a cured body, and a
cured state, that is now "free" of disease. For the players, the audience, and,
indeed, for everyone in England in 1606, this was an extremely significant,
though ironical, announcement. Chambers, quoting the plague records for that
year, gives depressing figures of death:

> The deaths reached 33 on 10 July and 50 on 17 July, rose to a maximum of
> 141 on 2 Oct., and remained, but for one or two weeks, above 40 to 4 Dec.
> and above 30 to the end of the year. The total, for 121 parishes, was 2,124.
> (Vol. IV 1923, 350)

As the stage rhetoric of well-being counters the dreadful reality and tempers it
within the make-believe world of the theatre, it temporarily "cures" all who are
still in the enclosed space of the playhouse by generating the unreal but therapeutic experience of a "free" time. The rhetoric of the desire for health and wellness
in *Macbeth* could be as contagious as the rhetoric of sickness that pervades the
play. It is precisely with this rhetoric that *Macbeth* replies back to antitheatrical
misgivings against the theatre, particularly to suspicions that foul and nefarious business might have "infected" the vulnerable audiences *inside* the public
playhouses.[24]

The dynamics of sickness and health in *Macbeth* are complex and are produced by the reciprocity of play and audience. Meanings and implications are
always fluid, never stable; and Shakespeare's *Macbeth* has held a rich variety
of meanings and implications for generations of audiences and readers across
over four centuries. Critical approaches have evolved, the study of literature
itself has required legitimization, and the influx of a host of literary and cultural theories has necessitated fresh, alternative readings of literary texts. The
material conditions that surrounded the production of *Macbeth* in 1606—James's
kingship, the question of the union of England and Scotland, popular discourses
on witches and witchcraft, the early modern understanding of the masculine
and the feminine, the Gunpowder Plot, theories of equivocation, Father Henry
Garnet's trial, and, of course, the devastation caused by the plague—were vastly
different from the socio-cultural and socio-political contexts within which the
play is performed and read today. The complex dynamics of sickness and health
in *Macbeth* in plague-ridden early seventeenth-century England, though lost in
large measure in modern-day performances and acts of reading, retains the

potential to be called up once more in the early twenty-first century by a world bruised and reeling under multiple waves of the Covid-19 pandemic. The reciprocity of play and audience is an enduring quality of live theatre, and it may require the experience of being in the audience for a production of *Macbeth* more than the solitary experience of reading to evoke, recognize and make sense of the play's discourses on sickness and health that relate to pressing early twenty-first century concerns.

Notes

1 This has been pointed out by Infusino, Win and O'Neill who also touch on the presence of the observations of older classical and Islamic researchers such as Galen and Avicenna in Mondino's work. Further, they mention the influence of the Salernitan school of anatomy on the treatise. See "Mondino's Book and the Human Body," 71–72.

2 Chalk and Floyd Wilson begin their "Introduction" by mentioning the absence of germ theory among the early moderns. For a short but helpful account of the theory of the humours, see Doran (1916, 422). Doran briefly illustrates Shakespeare's use of the theory with examples from *Love's Labour's Lost, 1 Henry IV, Troilus and Cressida, Much Ado about Nothing, Romeo and Juliet, King John* and *Richard II*.

3 Mortimer speaks of the generally abysmal state of hygiene in Elizabethan England. He speaks of vulnerability to illness, of "Nauseating smells and sights", and of the daily deaths "from unknown ailments", and states that people were tolerant of "Noisome smells and noxious fumes". See Mortimer, *The Time Traveller's Guide to Elizabethan England*, 264 and 266.

4 Jorden notes that the disease known in England as "the Mother" or "the Suffocation of the Mother" is also known by other names, among which are *Passio Hysterica, Suffocatio*, and *Praefocatio*, and asserts the "the perturbations of the mind are oftentimes to blame both for this and many other diseases. For seeing we are not masters of our own affections, we are like battered cities without walls, or ships tossed in the sea, exposed to all manner of assaults and dangers, even to the overthrow of our own bodies". For an extract from Jorden's work, see Carroll, *Macbeth: Texts and Contexts*, 354–357.

5 All quotations from Shakespeare are from *William Shakespeare: The Complete Works (Compact Edition)*, edited by Stanley Wells et al. (1988).

6 Moschovakis, while acknowledging uncertainties "over whether or not *Macbeth* upholds a *dualistic* view of morality: one which measures human actions and objectives by their worth relative to polar opposites of 'good' and 'bad'", proceeds to trace what he sees as an evolution, in critical reception, from the dualistic *Macbeth* toward its opposite, which he calls the "problematic" *Macbeth*. See Moschovakis, "Introduction: Dualistic Macbeth? Problematic Macbeth?" in *Macbeth: New Critical Essays*, edited by Nick Moschovakis, 1–72.

7 Moschovakis refers to McCoy's argument that one need not think in terms of the moral absolutes of good and evil while responding critically to *Macbeth*. He says that McCoy "reasserts the case for a *Macbeth* that is *relatively* dualistic but leaves some room for ethical and ideological 'ambiguity'". See McCoy, Richard C. "'The Grace of Grace' and Double-Talk in *Macbeth*." *Shakespeare Survey* 57 (2004): 27–37.

8 Doran informs us that in Shakespeare "'Distemper' and 'distemperature'alike are used for disease or indisposition in general". See Doran (1916, 434).

9 See, for example, *Julius Caesar* for Casca's mention of strange occurrences (I.iii.9–13, 15–32), Calpurnia's recounting of a catalogue of "most horrid sights" to Caesar (II.ii.13–26), and Caesar's description of Calpurnia's dream to Decius Brutus (II.ii.76–80). All these strange "events" immediately precede Caesar's assassination in the play.

10 For a detailed and illumination discussion on the date of Shakespeare's composition of *Macbeth*, see Leeds Barroll, *Politics, Plague and Shakespeare's Theatre: The Stuart Years*, 133–153. Baroll reaches the conclusion that "the dating of Macbeth defies final resolution and the methodologies commonly used for the task are seriously flawed, subject to the schematics of a narrative urging the consistent and definable development of Shakespeare as a playwright and the steadiness of his dramatic production. But these developmental assumptions or expectations are challenged by many historical texts, particularly those containing plague figures" (151).

11 For an account of some of the worst diseases in Shakespeare's London, see http://www.shakespeare-online.com/biography/londondisease.html.

12 The word "plague" occurs 13 times in *1 Henry IV*, 8 times in *King Lear*, 12 times in *Timon of Athens*, and 10 times in *Troilus and Cressida*, besides occurring less frequently in some of the other plays in the canon. Please visit the online Shakespeare concordance at https://www.opensourceshakespeare.org/concordance/findform.php.

13 Doran draws our attention to this strange fact at the beginning of his elaborate discussion on the figure of the surgeon in Shakespeare's England. See Doran (1916, 422–428).

14 Abhijit Sen observes that Banquo and Duncan are "mistaken" in their "assessment because the castle has now become the hatchingground of treachery". See Sen (2009, 34).

15 Nicholas Brooke glosses "delicate" as "delightful, charming (with connotations of sensuous relaxation) and says that "This sense is still common in USA". See Brooke (1990, 116).

16 Jaecheol Kim offers an interesting perspective by claiming that "*Macbeth* can be situated as a contribution to Jacobean *immunity* politics because Shakespeare conflates political and medical discourses" in the play and goes on to explain that "Immunity is a concept that weds biopolitics with political theology". See Kim (2020, 69).

17 Brooke reminds us that "Old Seyward" was one of the sons of the Earl of Northumberland, "and a strong supporter of Edward the Confessor". See Brooke (1990, 188).

18 Brooke notes that James himself attempted to cure by touch on some occasions but did so very reluctantly. Brooke also informs us that James "expressly rejected the suggestion of miracle, which Shakespeare retained" in Malcom's words IV.iii.148. See Brooke (1990, 72).

19 See Pettigrew, *Shakespeare and the Practice of Physic*, 83. For Pettigrew Macbeth metamorphoses into "a synecdoche for Scotland itself, a kingdom of incurable disease", a patient.

20 See Chalk and Floyd-Wilson (2019, 1). See also Barroll (1991, 70–116) for a very exhaustive account of, among other things, the different variations of plague, their causes, the relationship between infectious diseases and the theatre, and the measures adopted by the London authorities to combat the menace of pestilence.

21 E. K. Chambers discusses Gosson's antitheatrical writing and offers an analysis of the Puritan resentment against the theatre and the Humanist "apologies" which emerged in response to Puritan attacks. These apologies, Chambers notes, were not very adequately convincing replies to the literary war launched on the theatre through Puritan antitheatrical writing. See Chambers (1923, Vol. I, 254–268).

22 Leah Marcus, calling antitheatricality "a phenomenon inextricably linked to theatricality itself", draws attention to the fact that "the theater and the antitheatricalists of the era are often hard to distinguish: Many of those who joined the pamphlet campaign against plays were themselves associated with the theater – or associated themselves with it through the very writings that attempted to suppress it". See Marcus (2017, 185–186).

23 Chalk and Floyd-Wilson interpret one major strand of antitheatrical reasoning when they write that the theatre's "histrionic 'evils' might be spread by the playgoers

themselves, as they become unwitting vectors of the contagion through imitation."
See Chalk and Floyd-Wilson (2019, 2–3).
24 Leah Marcus refers to the belief about the vulnerability of audiences in the enclosed
space of the public playhouses. Taking note of what she calls "a vitalist materialist
belief in the ability of elements of a community to influence other elements through
the power of emotional contagion", Marcus says that audiences in the public playhouses were more "captive to the performance than had been the case with the earlier
open, street-based forms of theater". See Marcus (2017, 184).

References

Barroll, Leeds. 1991. *Politics, Plague, and Shakespeare's Theatre: The Stuart Years*. Ithaca. Cor-
nell University Press.
Brooke, Nicholas, ed. 1990. *The Tragedy of Macbeth*. Oxford: Oxford University Press.
Carroll, William C., ed. 1999. *Macbeth: Texts and Contexts*. Boston: Bedford.
Castiglioni, Arturo. 1947. *A History of Medicine*. Translated by Edward Bell Krumbhaar.
New York: Alfred A. Knopf.
Chalk, Darryl and Mary Floyd-Wilson, eds. 2019. *Contagion and the Shakespearean Stage*.
Palgrave Studies in Literature, Science and Medicine. Gewerbestrasse: Palgrave Mac-
millan. Accessed May 18, 2021. https://doi.org/10.1007/978-3-030-14428-9_1.
Chambers, E. K. 1923. *The Elizabethan Stage*, Volumes I-IV. Oxford: Clarendon Press.
Cole, Lucinda. 2010. "Of Mice and Moisture: Rats, Witches, Miasma, and Early Modern
Theories of Contagion." *Journal for Early Modern Cultural Studies* 10, no. 2 (January)Mort:
65–84.
Dekker, Thomas. 1603. *The vvonderfull yeare. 1603 Wherein Is Shewed the Picture of London,
Lying Sicke of the Plague. At the Ende of All (Like a Mery Epilogue to a Dull Play) Certaine Tales
Are Cut Out in Sundry Fashions, of Purpose to Shorten the Liues of Long Winters Nights, that Lye
Watching in the Darke for vs*. Pages unnumbered. Accessed February 16, 2022. https://
quod.lib.umich.edu/e/eebo/A20094.0001.001/1:5?rgn=div1;view=fulltext.
Doran, Alban H. G, 1916. "Medicine". In *Shakespeare's England: An Account of the Life and
Manners of His Age*, edited by Walter Raleigh, Sidney Lee and Charles Talbut Onions,
Volume I, 413–443. Oxford: Clarendon Press.
Durant, Will. 1953. *The Renaissance: A History of Civilization in Italy from 1304–1576 A.D.*
New York: Simon and Schuster.
Empson, William.1986. *Essays on Shakespeare*. Edited by David B. Pirie. Cambridge: Cam-
bridge University Press.
Infusino, Mark H., Dorothy Win and Ynez V. O'Neill. 1995. "Mondino's Book and the
Human Body." *Vesalius* 1, no. 2: 71–76.
Jewel, John. 2019. *An Homily against Disobedience and Willful Rebellion (1571)*. Last Modified Jan-
uary 11, 2019. https://internetshakespeare.uvic.ca/doc/Homilies_2-21_M/section/
The%20First%20Part/index.html.
Kim, Jaecheol. 2020. "'Let's Make Us Medicines of Our Great Revenge'': Medicine and
Sovereignty in *Macbeth*." *The CEA Critic* 82, no. 1 (March): 69–84.
Marcus, Leah S. 2017. "Antitheatricality: The Theatre as Scourge". In *A New Compan-
ion to Renaissance Drama*, edited by Arthur F. Kinney and Thomas Warren Hopper,
182–192. Oxford: Wiley Blackwell.
Mortimer, Ian. 2013. *The Time Traveller's Guide to Elizabethan England*. London: Vintage.
Moschovakis, Nick, ed. 2008. "Introduction: Dualistic *Macbeth*? Problematic *Macbeth*?".
In *Macbeth: New Critical Essays*, edited by Nick Moschovakis, 1–72. New York: Routledge.

Pesapane, Filippo, Stefano Marcelli and Gianluca Nazzaro. 2015. "Hieronymi Fracastorii: the Italian scientist who described the 'French disease.'" *Anais Brasileiros de Dermatologia* 90, no. 5 (September to October): 684–686.

Pettigrew, Todd H. J. 2007. *Shakespeare and the Practice of Physic: Medical Narratives on the Early Modern English Stage*. Newark: University of Delaware Press.

———. 2016. "Medical Practices." In *The Cambridge Guide to the Worlds of Shakespeare: Shakespeare's World, 1500–1660*, Volume I, edited by Bruce R. Smith, 811–815. New York: Cambridge University Press.

Sen, Abhijit, ed. 2009. *Macbeth*. Delhi: Pearson.

Stallings, A. E., trans. 2007. *The Nature of Things*. London: Penguin Books.

Tomaszewski, Lisa A. 2008. "'Throw Physic to the Dogs!' Moral Physicians and Medical Malpractice in *Macbeth*". In *Macbeth: New Critical Essays*, edited by Nick Moschovakis, 182–191. New York: Routledge.

Traister, Barbara Howard. 2004. "'Note Her a Little Farther': Doctors and Healers in the Drama of Shakespeare." In *Disease, Diagnosis, and Cure on the Early Modern Stage*, edited by Stephanie Moss and Kaara L. Peterson, 43–52. New York: Routledge.

Wells, Stanley, Gary Taylor, John Jowett, and William Montgomery, ed. 1988. *William Shakespeare: The Complete Works (Compact Edition)*. Oxford: Clarendon Press.

11 Their Mother's Gardens

Epidemic, Healing, and Motherhood in *Year of Wonders* and *Hamnet*

Chandrima Das

Periods of great historical and political upheavals like wars, revolutions, and, epidemics often put women in a double bind. They are expected to both conform to their traditional societal roles as caregivers, and simultaneously break away from those roles and become providers and wage-earners in families ravaged by death and diseases. In the context of the present times, multiple recent studies undertaken by sociologists have noted the alarming rise in the number of cases of domestic violence against women in India during the COVID-19 Pandemic and the subsequent economic and social turmoil (Maji, Bansod, and Singh 2020; Krishnakumar and Verma 2021).[1] Women, who have been victimized and batteredalmost as a matter of routine during times like these, have also historically fulfilled another function—that of healers, healthcare workers, and nurturers. This chapter will look closely into two historical novels set in the sixteenth- and seventeenth-century England which intertwine the themes of disease, bereavement, and healing, and foreground the role of women as repositories of traditional knowledge passed from one generation to the next. Geraldine Brooks' *Year of Wonders* (2001) and Maggie O'Farrell's *Hamnet* (2020), set some 60 years apart in the late sixteenth and middle seventeenth centuries, explore these themes and foreground the contradictions inherent in the society's conceptualization of what the role of a woman should be in times of dis-ease. The idea of esoteric knowledge being passed on from one woman to another has been explored in texts as diverse in their intended readership, and genre as Sally Gardner's historical fantasy for young adult readers *I, Coriander* (2005), Terry Pratchett and Neil Gaiman's fantasy novel *Good Omens* (1990), and Hansda Sowvendra Shekhar's *The Mysterious Ailment of Rupi Baskey* (2014). *Year of Wonders* and *Hamnet* also envisage an unbroken tradition of knowledge of traditional medicines and healing within an exclusively female domain, it is, as it were, a matrilineal tradition women share and pass on to the next generation. These two texts seek to re-inscribe the function of women from that of victims of diseases and domestic and/or societal abuse, to the role of the healer of the same diseased bodies, and the dis-eased society. The knowledge that enables them to do so is not the institution-imparted knowledge that was the sole preserve of men in the centuries under consideration, this stream of knowledge flows unbroken from woman to woman from one generation to the next.

DOI: 10.4324/9781003300762-13

The concept of 'Healing"—a word derived from the Anglo-Saxon term "haeling", encompasses more than the idea of merely treating or, even curing a disease. Healing has the added connotation of making someone—or something—whole again, to restore the ailing body and mind to full health. The two novels that we are going to look into in this chapter, embrace this very idea of healing as making someone/something wholesome again. The healers and the wise women we will meet in the course of these narratives, not only survive the bubonic plague and endure the agonies of losing their children to the dreaded disease, but also mend and nurture new relationships and point toward a future that holds the promise of a more wholesome life. Accusations of witchcraft followed closely on the heels of such powers and knowledge, and surely enough, it is again the women learned in their traditional arts who are the victims.

In their classic work *Witches, Midwives and Nurses: A History of Women Healers* (2010, originally published in 1973), Barbara Ehrenreich and Deirdre English attempt to formulate a concise answer to the fundamental questions about the identity and "crime" of women designated as witches. They go on to assert that

> Undoubtedly, over the centuries of witch-hunting, the charge of "witch-craft" came to cover a multitude of sins ranging from political subversion and religious heresy to lewdness and blasphemy. But three central accusations emerge repeatedly in the history of witchcraft throughout Northern Europe: First, witches are accused of every conceivable sexual crime against men. Quite simply, they are "accused" of female sexuality. Second, they are accused of being organized. Third, they are accused of having magical powers affecting health—of harming, but also of healing. They are often charged specifically with possessing medical and obstetrical skills.
>
> (Ehrenreich and Deirdre 1973, 39)

It is within these three parameters elaborated above—the sexual agency and liberty exercised by the putative "witches"; their organized system of passing on knowledge and power; and their healing practices that we will read the two novels in this chapter. It is hoped that in these uncertain times when women particularly are subjected to abuse and violence in the middle of a worldwide saga of disease and woe, the narratives of these remarkable—albeit fictional—women's struggle to move away from illness and health, both in the bodies of those they love, and the body of the society that they inhabit, might resonate with the lived experience of many women, almost 400 years after the action of the novels take place.

I

Geraldine Brooks' *Year of Wonders* is set in the years 1665–1666, the year of the Great Plague of London. The Bills of mortality published by the various London parishes during the Plague record a total number of 68,596 deaths, the number constitutes approximately 15 per cent of the total population of the metropolis in 1665–1666 (Shannon and Cromley 2015, 254). The plague mostly ravaged the city and its outlying parishes, hence giving the phenomenon the name, it has ever since been known by. Brooks, however, presents us with the remarkable story of a small village named Eyam in Derbyshire—still known as the "Plague Village" in the county—the inhabitants of which imposed upon themselves extremely stringent quarantining norms so that the spread of the disease could be checked. It is around this remarkable tale of resilience and prudence of a group of villagers that Brooks weaves a fascinating narrative of disease, healing, and motherhood with three women at its center.

Anna Firth, the first-person narrator and the protagonist of the novel, is a young widow with two sons. Anna works as a maid-servant at the local rectory inhabited by Reverend Michael Mompellion and his young childless wife Elinor. At the edge of the village, in a "lonely dwelling" at the side of the hill, is the cottage of the Gowdies, Anys, and Mem. The evidently poor niece and aunt live in a cottage "so ill-built that the thatch sat rakishly atop the whole like a cap pulled crooked across a brow" (2001, 50). The Gowdies however, are rich in a different way, they have their herbal garden and are practiced in the art of healing and midwifery. Anys, who is not much older than Anna, tells the latter about the garden adjacent to their dwelling:

> We do not even know the name of the wise woman who first laid out these beds, but the garden thrived here long before we came to tend it, and it will go on long after we depart. My aunt and I are just the latest in a long line of women who have been charged with its care.
>
> (2001, 51)

Like Anys, Elinor Mompellion is also partially learned in the herbal lore of medicinal plants, unlike Anys however, her learning has come from books that she had had access to as a young and wealthy noblewoman. The three women between themselves create an interesting triad. Since the local landlords, the Bradfords are mostly absent and are not even remotely interested in the well-being of the villagers, it is the rectory that becomes the center of the communal life of the village. With the rectory at the center, Elinor as its mistress, and the Gowdies' cottage at the very edge of the village, Anna becomes a bridge between the two. In terms of sexual agency and in relation to the question of maternity, the three women offer three completely different possibilities. Anna had been married at 15, and after giving birth to two sons in quick succession has been widowed at the age of 18. Elinor Mompellion's seduction by a rakish neighbor had led to a pregnancy that Elinor herself had terminated in a way that made it impossible for her to bear children in the future. Her husband, though apparently in love with his wife and in full possession of the facts of her previous misfortune, refuses to consummate their marriage as a form of a protracted punishment for her youthful dalliance. Anys, on the other hand, has no desire to marry and begin a family of her own. As she tells Anna, she has no intention of becoming "any man's chattel" (2001, 54). She pays heed to her physical desires and fulfills them without any notion of further commitment.

Another thread that connects these three women who occupy very different places within the social and economic hierarchy of the village is that all three of them grew up without the care and protection of their biological mothers. Anna's mother died in childbirth, and the four-year-old girl had witnessed the barber-surgeon at work whose intervention had caused excruciating pain to the mother and resulted in a still-birth of a mutilated baby, an image that haunts her even in her adult life. Her stepmother Aphra—to whom we will return in the course of this chapter—had treated her more as a liability than a daughter. Anys came to reside with her aunt as a young orphan and was brought up by Mem Gowdie, and together they comprised a unit of what would have been called the "wise women" of the village. Elinor lost her mother at a young age and rues the lack of maternal restraint that might have saved her from the misfortune of seduction and eventual abandonment.

With the outbreak of the bubonic plague in the village and the self-imposed isolation planned by Michael Mompellion, the little village becomes a completely insular, closed society. Death, grief, and privation eventually led to accusations of witchcraft against Mem and Anys.

While collecting data for his sample study on witch-persecution in Tudor and Stuart England- focusing on the county of Essex—Alan Macfarlane in his 1970 classic work *Witchcraft in Tudor and Stuart England: A Regional and Comparative Study*, notes an important socio-economic factor underlying the sudden increase in the cases of witch-hunting during the period. He goes on to elaborate upon the said factor

> Witchcraft prosecutions in Essex centred on the relationship between middling to rich villagers and their slightly less prosperous and older neighbours. These neighbours were usually women, and often widows. It seems, therefore…two other problems were of particular importance in witchcraft accusations: the first was that of poverty, the second was that of the old.
>
> (Macfarlane 1970, 205)

Mem Gowdie is, of course, both old and poor and is an easy scapegoat for such accusations considering her status as a healer. When Mem is attacked by a mob of hysterical villagers, Anys is drawn into the melee in her attempt to save her aunt. The wrath of the mob substitutes the niece for the aunt and the accusations against her are again the oft-repeated ones of consorting with the devil, of sexual deviance. Moments before her death by strangulation, Anys not only shouts defiance at the face of her tormentors but also conjures up an image of a witch's sabbath participated in by not only her, the alleged witch but also all the married women present in the crowd. Her declarations bring to the fore the suspicions of the husbands, the vague fear surrounding the idea of female sexuality itself. It is as if, Anys emasculates the men who pretend to know her true nature with her cutting remarks—"For I have not laid with [the Devil] alone! No! I tell you now, I have seen your wives lie with him!… He is a stallion amongst geldings compared to you" (2001, 93). Even in the face of death, she retains and exercises her sexual agency by shouting defiance at the face of her accusers.

It is after Anys' and Mem's death that Elinor and Anna are forced to take over some of the tasks the healers used to fulfill within the village community. Anna, already skilled in birthing lambs, accompanies Elinor to the houses of pregnant women in need of a midwife. Together, they tend the abandoned herbal garden of the Gowdies, and grow their own herbs in the rectory. The traditional knowledge of the Gowdies' is supplemented by Elinor's books on herbs and medicines. Historically, the Post-Reformation Church had been at the forefront of the persecution of so-called witches in the sixteenth and seventeenth centuries, but with the presence of the rector's wife who is also skilled in the practice of plant-based medicines, even the very precinct of the church is pressed into the service of traditional remedies. The Latin word "spiritus", which means "breath" or "soul" and is the root word for "inspire", seems an apt description of the way Anys's disembodied soul guides Anna and Elinor in their work. While acting as a midwife for the first time in her life, Anna not only feels the presence of the deceased wise woman by her side but also repeats the same incantation she had heard her chant—"May the seven directions guide this work. May it be pleasing to my grandmothers, the ancient ones. So mote it be" (2001, 84, 122). By uttering the same incantation, Anna creates a bridge between the living and the dead, between the present generation of healers and their metaphorical grandmothers who have been learned in the same art.

Anys and Mem had been haunted by the specter of their poverty, age, and sexual agency. The challenges facing Anna and Elinor are of a different order altogether. Apart from the ministrations of the midwives and wise women, people in the early modern period had recourse to trained physicians, surgeons, and apothecaries. The services of the physician were often too expensive for the poorer people, and apothecaries were mostly located in cities and towns. Anna's mother was a victim of a barber-surgeon's mistreatment, whereas the physicians, on the rare occasions they did come to the "Plague Village", did more evil than good. But their real challenge comes from an impostor who claims to be the spirit of Anys Gowdie and feeds off the fear of the semi-destitute villagers and had begun a thriving business of selling spells and talismans. Keith Thomas, in his seminal study *Religion and the Decline of Magic* (1971, 1991), quotes from a remedy for toothache by an Elizabethan wizard. The remedy consisted of writing the words "in capital letters, AAB ILLA, HYRS GIBELLA, which he swears is... the names of the three spirits that enter into the blood and cause rheums, and so consequently the toothache" (Thomas 1991, 197). Elinor finds a piece of paper with exactly the same inscription on a grieving mother who has just lost her infant daughter to the plague. Elinor has been told that—"A 'witch' gave it her. The ghost, as she said, of Anys Gowdie. The ghost told her the words were Chaldee—a powerful spell from sorcerers who worshipped Satan, naked and painted with snakes, at each full moon" (2001, 211). The name and reputation of the wise woman, the healer, and the practitioner of what was known as "white magic" were being abused by an impostor, someone definitely acquainted with the practices of black magic. The empirical knowledge of the Gowdies, and of Anna and Elinor after them, was being challenged and undermined by someone determined to profit off of the fear of the villagers. As it turns out, the impostor is none other than Aphra, Anna's stepmother, who in a fit of insane rage would eventually murder Elinor Mompellion in full public view.

That the theme of motherhood is intertwined with the theme of healing in the novel becomes evident when we compare Aphra with Anna. The former had been an unkind mother to both her stepdaughter and her biological daughter, whereas Anna had loved her two sons and tried to hold on to their memory as long as she could. Her eventual escape from the village, and metaphorical emancipation from the apparitions of the past come when she decides to take for herself the unwanted and illegitimate baby daughter of Lady Bradford. Anna's escape is also a foray into a much more advanced world of medical science. She embarks upon a journey to Venice but decides to disembark at the port of Oran in Algeria instead.[2] She enters the harem of Ahmed Bey, a celebrated physician, and becomes his disciple, assistant, and wife, "in name". In her new life, in a new climate and a new culture, Anna is able to fulfill her destiny as a female physician to women who would not be allowed to be attended by male physicians. Not only does she now learn new advances in medicine and hopes "to accomplish a worthy life's work" in Oran (2001, 302), but she is also accompanied by two baby girls. The first one is the illegitimate daughter of Lady Bradford, whom Anna who is now called Aisha, meaning "Life", but also her own daughter, born out of her union with Michael Mompellion after the death of Elinor, and this daughter of hers is also called Elinor. The triad that Anys, Anna, and Elinor had once formed, dissolves and rearranges itself in the form of a new one, with Anna and her two daughters, Aisha and Elinor.

Anna's survival and her eventual settlement in a new home, in a different continent is also a rite of passage. The young widow of Sam Firth, her miner husband; the lover of Michael Mompellion, the underlying cruelty of whose nature she comes to understand during their brief relationship, finds herself settles within a family where she can exercise her talents and learn the art of healing while raising her two daughters. It is a passage from sickness to health, and also from menial drudgery as a miner's wife/ servant at the rectory to a skilled physician.

II

In her book *Shakespeare's Wife*, Germaine Greer makes an interesting observation about the given name of the woman most of whose life is still shrouded in mystery and speculation. Greer writes,

> The given name of the woman who married William Shakespeare in 1582 is as unstable as her surname. The only evidence that Richard Hathaway alias Gardner of Shottery had a daughter called Ann is a reference in his will to a daughter called Agnes. Scholars have demonstrated convincingly that in this period Agnes and Ann were simply treated as versions of the same name, pointing out dozens of examples where Agnes, pronounced "Annis", gradually became "Ann".
>
> (2007,12)

If "Agnes", "Annis", "Ann"—and as Greer goes on to point out—and "Anna", as a shortened form of "Hannah", were used almost interchangeably in the Tudor and Stuart periods, we can draw an interesting connection between Anna Firth and Anys Gowdie on the one hand, and Agnes Shakespeare on the other. Maggie O'Farrell's 2020 novel, *Hamnet*, provides the readers with a fictionalized account of the day-to-day life of the Shakespeare household, primarily focusing on his wife and the death of their teenage son Hamnet of bubonic plague in 1596.

Our discussion of the novel will not be an attempt to establish the historical accuracy, or the lack thereof of the events and characters it depicts, on the contrary, as we had done with *Year of Wonders*, it is the intertwined themes of disease, healing, and motherhood that will be examined in some detail. However, we will take a brief look at the common perception about the Shakespeare's marital life in order to understand the implication of re-casting Agnes Shakespeare as a healer and a wise woman in Farrell's novel. It has been a long-established tradition in literary history to think of William Shakespeare's marital life as an unhappy one. In the absence of any concrete evidence in support of this hypothesis, his plays have been zealously searched and made to yield unflattering remarks about marriage, and especially of marriage to women older than the husband. Neither the fact that Anne/Agnes Shakespeare was eight years senior to her husband nor that she was left the second-best bed in the poet's will is proof enough that their married life was a miserable one. But the lore has continued to thrive, in literary histories, in historical fictions like Anthony Burgess's *Nothing Like the Sun*, and in representations of the poet's life in popular culture.

Contrary to these perceptions, what we *do* know about the woman who was married to the poet, paints a picture of an able and resourceful manager of household affairs and property-related matters. Lena Cowen Orlin (2014)[3] speculates on the basis of the life and works of the Quiney family, who were both neighbors and related by marriage to the Shakespeares (Judith Shakespeare, Hamnet's twin sister was married to one Thomas Quiney) that Anne, was more likely to be "a businesswoman of success" whose enterprising nature ensured that William Shakespeare could afford to buy shares in the Globe Theatre and landed property in Stratford (Orlin 448). When Maggie O'Farrell re-casts Agnes Shakespeare as a healer and a wise woman, she is curiously enough, both circumventing as well as teasing out a positive implication from the well-established but probably apocryphal reputation of Shakespeare's wife as a shrew. Accusations of witchcraft, of being able to perform both black and white magic have been routinely leveled against women who refused to conform to the societal norm of the submissive and docile daughter/wife. The double bind of womanhood that we have referred to at the beginning of the chapter might also be seen in the way femininity and female sexuality is culturally perceived. As Clarke Garrett noted in 1977,[4]

> In a world in which men make the rules, female sexuality creates a perpetual dilemma. As the vessels of the biological mysteries of menstruation and lactation, as creatures of sexual passion, women are mistrusted, but as mothers,

women are the nurturers and preservers of society... When a woman failed to maintain her reputation because of inappropriate female behavior, she faced not ostracism... but distrust, animosity and even fear.

(Garrett 1977, 466)

The Gowdies in Brooks's novel and Agnes Shakespeare in *Hamnet* embody this duality and draw upon themselves the accusations of being witches.

At the very heart of Farrell's novel, two consecutive chapters narrating birth and death underscore the continuous thematic movement of the narrative from past to present, and from birth to death. Like Anna Firth, Agnes Hathaway is brought up by an unloving stepmother after her biological mother dies in childbirth. Like Anys Gowdie, Agnes grows up at the very edge of the inhabited part of the village. The farmland where she resides with her brother, her stepmother, and stepsiblings, skirts the forest of Arden. For Agnes, the forest, with its teeming life-forms is the element that she identifies the most with. Her biological mother, Rowan, is an inscrutable mystery to her conventional neighbors as she "had appeared out of the forest and married one of their own, who went by the name of a tree" (2020, 48). It is from her mother when she was still alive and from one of her only friends, the widowed wife of an apothecary, that Agnes learns the rudiments of the art of healing. Like Rowan, Agnes also has a dubious reputation, her young suitor has heard the rumors about her—

She has a certain notoriety in these parts. It is said that she is strange, touched, peculiar, perhaps mad. He has heard that she wanders the back roads and forest at will, unaccompanied, collecting plants to make dubious potions. It is wise not to cross her as people say she learnt her crafts from an old crone who used to make medicines and spin, and could kill a baby with a single glance.

(2020, 37)

Here we have the usual paraphernalia that accompanies the idea of a witch. Agnes is skilled in making potions, she can both heal—and as her stepmother would claim—and harm living things. She is both sought after by her neighbors for her skilled potion-making, at the same time feared on account of her preternatural ability to look into people's hearts. She is also credited with the ability to make prophecies. In other words, she is an intuitive healer and a woman whose sympathies are aligned with the rhythms of the natural world. At the narrative center of the novel, the readers witness Agnes giving birth to her first child in the forest, immediately followed by an account of how the bubonic Plague that would claim the life of one of her twins travels from Alexandria to rural Warwickshire. It is the essential cycle of Agnes's life, the intertwining of birth and death, of disease and healing.

Like Anys again, Agnes is not afraid to assert her sexual agency. Knowing full well that her stepmother would never consent to her marriage to the "Latin Tutor" without a fixed trade or livelihood, Agnes contrived to get pregnant so that the objections of her family come to naught. In her new home, away from the farmland, she continues to make her healing potions and exerts a fascinating pull on the imaginations of her neighbors. However, her learning proves ineffectual against the dreaded disease, the pestilence which attacks first Judith, and then Hamnet. In spite of all her efforts, Hamnet succumbs to the disease, whereas Judith eventually recovers. The death of her son ushers in a period of protracted grieving for Agnes, it also lays bare the dis-ease that has crept into her marriage. It is during this period of grief that Judith—and not her firstborn daughter Susanna—starts learning about the various plants and their healing properties. Just as Agnes had once learned her art from her mother, Judith in her turn learns from hers.

Like *Year of Wonders*, *Hamnet* also charts a movement from despair and disease toward hope. Agnes travels to London to confront her husband about his new play—a tragedy—to which he has given the name of their deceased son. It is in the playhouse, and in the words of the ghost—"Remember me"—Agnes finds solace and proof that her husband has not forgotten her or their dead child. It is also a clear indication that the marriage which had been slowly disintegrating over the years is finally entering the phase of healing.

III

Do these two novels then, in their emphasis on the matrilineal traditions of the arts of natural healing and focus on motherhood re-affirm the tradition of essentializing women as being closer to nature, and men to culture and civilization? Or do they typify women as being *essentially* mothers, a gender role which as Adrienne Rich points out—"In the most fundamental and bewildering of contradictions… has alienated women from our bodies by incarcerating us in them?" (1995, 13).[5] I would like to argue to the contrary. Both the novels discussed in this chapter depict women who manage to form strong homo-social bonds irrespective of differences in class and social status. Though the protagonists of each are mothers, motherhood is neither the primary nor the only denominator of their identity. The notion that a mother should be tied to the domestic space, with motherhood as their only vocation, according to Rich, might be traced back to the nineteenth century (45). In the early modern period, in which both of these novels are set, women—unless they were noblewomen by birth or marriage—were almost always an integral part of the labor force. Anna Firth and Agnes Shakespeare, in addition to being mothers, find their vocation as healers. By the end of the novels, Anna and Agnes, both have established themselves as reputed women healers. We might also see the beginning of the process of history that would eventually relegate these women healers to the position of charlatans, negate their experience, wisdom, and knowledge, and ensure the final victory of the formally-trained medical professional, mostly men till the twentieth century.[6] Both novels, interestingly enough, also contain multiple episodes/accounts of gender-role reversals. Anna and Elinor dressed themselves up in the garb of male miners in an attempt to help an orphan girl extract lead from her father's abandoned mine, Micahel Mompellion fails to recognize his wife and their maid in the new attire they have donned. When the Latin Tutor, who would eventually become Agnes's husband (significantly, the poet is never referred to by name in the novel) sees her for the first time, he mistakes her for a young man because of her male attire and the fact that she was carrying a hawk in her arms. She appears more like a young farmer interested in hawking than the eldest daughter of the household. In his attempt to hoodwink death, Hamnet exchanges place in bed with his identical twin Judith and metaphorically re-enacts the numerous instances of cross-dressing that his father's plays are punctuated with. Even Agnes is baffled for some time while tending to her two ailing children. The women in these two novels both conform to and go beyond the circumscribed gender roles that contemporary society had delineated for them. They are healers, but not necromancers; their commitment is toward life, well-being, and health. Mem, Anys, Elinor, Anna— all would concur with Agnes that "If there is life, there is hope" (2020, 244).

Notes

1 For a detailed analysis of the rise in the incidence of domestic violence in India during COVID-19, please see Krishnakumar, Akshaya, and Shankey Verma. "Understanding Domestic Violence in India during COVID-19: A Routine Activity Approach". *Asian Journal of Criminology* 16, no.1 (Winter): 19–35 and Maji, Sucharita, Saurabh Bansod, and Tushar Singh. 2021. "Domestic Violence During COVID-19 Pandemic: The Case for Indian Women". *Journal of Community & Applied Social Psychology.* Early View: 1–8.

2 It is interesting to note that Brooks makes Anna find her destiny in Oran, a port city in Algeria. As Susan J. Rasmussen has noted, there was a long-established tradition of healing women and female herbologists in various Islamic groups in North-West Africa, most notably the Tuareg women of Niger.

3 Orlin, Lena Cowen. 2014. "Anne by Indirection". *Shakespeare Quarterly* 65, no.4: 421–454. https://doi. org/10.1353/shq.2014.0043. Orlin's essay follows the life and career of the matriarch of the Quiney family and draws a plausible parallel with that of Anne Shakespeare.

4 Garrett, Clarke. 1977. "Women and Witches: Patterns of Analysis". *Signs: Journal of Women in Culture and Society*, 3: 461–470.

5 Rich, Adrienne. 1995. *Of Woman Born.* New York: W. W. Norton & Company.

6 See Mary E. Fissell's Essay, "Introduction: Women, Health, and Healing in Early Modern Europe". *Bulletin of the History of Medicine* 82, no. 1 (Spring): 1–17.

References

Brooks, Geraldine. 2001. *Year of Wonders.* London: Harpers Collins.

Ehrenreich, Barbara, and Deirdre English. 1973. *Witches, Midwives & Nurses: A History of Women Healers.* New York: Feminist Press.

Fissell, Mary E. 2008. "Women, Health, and Healing in Early Modern Europe". *Bulletin of the History of Medicine* 82, no. 1 (Spring): 1–17.

Garrett, Clarke. 1977. "Women and Witches: Patterns of Analysis". *Signs: Journal of Women in Culture and Society* 3: 461–470.

Greer, Germain. 2007. *Shakespeare's Wife.* London: Bloomsbury.

Krishnakumar, Akshaya, and Shankey Verma. "Understanding Domestic violence in India During COVID-19: A Routine Activity Approach". *Asian Journal of Criminology* 16, no. 1 (Winter): 19–35.

Macfarlane, Alan. 1970. *Witchcraft in Tudor and Stuart England: A Regional and Comparative Study.* London: Routledge & Kegan Paul.

Maji, Sucharita, Saurabh Bansod, and Tushar Singh. 2021. "Domestic Violence during COVID-19 Pandemic: The Case for Indian Women". *Journal of Community & Applied Social Psychology* 32, no. 3: 374–381.

O' Farrell, Maggie. 2020. *Hamnet.* London: Tinder Press.

Orlin, Lena Cowen. 2014. "Anne by Indirection". *Shakespeare Quarterly* 65, no. 4: 421–454. https://doi. org/10.1353/shq.2014.0043.

Rasmussen, Susan J. "Only Women Know Trees: Medicine Women and the Role of Herbal Healing in Tuareg Culture". *Journal of Anthropological Research* 54, no. 2: 147–171.

Rich, Adrienne. 1995. *Of Woman Born.* New York: W. W. Norton & Company.

Shannon, Gary W., and Robert G. Cromley. 2013. "The Great Plague of London, 1665". *Urban Geography* 1, no. 30: 254–270.

Thomas, Keith. 1991. *Religion and the Decline of Magic: Studies in Popular Beliefs in Sixteenth- and Seventeenth-Century England.* London: Penguin Books.

12 "stand aside death...today is my day"

Contextualizing the Naga Esotericism in Easterine Kire's Novels

Nilanjana Chatterjee

I

The chapter aims at understanding the esoteric worldview of the indigenous Naga communities in India within the context of the present Covid-19 dystopia. The purpose of the engagement is for critical thinkers and researchers to have a deeper understanding of Naga indigenous perceptions of holistic healing practices, and to interconnect embedded esoteric consciousness with everyday pandemic unease with the self and the community and thereby formulate a transrational mode of improving individual and community wellbeing. Unrecovered esoteric knowledge of the Naga world informs the writings of Angami Kire. Her engagement in esoteric narratives, within the mainstream Indian Anglophone writings, visibilizes the alternative indigenous esoteric practices to survive political, environmental, individual, and biomedical crises. This chapter, therefore, identifies and contextualizes the esoteric elements in Kire's novels – a study under-noticed[1] by scholarly writers or critical thinkers on Kire. Versluis's defines esotericism:

> I use the word esoteric in a religious context to refer to individuals or groups whose works are self-understood as bearing hidden inner religious, cosmological, or metaphysical truths for a select audience. Such a definition can include al-chemical, magical, Masonic, or gnostic groups or individuals.
>
> (2004, 8)

Versluis differentiates esoteric knowledge from exoteric knowledge by ascribing esoteric knowledge to a select audience and exoteric knowledge to the general populace. Esoteric knowledge, therefore, includes an indigenous social-anthropologic sense of initiation as admission into a secret society which is embedded and is exclusively visible in cultural representations (like literature and art) – symbolically and literally.

Spiritual wellbeing among indigenous communities is integral to their everyday culture and informs the very perception of an ideal life (Chatterjee and Sharma 2018; James 2015; Ritskes 2011). The distinction between indigenous esotericism and a broader universal understanding of spirituality must be made

DOI: 10.4324/9781003300762-14

early on. Indigenous esotericism is intrinsically connected to the host culture and therefore necessitates a more systematic and organized critical approach (Fleming and Ledogar 2008). The study of indigenous esotericism in Indian Anglophone literatures – hitherto under-noticed in serious academic analyses – is an invisibilized and transrational mode of knowledge. Moreover, Naga indigenous esotericism – discarded and not just unnoticed or underrealized by the dominant modes of critical studies based on reasoning and cultural flattening – is a doubly marginalized mode of critical study. In the present moment of the postmodern critique of linear history and of contemporary engagement in indigenous culture studies, it is necessary to problematize the literary representations of indigenous esotericism in Indian Anglophone literatures, especially Naga Anglophone literature. The people of Nagaland have experienced severe phases of political subordination and cultural silencing: The greater the subordination received, the deeper have been the esoteric responses of the Naga communities and individuals. Naga oral literature thereby has emerged as a rich treasure trove of hidden indigenous esoteric knowledge and practices, which has been empowering its people to survive and resist powers beyond their control – the continued political and cultural uncertainties, on one hand, and the biomedical, environmental, and spiritual anxieties and crises on the other hand. In this context, Kire's Anglophone writings revive and visibilize – through strategic couching of the metaphoric language of vivid sensuous images – the hermetic tropes of epiphany, taboo, mystery, and initiation through mythic vision and spiritual intelligence. The Naga Anglophone literature in general – and Kire's writings in particular – is deeply rooted in Naga oral literature[2] and therefore reflects the protective and empowering esoteric wisdom and cultural practices and perpetuates them. The next segment analyses the narrative tools and explores the esoteric elements employed in Kire's novels to show how the Naga tribes' indigenous esoteric knowledge – pertaining to botanical healings, geographical reference points (both spiritual and imaginary) of legendary villages of the seers, eco ethical consciousness, food conservation techniques, everyday spiritual conditioning to survive battles (both internal and external) – offers individuals and their communities a sense of preparedness and the courage to fight back political, environmental, biomedical, and internal crises even in moments of overwhelming grief and fear. In doing so, the final segment intends to connect the esoteric realities of Kire's writings to the present biomedical and politico-economic crises, wherein individual or/and community wellbeing is/are at stake.

II

Finley's dissertation (2012, 12) analyses certain narrative techniques (for example, epic adventures of the protagonist culminating in the moment of initiation, transition from one state of consciousness to another, the tell-tale sign of initiation, sudden break in narrative continuity, and a formal gesture which replicates the initiate's solemn vow not to speak of esoteric mysteries which are themselves, in large part, incommunicable) in Lippard's *Paul Ardenheim* to explicate how Lippard effectively embeds American esoteric knowledge in it. Similar narrative strategies could be identified in Kire's novels, emphasizing the fact that her novels could be read as silent but powerful esoteric narratives wherein are couched strategic mediation of traditional esoteric myths and personal responses to cultural uncertainties. Literary Imagination and faith in Naga esotericism go hand in hand in Naga oral narratives, representing the broader implications of the external and internal crises of the Naga tribes since the nineteenth century unequal resistances to the British Imperial Army with spears and rocks (Gott 2011, 330) and even before that. In *Walking the Roadless Road: Exploring the Tribes of Nagaland*, Kire (2019b) makes a written documentation of the significance of the indigenous esoteric worlds in the everyday lives of Naga tribes for confronting the political, environmental, biomedical, and internal anxieties:

> The Naga mind accepts the parallel existence of the natural and the spiritual world. All tribes believe in life after death and coexistence of spirits with man … Though there is no spirit worship in the tribal religions, there is a practice of spirit appeasement or spirit propitiation if a member of the family falls sick after a trip to the deep woods.
>
> (2019b, 46)

Kire re-creates many of the Naga oral narratives in her novels by simultaneous representations of the natural world and the supernatural enchantment and makes the elements of esotericism relatable by unification of vivid imaginary and mythical landscapes with everyday dwelling, farming, hunting, weaving, fishing, and culinary practices of the Naga tribes. The readers can connect with the protagonists who set out to conquer the unattainable through perilous journeys – both within and without.

In Kire's novels, strengthening of mental health involves a simultaneous understanding of the self and the collective. The texts exhibit indigenous Naga cultural ideologies of honoring one's spirit through spiritual recognition of one's lineage and community. They acknowledge the power of benevolent selfless spiritual knowledge – absorbed from family and community and applied in everyday crises – above all other forms of power and strength. In *When the River Sleeps*, Kire (2014) transports the readers to a transrational world of dreams and shadow moments (between waking and dreaming) wherein Villie – the middle-aged lone forest dweller, hunter, and 'the official protector of the rare tragopan' (Kire 2014, 4) – undertook a death-dealing journey through the natural and supernatural lands of Nagaland in quest of the (almost) impossible: to wrest from the sleeping river the heart-stone that would empower him with esoteric knowledge (Dhanya and Bhattacharya 2019). In the unclean forest, when Vilie had to fight 'a dark indistinguishable shape' (Kire 2014, 82) and was almost petrified and devasted by fear and helplessness, he remembered the seer's words:

> Let your spirit be the bigger one. They are spirits, they will submit to the authority of the spirit that asserts itself.
>
> (Kire 2014, 83)

The very remembrance of the seer's words inspired Vilie to gather courage and a renewed mental strength and willpower. Consequently, the overpowering evil spirit appeared to reduce into a detestable entity which could be easily crushed under Vilie's feet. The seer's esoteric inspiration transformed Vilie into a hero and churned up in his human heart superhuman courage to strike back. Vilie cried: 'Mine is the greater spirit! I will never submit to you' (Kire 2014, 83). The spirit grew smaller in size and eventually flung itself against a tree trunk. At every step of his journey until he reached the Border Village, Vilie's acknowledgment and reverence for the inner spirit and esoteric consciousness, the land, and community, and for human life and spirits had been put to test. Kani, the headman of the Border Village warned Vilie:

> Remember when we are out at the sleeping river, there can be no room for fear. If you harbour fear, you are a dead man. If you came here after committing something terrible, like a murder or sending a man to his death by a false testimony, your spirit will not be able to outwrestle their spirits. Any evil action of yours will weigh on your conscience, and make you vulnerable to their onslaught. It is an attack, there's nothing gentle about it. So your protection is your own good heart and your clear conscience. Harbour no evil against any man when you are going on this trip.
>
> (Kire 2014, 93)

The moral and ethical cleansing of self and a sense of comradeship with the community were the basic requirements for undertaking the deadly journey. According to Kani, the true power of the heart-stone was the 'knowledge of the spiritual' (Kire 2014, 96), which offered power over the world of the senses and the world of the spirit. This interpretation transformed Vilie as an individual and his understanding of the quest for the heart-stone so much so that he realized he came very far from the man who had left his forest home. The transformed Vilie wanted to catch the sleeping river and seize the heart-stone in search of 'spiritual knowledge that sleeping river would give him if they [Vilie and Kani] found it' (Kire 2014, 96). As Vilie plunged into the sleeping river, the river flung him back like a bit of driftwood and the only weapon that helped him to survive was his mental courage and deep focus gathered from the spirit words that he had learnt from his community:

> Sky is my father, Earth is my mother, stand aside death! Kepenuopfu[3] fights for me, today is my day! I claim the wealth of the river because mine is the greater spirit. To him who has the greater spirit belongs the stone!
>
> (Kire 2014, 103)

It was then when the waters retreated, and Vilie came out safe holding the heart-stone. According to Kani, Villie could return from the sleeping river unharmed because of his unfailing 'faith' (Kire 2014, 108) in his esoteric consciousness. Besides the esoteric quality of the heart-stone, Kani explained to Vilie the difference between the bodily and the spiritual responses to the spirit encounters:

While the human spirit emerges as a triumphant, the flesh in his body struggles with its own memories of fear. On his homeward journey, Vilie fought the most fearful and selfless battle to save Ate – a Kirhupfumia[4] girl whom Vilie considered as his own daughter – from the spirits. Ate even 'slipped away [into death] for some time' (Kire 2014, 197), but Vilie held the heart-stone and shouted to the spirits using – 'His name [the name of the attacking spirit which is supposed to disempower the spirit]' (Kire 2014, 197). Once Ate came back to life, Vilie acknowledged 'the creator deity' (Kire 2014, 197) who had helped him in fighting back the spirits even when Vilie had been overwhelmed with grief. By the end of the novel, after Vilie's death, Ate realized the wisdom of the heart-stone:

> It [the stone] helps us discover the spiritual identity that is within us, so we can use it to combat the dark forces that are always trying to control and suppress us.
>
> (Kire 2014, 238)

However, Ate also understood that men who weren't initiated could not understand the stone's real worth and would use it to gain wealth and other material things.

Jakovljevic (2017) defined spirituality as a binding force that incorporates the notion of transcendental values and faith that offer a holistic understanding of self, people, nature, and the universe. This approach to holistic understanding connects individuals with kin, communities, and the world. Kire (2019b) in *Walking the Roadless Road: Exploring the Tribes of Nagaland* records, 'An Ao cannot conceive of a world apart from religion. The whole universe is sacred and filled with gods' (Kire 2019b, 76). The Ao worldview restores holistic wellness in everyday life by following certain esoteric practices:

> Believing that their [the spirits'] influence is real, man therefore tries to live aright so as not to incur the anger of spirits; he strives as far as possible to live out sobaliba[5], the principles learnt from the teachings of the morung[6]. Central to the concepts of sobaliba are indispensable features that prompt a man to put others first, live a life of compassion, integrity and thoughtfulness, combined with the qualities of industriousness, hospitality and respect for all members of the village. It encompasses values such as being unselfish, self-effacing and honest, avoiding adultery and obeying the customary practices of the tribe.
>
> (Kire 2019b, 77)

The Ao people aspire to practice this everyday spirituality to die a good death and avoid apotia (cursed and therefore dreaded) death (for example, death caused by wild animals, snakebites, falling off cliffs or trees, drowning, getting burnt or dying in childbirth).

In *Don't Run, My Love*, Kire (2017) merges the everyday lives of the natural and the supernatural world of the two woman-farmers of Kija - Atuonuo and her widowed mother Visuenuo and in so doing, she strategically embeds the esoteric perceptions of the ancient Angamis. Atuonuo's uncertain love for Kevi, a *tekhum-iavi*,[7] followed by an intense fear of falling in love with a weretiger, led Atuonuo and Visuenuo to set out from Kija for the Village of Seers. The Village – the cradle of ancient esoteric knowledge – could be as far or as near as a seeker would want it to be. To a mere visitor, it would be 'the furthest point on earth' (Kire 2017, 79). This was an uncharted village – more powerful than the legendary village of Meriezou (the seat of Angami culture and the birthplace of many famed seers):

> What was the truth? No human could tell and it was pointless to try to situate it in a fixed location because it was inarguably the most powerful village, the village that held answers for all the problems that man could encounter in his physical existence. And by virtue of that power, the village was quite capable of shifting location as it pleased.
>
> (Kire 2017, 82)

Time and again Kire informs that the Village and its esoteric values, practices, and antidotes are unknowable, unmappable, and almost impenetrable. The empty streets with few humans passing without a word, or the rough dangerous steps to the old seer's house heighten the potential of indigenous esoteric unknowability. The great wood apple tree served as the gateway to the spiritual village which marked the boundary between the natural and the supernatural. The path from here was swampy and dark and the sights and sounds it offered were to be strictly ignored. The journey through the lonely path was a litmus test of the seeker's integrity, faith, determination, and need for esoteric knowledge.

Indigenous people consider the everyday natural world as the manifestation of divine power and therefore revere the elements of nature as their true guide or teacher (Kechutzar 2008). Kire (2019b), in *Walking the Roadless Road: Exploring the Tribes of Nagaland*, records that the Chakhesang culture believes in the omnipresence of the divine spirit that guides people's actions – 'especially those of an ethical nature—in their daily lives' (2019b, 86). Ancient Konayaks worshipped the natural world by worshipping the sun, the moon, stones, rivers, jungles, and trees as each possessed spirit (2019b, 121). Vilie's mother, in *When the River Sleeps*, educated Vilie to acknowledge the provider while taking firewood, hunting forest animals for food, or gathering herbs from the forest, and in this way helped in building the collective consciousness (Kire 2014). Vilie therefore pronounced a prayer thanking the provider on such occasions, *Terhuomia peziemu* (Kire 2014, 80) – e.i. thanks to the Ukepenuopfu[8] and this can be regarded as a form of totemism wherein people, trees, animals, and places are interlinked to form a complete whole. In fact, totemic ways of interconnectedness are based on a value system that recognizes an interdependence between the species and the totemic site (Grieves 2008).

The Naga indigenous people – as represented in Kire's novels – are geographically and intellectually closer to the forest and therefore possess unique knowledge of the sacred medicines, spiritual values, and rituals to survive the diseases and wounds caused by the neighboring woods. Vilie (Kire 2014) was aware of certain esoteric healing practices. He remembered the names of curative herbs – advised by an old man of his community – without which he wouldn't be able to survive in the deadly forests: Ciena (bitter wormwood used to staunch blood from small cuts and believed to have supernatural properties) and Tierhutiepfu (amaranth) (Kire 2014, 32). For curing victims of tiger attack, indigenous people would apply vilhuu nha (redflower ragleaf) paste (Kire 20014). They considered Japan nha (crofton weed) paste as an effective antidote for curing malaria patients (Kire 2014). For malaria fever:

> … the people from his [Villie's] village who used to fall sick when they wandered into *Rarhuria*[9] while out hunting or cutting wood. To cure them the seer would give them a drink made of ginseng and *tsomhou* [nutgall tree] the wild sour seed that grew on trees. Stir a little honey and the mixture would go down easily.
>
> (Kire 2014, 53–54)

In fact, the non-Christian Nagas would offer chicken sacrifices for the sick member of the community. The community would bring a chicken into the forest and announce, "Life for life" (Kire 2014, 54). Eventually, the chicken would be released which would be eaten by a wild animal in the woods. However, the Christian Nagas believed that Jishu (or Isu) had been sacrificed for everyone's disease on the earth (Kire 2018). Vilie was also aware of the traditional indigenous esoteric values of enhancing individual energies during food crisis:

> All hunters knew that if they found food after a long period of starvation, they should eat slowly, masticating their food properly to help their digestive organs. "You can eat yourself dead!" the older hunters would warn when they were teaching younger hunters about this.
>
> (Kire 2014, 55–56)

During his journey into the forest, Vilie – suffering from acute illness, body ache, fatigue, and fever – realized that the simple knowledge of eating food, according to the indigenous Naga esoteric practices, could provide him with a renewed energy and vigor. Although he was dying with hunger, Vilie strategically ate certain portion of his food and rested, and repeated the process. He was taught by his mother the wisdom of eating food – 'food eaten slowly stayed in your stomach longer' (Kire 2014, 56). Vilie could fight and survive the deadly fever (even without the seer's anecdotes) and the food crisis in the woods – that too singlehandedly – because he had revered the wisdom of the esoteric values infused by the family and community. The Naga indigenous esoteric healing practices also provided remedies for mental illness: When Vilie felt nauseous and dropped to his knee due to an intense sense of guilt that continued to disturb him since Pehu's death in the hands of Hiesa, Ate treated him with a unique Kirhupfumia antidote – a mug of bitter bark juice. After drinking the juice, he was able to build a memorial for Pehu and felt 'the despondence lift from his spirit' (Kire 2014, 178). In fact, the indigenous people could survive the political turbulences partly because of the esoteric faith and practices which influenced the indigenous culture and in turn got influenced by transcultural and transreligious interactions.

Kire, in '2016 Gopinath Mahanty Lecture,' identifies the three phases of political subordination: The first phase includes the American missionaries' cultural intrusion in the 1860s; the second phase includes the political turmoil during British imperialism in 1919, the World War II and the Battle of Kohima in 1944; and the third phase begins with the post-independent period under the shadow of cultural homogenization (Patton 2019). In this context, the Naga indigenous esoteric knowledge has been a fluid concept wherein history and culture, memory, and trauma – of the individual and the community – appear to transform and transcend the ancient pre-Christian notions of esoteric warnings and fear, sense of (un)belonging and (un)protectiveness. In the late nineteenth century, the British Imperial Army was fiercely resisted by Angami warriors of the Khonoma village. As a result, burning of houses and villages of the Naga rebels became the 'standard practice of [British imperialistic] punishment' (Kire 2018, ix). Eventually, the villages (for example, Piphema, Meriema, Sechuma, Tsiepama, Pfuchama, Kigwema, Viswema, and Jotsoma) that united in the uprising against the Kohima garrison met with similar destructive consequences (Kire 2018, xiv). Kire (2018), in *Sky Is My Father: A Naga Village Remembered*, narrativizes the esoteric life that sustained the freedom-loving villagers of the Khonoma during the toughest of British colonial encounters. The novel explicates Piano's recollection of the childhood days when she observed from a safe distance the Terhase ritual – the ritual of making peace with the spirits following the path of honesty:

> The Thevo priest, an old man with fierce eyes, called loudly: *Spirit Vo-o, we were wondering where you were but here you are. We have come to solicit peace between man and spirit. Let there be no destruction and calamity, no death and disease and plague. Who is honest, you are honest. Who is honest, I am honest. We will compete with each other in honesty.*
>
> (Kire 2018, 14)

Piano, like other members of the village, was initiated in pre-Christian esoteric practices by her father. She devoutly observed the Genna days[10] to protect the fertility of the agricultural fields. Willaert (2020) records that William McCulloch (the British political agent) in 1859, recorded how people of Manipur and Naga Hills (the present-day Nagaland, Manipur, Assam, Arunachal Pradesh, and Myanmar) practiced Genna to fight smallpox and cholera (new diseases transmitted as a part of British colonizing project). Here, Willaert points out, Genna is a form of worship which 'served multiple purposes including preventing epidemics, natural disasters, and unforeseen circumstances' (2020). The esoteric practices related to Genna were sustained through strict customary laws and beliefs at the village level. Child Piano's father would warn, "*If you break the taboos, you break your-self*" (Kire 2018, 14). Love and responsibility toward one's clan was inculcated in children by the family (for family is the smallest unit of the community). Piano's son Levi was taught by his parents the spiritual and moral obligations to protect and safeguard the self and the community and to participate in meaningful ways at the community feast:

> This is the key to right living – avoiding excess in anything – be content with your share of land and fields … When you are older and your hearts are strong within you, you will take on the responsibility of guarding the village while others will go out to earn a great name for our village … Never be arrogant, respect yourself sufficiently so that you can fulfil the responsi-bilities of manhood … A real man does not need to roar to show that he is a man.
>
> (Kire 2018, 30)

The dwellers of Khonoma followed certain esoteric principles while mourning the death of the loved ones. The inconsolable Lato, Levi's brother, was asked by old Kovi to control his emotions for his dead mother, Piano: "My son, you will grieve the spirits, please cease, we must not mourn the dead to excess" (Kire 2018, 114). In fact, Lato was inspired to draw solace from the faith in afterlife – a wonderful reunion awaiting Piano with her warrior husband.

Kire (2018), in the novel, records spirit-sighting at the Kohima village dur-ing the 1890s wherein a non-Christian British soldier – appointed to guard the deeply religious white teacher and medical practitioner, Dr. Sidney Rivenburg – confessed to Rivenburg the nightly visitations of 'a spirit that grew larger and larger till he stood as big as a mountain before he disappeared' (Kire 2018, 117–118) from near the water source. However, as Rivenburg accompanied the guard to the water source, 'the spirit miraculously grew smaller' and disappeared, lead-ing the non-Christian soldier to believe in Christian esoteric knowledge to combat spirits in Kohima village. The Christian value system metamorphosed the pre-existing non-Christian indigenous Naga esoteric sensibilities – sometimes with cultural resistance. Levi's son, Sato, wished to be a follower of Isu (Christ) but Levi conducted Sato's initiation into manhood in person at the indigenous festival of Sekrenyi (an important annual festival of the Angami Nagas to renew and purify the self and the community by cleansing the body and the soul) by cutting a sec-ond chicken to perform the ritual of pulling out the intestines from it (Kire 2018, 121). Though Sato was internally tormented – as if 'being pulled in two directions, by two almost equal forces' (Kire 2018, 122), his initiation into manhood and into the Khonoma clan offered him 'a sweet calm' (Kire 2018, 122). The esoteric con-sciousness in him was a fluid transrational transreligious transcultural entity that led him to believe that two religions weren't opposed to each other:

> He thought of Isu on the cross as a chicken sacrifice much greater than all the chicken sacrifices the Angamis had made. Isu [Jesus] was the chicken

being sacrificed, for man to be free from disease, and all the ailments the spirits could bring upon him ... How Sato wished that his father would come to see that the new religion was really a fulfillment of the old – answering the questions that the old was struggling with, and giving meaning to the feasts, and to life as the village knew it and lived it.

(Kire 2018, 123)

However, the mediation of non-Christian (old ways) and Christian (new ways) concepts of esoteric consciousness were not always compatible with each other. While Sato's father was deeply wounded by Sato's conversion, Sato's mother was worried about the conflict between the 'old' and 'new' esoteric perceptions of her afterlife reunion with the spirit of her dead husband in a land of (un)happiness. She was equally perturbed by 'a treacherous sense of liberation ... a release from the constant tension of living with the man [Levi after Sato's conversion] he had become' (Kire 2018, 144). Sato comforted his mother by differentiating between the old and the new ways:

It [the old religion] says that life is unpredictable and hard, and man should harden his heart and bear all of his misfortunes with fortitude ... Isu says that his followers are blessed with his protection – they are free from uncertainty and fear – they walk in love and light all of their lives.

(Kire 2018, 144–145)

Though Sato remained apparently unperturbed by the 'new' and the 'old' esoteric ways of living as he seemed to have (meaningfully) negotiated between the two, he suffered from a continuous self-reproach since his conversion, blaming himself for his parents' sufferings. Indigenous Naga esoteric knowledge underwent cultural and religious metamorphoses during and after the British colonization of India. Moreover, it underwent further modification due to Nagaland's exclusive political and territorial complexities during and after the Battle of Kohima (from April 4, 1944, to June 22, 1944).

In *a respectable woman* (Kire 2019a), Kire records that during and after the Second World War in 1944, the people of Kohima experienced strange spirit-sightings. In this connection, she refers to the spirit-sightings by Ania Nisou (Kire 2019a, 176). Since spirit-sighting is a fluid transcultural experience deeply connected to the Naga everyday (and therefore hidden) responses to the political anxieties and uncertainties, The Angamis – familiar with spirit-sighting – continued to sight spirits after the Second World War but in slightly different forms. Kire points out in *a respectable woman*:

People claim that spirits have favourite haunts such as village ponds, the village gate, big boulders, great trees, abandoned house and gullies, and graveyards. After the war, the new spirits that were sighted were the spirits of the soldiers who died in war.

(Kire 2019a, 176)

As the Japanese invaded the Naga hills in 1944, there was a mass evacuation of people from Kohima village to other villages. The evacuation of families to nearby shelters and their return almost after two months to the same but different space led to silent helpless suffering for years. The sense of deterritorialization and uprootedness from one's own home and hearth, and the familiar topography led to spirit-sighting at former Garrison Hill 'known for its ghost soldiers' (Kire 2019a, 4), or at War Cemetery. The trauma was so intense that an Angami woman experienced nightly visitations of her Sikh spirit-lover from the grave of the Sikh soldier (Kire 2019a, 5). In the face of political devastation, Kire records the invisible Naga voices of 'the human struggles that our people endured' (Kire 2019a, 6) and the Naga esoteric consciousness was integral to the human struggle to endure deep wounds of the Battle of Kohima (both within and without, during and after the battle). After the ravages of war and imposed peace, as Kohima village has grown into a multicultural modern town and as the memory and trauma of the Battle of Kohima (at the individual level and at the community level) have apparently faded away, Kire wishes to preserve the indigenous survival strategies:

> Hopefully there will be some wise children in Uvi's generation who will see to it that the legacy upon which their civilisation has been built is not completely wiped out.
>
> (Kire 2019a, 177)

To indigenous people, 'community means the living, the unborn, the dead, and nature as a whole' (Wangoola 2000, 271). Indeed, the indigenous ways of dwelling, knowing, and being is informed by the simplicity and complexity of their psycho-spiritual-socio-ecological cosmological worldview (Rowkith and Bhagwan 2020). In the context of Naga indigenous people, each strand of the community is interwoven by esoteric values, faith, and rituals which help the individual and the community to sustain and thrive through political, medical, religious, or environmental crises.

III

The Naga indigenous esoteric responses to the environmental, cultural, and political metamorphoses are mediated by their esoteric interpretations and practices. The Indian indigenous people – around 7 per cent of the Indian population[11] – have been able to fight back the Covid-19 virus and its economic impact due to climate-resilient and nature-based lifestyles (Basu 2020): The natural diets have strengthened their immune system and the healing power of the forest resources (for example, honey, curative flowers, and herbs) and the local herbaceous plants have helped to combat the virus away. Moreover, the sustainable ways of natural resource management (preservation of forests and protection of wildlife) have allowed them to cope with the food and medicinal crises. The Indian indigenous communities have used the powers of spiritual healing rituals as a part of holistic healing and wellbeing. Dr. Jayalal (President of the Indian Medical Association), in an interview, mentions, "I personally think that during this time, people have prayed and worshipped more than ever" (Lee 2021). The present chapter, in this context, has explored the indigenous esoteric values and rituals in Naga communities as strategically represented in Kire's novels. Willaert (2020) explicates how the pre-Christian concept of Genna – lockdown practiced for days or weeks – was used by the Naga tribes during the colonial days of fearful epidemics to control further spread of smallpox and cholera. Indigenous people demonstrate esoteric consciousness through several ways, which include the practice of taboos, sustainable ways of natural resource management, and rituals. The Naga esoteric healing remedies involving natural resources, the sustainable ways of maintaining food security, the old and new ways of fighting spirits, the prayers, and simple everyday acts to strengthen body and mind, and the taboos imposed by the community are integral to the wellbeing of the Naga self and the communities. Kire's esoteric novels delineate the horrors and trauma of the dis-ease with the self and the society. The transrational concepts of (mostly non-Christian) Spirit-sightings, omen, and dreams[12] by the Naga tribes are deeply rooted in their lived environmental, cultural, and political transitions and adaptations. This unique indigenous knowledge, which Kire documents in her novels, has been strategically transmitted from one generation to another through repetitive oral narratives couched in folklores to educate, instruct, warn (and entertain) young indigenous tribes by the old indigenous tribes since ages about the transrational ways of restoring and expanding the notions of wellness and mystical past.

Notes

1 Apart from writing book reviews (Shekhar 2017), academic scholars have engaged in critical analyses of Kire from mythic (Mandal and Singh 2019), theological (Babar 2019; Bhattacharya 2020), postcolonial (Bhumika 2019), pre-pandemic spiritual (Manickam and Balakrishnan 2019), ecocritical (Karki 2019), diasporic (Barman 2020) and netnographic perspectives (Chatterjee 2022).

2 Some of the eminent anglophone writers from Nagaland are Easterine Kire (1959–), Monalisa Changkija (1960–), Temsula Ao (1945–) and Vishu Rita Krocha (1983–). Patton (2019), in "Contemporary Naga Writings" Reclamation of Culture and History through Orality", points out that one of the chief reasons for the Naga writers to write is the 'overpowering' urge to archive their culture for future dissemination.

3 Kepenuopfu is referred to the birth-spirit, the supreme God worshipped by the Tenyimia in the old religion. The same name is used for the Christian God (Kire 2014, 243).

4 Kirhupfumia is a minority group of Naga women thought to have the power of maiming, blinding, or killing people simply by pointing at them with their fingers (Kire 2014, 244).

5 Sobaliba is the indigenous notion of the true solutions that a community invents to adapt to their natural and social environment (Verhelst 1990, 3).

6 The Morung is a key educational institution of the Nagas, and the centre for social life of the unmarried male members of the Naga society. Here, the young boys are tutored by the elders about the social practices, cultural ideologies, and esoteric values.

7 Tekhumiavi, meaning weretiger, is a phenomenon amongst the Tenyimia people where certain members of the tribe transform their spirits into tigers (Kire 2014, 242).

8 Ukepenuopfiu – the other name for Kepenuopfu – is referred to the birth-spirit, the supreme God worshipped by the Tenyimia in the old religion. The same name is used for the Christian God (Kire 2014, 243).

9 *Rarhuria* is referred to as the unclean forest.

10 Genna Day is a day declared as a no-work day. It is a taboo to work on genna days and the cultural belief is that those who violate genna days are punished with injuries and accidents that have even resulted in death (Kire 2014, 243).

11 Seven per cent of the Indian population has been recognized as tribals (Chatterjee and Sharma 2018).

12 Since Indigenous people draw knowledge from elements of nature and environment, their esoteric sensibilities include omen, dreams, and divination (Kechutzar 2008).

References

Babar, Aniruddha. 2019. "A Peek into Spiritual World of the Nagas through the Eyes of Easterine Kire." *Tetso Interdisciplinary Journal* 7. https://ssrn.com/abstract=3607864.

Barman, Resha. 2020. "Challenging the Stereotypes: Diasporic Writers from India's Northeast." In *Re-theorising the India Subcontinental Diaspora: Old and New Directions.* Edited by Nilanjana Chatterjee and Anindita Chatterjee, 174–187. Newcastle upon Tyne : Cambridge Scholars Publishing.

Basu, Moushumi. December 7, 2020. "To Ward Off Pandemic, India's Indigenous Tribes Find Remedies in Forests." https://cc.bingj.com/cache.aspx?q=Moushumi.+December+7%2c+2020.+"To+ward+off+pandemic%2c+India's+indigenous+tribes+find+remedies+in+forests."+&d=4656818585404083&mkt=en-IN&setlang=en-GB&w=Gz7aSyFs2LRFrTeUIVeTFHdPdvFv25Ut. Accessed December 21, 2021.

Bhattacharya, Panchali. 2020. "Reviving the Indigenous Knowledge of the Tenyimia Nagas in Easterine Kire's *When the River Sleeps.*" *Humanities & Social Sciences Reviews* 8(1), 751–758.

Bhumika, R. 2019. "Engaging with the specific realities of postcolonial literatures: a discussion of the complex socio-cultural and political contours of contemporary Naga literature in English." *Asian Ethnicity* 22(4): 1–17. DOI: 10.1080/14631369.2019.1677453.

Chatterjee, Nilanjana. 2022. "The E-turn of the Naga English Writings: Easterine Kire and Culture Production." Sahapedia. https://map.sahapedia.org/article/The-E-turn-of-the-Naga-English-Writings:-Easterine-Kire-and-Culture-Production/11621.

Chatterjee, Subhasish, and Rahul Sharma. 2018. "Belief of Tribal's in Supernatural Power and Its Relation with Religious Life (with Special Reference to Indian Tribal Society)". *International Journal of Research and Analytical Reviews* 5, 48–55.

Dhanya, A.P., and Sudakshina Bhattacharya. 2019. "The Praxis of the Wedded Mystic: A Divergent Reading of Easterine Kire's Novel *When the River Sleeps.*" *Rupkatha Journal on Interdisciplinary Studies in Humanities* 11(3), 1–12. https://dx.doi.org/10.21659/rupkatha.v11n3.05. Accessed November 3, 2021.

Finley, Lana Louise. 2012. "Occult Americans: Invisible Culture and the Literary Imagination." PhD diss., University of California.

Fleming, John, and Robert J Ledogar. 2008. "Resilience and Indigenous Spirituality: A Literature Review." *Pimatisiwin* 6(2), 47–64. PMID: 20963185; PMCID: PMC2956755.

Gott, Richard. 2011. *Britain's Empire: Resistance, Repression and Revolt.* Brooklyn, NY: Verso.

Grieves, Vicki. 2008. "Aboriginal Spirituality: A Baseline for Indigenous Knowledge Development in Australia." *The Canadian Journal of Native Studies* 28, 363–398. http://www3.brandonu.ca/cjns/28.2/07Grieves.pdf. Accessed May 22, 2021.

Jakovljevic, Miro. 2017. "Psychiatry and Religion: Opponents or Collaborators?." *Psychiatria Danubina* 29, 82–88.

James, Lovely Awomi. 2015. "Indigenous Spirituality: Insights for a Life-Affirming and Life-Sustaining Economy of Life." *The Ecumenical Review* 67, 203–208. Accessed December 12, 2021. Indigenous Spirituality: Insights for a Life-Affirming and Life-Sustaining Economy of Life - James -2015- The Ecumenical Review - Wiley Online Library.

Karki, Rebecca. 2019. *Theoretical Perspectives on Easterine Kire's Writings in English.* M.Phil. Sikkim University. http://dspace.cus.ac.in/jspui/handle/1/6334.

Kechutzar, Sashikaba. 2008. "Omen, Divination and Dream (Tatakrutsu, Antokdangba/ Amsu and Pongmang): Medium for Divine Revelation." *Garnering Tribal Resources for Doing Tribal Christian Theology.* Edited by Razouselie Lasetso. Tribal Study Series No. 16. Jorhat: ETC Programme Coordination.

Kire, Easterine. 2014. *When the River Sleeps.* New Delhi: Zubaan.

———. 2017. *Don't Run My Love.* New Delhi: Speaking Tiger.

———. 2018. *Sky is My Father.* New Delhi: Speaking Tiger.

———. 2019a. *A Respectable Woman.* New Delhi: Zubaan.

———. 2019b. *Walking the Roadless Road: Exploring.* New Delhi: Aleph Book.

Lee, Morgan. March 30, 2021. "An Indian Christian Doctor Sees Covid-19's Silver Linings." https://www.christianitytoday.com/ct/2021/march-web-only/india-covid-19-pandemic-medical-association.html. Accessed April 16, 2021, November 18, 2021.

Patton, Jasmine. July 26, 2019. "Contemporary Naga Writings' Reclamation of Culture and History through Orality." www.thecuriousreader.in. Accessed February 11, 2020.

Ritskes, Eric. 2011. "Chapter Twenty-Six: Indigenous Spirituality and Decolonization: Methodology for the Classroom". *Counterpoints* 379, 411–421.

Rowkith, Shannal, and Raisuyah Bhagwan. 2020. "Honoring Tribal Spirituality in India: An Exploratory Study of Their Beliefs, Rituals and Healing Practices." *Religions* 11(11), 549. https://doi.org/10.3390/rel11110549.

Shekhar, Hansda Sowvendra. 2017. "When a Writer Reads Another, It Can Sometimes be Love (and Envy) at First Sight." https://scroll.in/article/827791/when-a-writer-reads-another-it-can-sometimes-be-love-and-envy-at-first-sight.

Verhelst, Thierry G. 1990. *No Life Without Roots: Culture and Development.* London: Zed Books Ltd.

Versluis, Arthur. 2004. *Restoring Paradise: Western Esotericism, Literature, Art, and Consciousness.* Albany: SUNY Press.

Willaert, Rita. July 3, 2020. "Traditional Lockdown Practices in the Naga Highlands." The Indian Forum. https://www.theindiaforum.in/letters/traditional-lockdown-practices-naga-highlands. Accessed January 31, 2022.

13 Dis-ease, Dis-order and the Refugee Experience

Appraising South Asian Partition Narratives

Debasri Basu

Introduction

British India, colonized by the East India Company in the eighteenth century and the British imperial government a century later, ultimately gained its freedom in August 1947. However, this political liberty came saddled with the Partition[1] of the subcontinent because of religious antagonism, leading to the independence of India and the creation of Muslim-majority Pakistan. While hundreds of thousands were killed, abducted, raped, and mutilated in this socio-political cataclysm, there were others who had to bear an indirect form of violence: sickness on account of physically rigorous journeys during the migration process across newly demarcated international borders, compounded by dearth of proper food, potable water, and medical facilities. They became easy victims of a gamut of diseases, leading to further loss of lives. Creative writers have striven to represent the untold miseries of these infirm men and women through their literary works, and this chapter analyzes three such fictional texts: "The Crystal Goblet" by Ritwik Ghatak, "Ya Khuda" by Qudrat Ullah Shahab, and "Hope" by Mohinder Singh Sarna. These stories, originally written in various vernaculars and subsequently translated into English, highlight the plight of those caught in the Partition maelstrom, while simultaneously showcasing the artistic response of their writers to this catastrophe. The governments in both India and Pakistan proved pitifully inadequate in providing relief and rehabilitation to the throngs of refugees arriving for months after the split, and the present chapter intends to explore how disease and death prowling the refugee convoys and camps underscore the general state of disorder in the subcontinent in the aftermath of its fateful vivisection.

Partition Violence and Migration

The movement of religious minorities to comparatively safer havens had started in the wake of the Great Calcutta Killings of August 1946,[2] much before the official division of the subcontinent. It went on intermittently throughout the succeeding months, to reach its apex the next year. Once the Mountbatten Plan[3] was announced on June 3, 1947, confirming the imperial government's decision

DOI: 10.4324/9781003300762-15

to partition the land, savagery took a record leap and hundreds of thousands were murdered or maimed in August-September.[4] It resulted in a stupendous rise in the influx of refugees on both the western and eastern sectors of the Indo-Pakistan border, continuing unabated for months thereon. Historian Mushirul Hasan (1997, 47) has estimated that this Partition resulted in almost twelve and a half million people, amounting to approximately 3 per cent of the population of undivided India, being displaced. The unofficial numbers could be more, as many of them remained undocumented, or were deprived of the "refugee" status on various, often flimsy, grounds.

Moreover, the monsoon and winter of 1947 were exceptionally severe in the northern parts of the subcontinent, and the resultant heavy rainfall (Pandey 1997, 2270) followed by the harsh cold (Chattha 2018, 277) aggravated the situation. The direct consequence of this insidious combination of manmade and natural adversities had to be borne by the refugees on both sides of the border. Even if spared from the enemy's sword or bullet, many of these ill-fated men and women contracted infections of all sorts during their journeys from their native places to their purported 'homeland'. While those hailing from the economically upper and middle classes could avail of faster modes of conveyance like trains and steamers, the poorer sections had no other option but to walk on foot or at the most travel by bullock-cart, unless they found themselves in the fortuitous position of being transported by military trucks once the 'exchange of populations' was taken up at the governmental levels. Such official arrangements, however, took place only on the western sector; Bengali refugees were extended no such assistance. Even so, these transport services proved to be few and far between, and most of the evacuees had to go through a laborious experience while fleeing for their lives. This became all the more cumbrous due to the fact that many of them were also carrying their belongings, no matter how meager, on them. U. Bhaskar Rao (1967, 16), who penned *The Story of Rehabilitation* recounting the authorized Indian version of the post-Partition migration, has stated that "at times, the caravans of the refugees could be as long as 240 kilometres with 50,000–60,000 refugees". In this context, he concedes that "often the sick and the feeble-bodied were abandoned by the roadside. So were the dead, with none to mourn them or perform obsequies. The living had no time for the dying and the dead" (Rao 1967, 17).

There was little in terms of relief and support to these refugee columns during their arduous travels, a fact also confirmed by Mohinder Singh Randhawa (1954) in *Out of Ashes: An Account of the Rehabilitation of Refugees from West Pakistan in Rural Areas of East Punjab*. This narrative, similar to Rao's book mentioned above, but framed in a regional setting, details the toils of refugees coming to the Indian side of Punjab. He goes on record to state that most of these people

> looked to their own selves, as few showed pity for age or sex, and many aged or infirm persons who could not walk were deserted by their relations and left to die on the roadside. Mothers threw their newborn babies in bushes along the roadside and left them to die. The urge among the columns was to

escape Pakistan and to cover the journey in the quickest possible time. Such a quick exit was possible only if one had the physical ability or the means to possess sturdy bullock carts. The ones who possessed bullock carts could place their bundles in the carts to gain speed, while others not so fortunate carried them on their heads. Among them were landless Harijans, and village workers, who did not possess any bullock carts of their own, and were accompanying their co-villagers.

(Quoted in Kaur 2007, 73–75)

Malnutrition, fatigue, and paucity of medical amenities contributed greatly to their escalating death count, and the authorities failed miserably in rising to the occasion and offering relief to these hordes. The Indian government initially opened some Transit and Relief Camps in different parts of East Punjab, Delhi, and West Bengal to offer temporary accommodation to these teeming millions. However, the hardships of these refugees did not end with their arrival at such supposed havens. Provisions were piteously small in these camps, and the exhausting circumstances often affected the health of the dwellers.

Contagion in the Times of Partition

The dismal state of hygiene and sanitation in refugee camps caused diseases to spread rapidly, and epidemics were not unheard of during these tumultuous times. Ritwik Ghatak[5] poignantly captures the anguish of bereaved and dispossessed refugees in his short story "The Crystal Goblet", focusing on the taint of cholera which was widespread at such sites. The narrator, a civil servant visiting Delhi to attend a family function, was struck by the sight of "bands of displaced, homeless refugees" (Ghatak 2012a, 295) dotting the streets and railway platforms of India's capital. On a whim to have a look at "this new tribe of beggars" (Ghatak 2012a, 296) from close quarters, he sauntered along a road to a refugee camp located outside the city limits, and was handed down a lesson in humility. The place was basically a slum, hurriedly erected out of dried-up stalks of crops in the middle of a field. He felt dazed by the absence of even the bare necessities of a civilized life: "Filthy, tattered clothes and despairing looks made up a stark picture of naked pauperism. How the meagre straw thatching could ward off the sharp sting of the January cold was certainly something one could make the subject of research!" (Ghatak 2012a, 296).

The unnamed narrator soon learned that a cholera epidemic was at that time rampant among the camp-dwellers, and noticed a group of nurses caring for the patients. Inoculation was being carried out in one of the rooms, and he saw a girl there "smeared with vomit" and flies "swarming around her" (Ghatak 2012a, 296). His attention was abruptly redirected towards "a heart-rending wail" rising from another room, and he proceeded there along with some of the other bystanders to explore the source of the sound which had, by then, turned into "a stifling sob" (Ghatak 2012a, 296). They discovered a young woman groaning over the gasping body of a beautiful child. She was crying out "Mera munna, mera lal" (Ghatak 2012a, 297) from time to time; literally meaning 'My son, my boy', her words were common terms of endearment in her native Hindustani language. According to the narrator, the mother "must have been pretty some time in the remote past; now she looked unclean and had a pained and panic-stricken expression on her face" (Ghatak 2012a, 296). When the doctor checked the pulse of the child and shook his head, it became evident that the boy had become yet another statistic in the colossal human tragedy that was the 1947 Partition.

The remaining part of the story reveals how even such a tragic incident as the untimely loss of a child could be rendered absurd by the uphill task of survival. The narrator was surprised to find the mother quickly picking up the blanket her son had earlier kicked away, and making her way out of the room. She settled in a corner of the verandah, having wrapped herself up in that blanket without delay. By then the doctor was asking for the parent of the child, while a couple of orderlies had put the corpse on a string cot to bring it outside. The mother looked up nervously at them, her lips "slightly apart as if she wanted to cry her heart out. But she stifled her sobs by pressing her mouth with her two dirty, petal-like hands" (Ghatak 2012a, 298). The narrator, astonished at this response which was so divergent from her previous hysteric laments, felt compelled to offer words of consolation and in the process, accidentally fingered the corner of her blanket. This had an instantaneous reaction from the mother who jerked away like a flash and mumbled: "Don't, don't, ...take that – I feel cold" (Ghatak 2012a, 298). When the narrator assuaged her fear and explained that he was not part of the camp staff, she disclosed: "They'll take it away if they come to know who the blanket belongs to...in these terribly cold days" (Ghatak 2012a, 298). She was apprehensive that the "germ-ridden rug" would be disposed of once the blanket's antecedents were known. Her words expose the stark reality of women and men who found themselves in the same miserable situation by quirks of fate, and the narrator, after overcoming his initial shock, comprehended this grim truth: "She must have witnessed that happen to others....Those who are interested in taking, merely take without wanting to give anything back in return" (Ghatak 2012a, 298). Along with him, the reader too realizes that having become indigents all of a sudden after communal riots robbed them of their belongings, these people were now living in a strictly Hobbesian state where there were no enforceable criteria of right and wrong. Even death had lost its sting in the struggle that was waged day in day out, and the refugees took for themselves all that they could without any thought to gentility and discretion.

Such dreadful conditions were not confined to India's capital city or other places in north India but stretched to the east as well. Similar scenes were to be found in West Bengal which had the unenviable distinction of receiving Partition refugees in multiple phases long after 1947 owing to waves of violence against religious minorities in East Pakistan (Sinha 2015, 823). These hapless millions were harbored in different types of refugee camps – Transit and Relief Camps, Work-site Camps, Colony Camps, and Permanent Liability camps [later called 'Homes of Infirmities'] – set up by the West Bengal government at various places across the state. A range of ailments from cholera and small pox to tuberculosis, malaria, dysentery, amebiasis, diphtheria, pneumonia, asthma, kala-azar [black fever] and scabies besieged the refugees there, apart from the common complaints of malnutrition and fever (Sengupta Chatterjee 2015). Lack of proper sanitation turned these environs hellish, with historian Joya Chatterji (2007, 1011) mentioning one such camp located at Jirat in Hooghly district where "during the monsoon, the flooded lavatories polluted the surrounding area and water in the tanks". Irregular disposal of corpses compounded matters, for often the dead were not cremated in a timely manner but stocked in a pile to be disposed of only once a week when a truck came to take them to the crematorium. The camp inmates were forced to carry out their daily activities in the same premises, causing further spread of disease among these refugees as also the local residents.[6]

Disease and Death in Refugee Camps

The scenario across the border in Pakistan was comparable, with reports of a host of maladies plaguing the refugees. Partition scholar Ilyas Chattha (2018, 274) states that "[i]n addition to the mass killings of hundreds of thousands, thousands of people died of starvation, exhaustion, cholera and grief". The country's Finance Minister Ghulam Mohammad too admitted to this dismal situation while referring to refugees pouring into Lahore: "They are growing too weak to move. Most of them are moving on foot without any supplies. We learn that they are dying at a rate of about a thousand a day" (quoted in Chattha 2018, 275). Qudrat Ullah Shahab's[7] short story "Ya Khuda" [O God] portrays these harrowing issues through the experiences of women, children, and the aged. Originally written in Urdu and later translated into English by Faruq Hassan, it is the tale of Dilshad, a young Muslim woman hailing from Chamkor village in Ambala district of East Punjab. Her father Ali Bakhsh, a mullah, had already been killed by the Sikh miscreants who formed a majority there, and she too suffered sexual abuse at the hands of these perpetrators. For her, as with countless other Indian Muslims, the vision of West Punjab in the newly founded Pakistan had come accompanied with the promise of "a life of dignity and comfort" (Shahab 2005, 276). Eventually, she managed to escape the clutches of her captors and boarded a train traveling to the "west", signifying her cherished homeland. By this time she was pregnant, an outcome of the prolonged sexual violence inflicted on her body. During this journey, she experienced labor pains and gave birth to a daughter in the railway compartment. When the train reached its terminal station, she discovered that it was Lahore – a city located a few kilometers into West Pakistan. However, her hopes were rudely dashed right at the very outset when a sweeper woman hurled expletives at her: "The slut. Polluted the whole compartment; couldn't even wait; gave birth right here…" (Shahab 2005, 278). Unable to find much succor from the passersby on the platform, she got branded as a *Mohajir* and was urged by them to go to the *Mohajir* Camp.

Till then, Dilshad had no clue about the import of the term *Mohajir* – a word derived from the Arabic *muhājir* denoting a 'migrant' with a religious undertone. It is associated in early Islamic history with the migration of the Prophet from Mecca to Medina. Muslims who relocated from India, mainly from Punjab, United Provinces, and Bihar, came to be known by this name in Pakistan. Incidentally, Lahore had harbored the largest refugee camp in West Pakistan as the city became the entry point for most of the migrants and evacuees taking flight from East Punjab. Beleaguered with the huge inflow of refugees, the state of affairs there too was far from ideal, notwithstanding the fact that this country had been promoted by the Muslim League leaders as the panacea for all ills supposedly afflicting the Indian Muslim populace before the Partition. Alluding to interviews and diaries of volunteers who worked in refugee camps of Lahore, Chattha (2018, 275) reminds that "[a] great number of refugees died of cholera, malaria, diarrhoea and respiratory diseases. Many wounded died because they could not receive any immediate medical treatment". In an attempt to contain the spread of infection, the authorities even established a separate Cholera Camp at Kasur near Lahore (Chattha 2018, 278). The wretched condition of a similar refugee camp in Lahore is described in Shahab's story where Dilshad heads to from the railway station. After providing her name and family details to the clerk, she looked around the premises which were to be her initial home in Pakistan – the "land of the pure". Shahab's portrayal of the camp is bleak enough to indicate the shabby living conditions of its inhabitants; measuring around 800 by 500 feet, it was "a yard surrounded by barbed wire all around under an open sky" (Shahab 2005, 285). Dilshad found an empty space where she could rest for the night but was not able to eat or sleep like the others since she carried no possessions. An elderly man took pity on her destitute state and lent his bowl so that she may collect food from the camp kitchen. He also informed her about the clothes store near the kitchen from where she could borrow bedding and warm apparel for her infant. The store at the camp was surprisingly well-stocked: "Quilts lay in piles inside a tent; also black, red and brown blankets. In one corner there was a small heap of woolen clothing – sweaters, waistcoats, shawls" (Shahab 2005, 287). But the store clerk curtly turned her away, citing that the Office was closed and that she should come back the next morning at 8. Dilshad pleaded her situation, informing that she had no warm attire, but the clerk remained unmoved, maintaining that "[n]obody will die" (Shahab 2005, 287) – an assurance that proves to be painfully hollow once the plot unfolds. When she beseeched again, the man got annoyed and gruffly dismissed her.

The atmosphere grew colder, and the ensuing lines of the story relate in agonizing detail its punishing effect on those like Dilshad who had to fend it without the requisite accoutrements:

> As the night advanced, the cold started becoming unbearable, and gradually it began to seem as if the whole universe was freezing up. Blasts of cold hit the body like arrows, and moisture in the ground pricked it like thorns.
>
> (Shahab 2005, 287–288)

Dilshad's teeth clattered in the extreme cold, and she sat holding the baby wrapped in the woolen flannel close to her breast. In an effort to generate some heat from movement, she at times sat up or began walking. Sadly, none of these measures were helpful enough and the cold steadily crept into her bones. With every ticking minute, she became afraid that "she would freeze like an ice cube and fall down" (Shahab 2005, 288). To make matters worse, it started raining after a while, and Dilshad felt as if the raindrops were shots from an air gun or scimitars of the Sikhs like Amrik Singh, Tarlok Singh, Surmukh Singh, and Darbara Singh who had sexually assaulted her in Chamkor. With the passing hours, the rainwater began to seep through her daughter's clothes and the baby started shivering. It seemed as if nature too had transformed into a malicious force during those distressing times and joined hands with the vicious men in an unholy alliance to inflict cruelties on Dilshad and her ilk.

The severe weather resulted in a similar plight for the old man who had earlier shown kindness to Dilshad. He had just one blanket and had utilized it to cover his young grandchildren Mahmood and Zubeida. Wrapped in only a thin soiled bedsheet, the man lay on the ground tossing and turning during the night, and by the time Dilshad thought of seeking his permission to use a part of the blanket to cover her daughter, life had already left his aged, frail corporal form. The grandfather had gone "beyond any concern for heat and cold. Blood had already frozen in his veins; his body was stiff like an iron rod" (Shahab 2005, 289). As it emerged, his was not the sole fatality in this dark and inclement night, for a little ahead of them was another young woman trying hard to transfer the warmth of her body into her four-year-old girl. Like Dilshad and her daughter, they too had neither quilt, nor a blanket, nor any sheet. The girl was breathing with extreme difficulty, her chest wheezing and whistling when she drew each breath. As the temperature plummeted, these sounds turned into "a ringing of bells, as if the angels of life and death were locked in a mortal battle" (Shahab 2005, 288). In a desperate attempt to provide her daughter warmth, the mother looked around and then, hesitatingly, took off her clothes to wrap them around her sick girl. A shaft of lightning during the rains showed the naked body of the young woman to the world, the cruel irony not lost on the readers that piles of quilts and blankets were lying unutilized in the nearby tent. The author remarks sardonically that the "bare body of that woman was the worst insult to all that had been achieved by mankind; it darkened the face of the night even more" (Shahab 2005, 289).

Shahab's depiction of this scene is, without a doubt, intended to expose the brazen callousness of such camp personnel who were negligent of their duties and turned a blind eye to the suffering of these hapless refugees. Incidentally, it offers a close resemblance to the words of Ali Muhammad Khan, the then-president of the Muslim League branch in Great Britain, who had visited Lahore on a fact-finding mission. Having completed his three-week tour of the districts in West Punjab, he deplored in an interview:

> "What I have seen of the refugees has shattered my nerves and I believe my report to my organization will go a long way in opening their eyes with regard to the utter callousness and demoralization of the administration in

West Punjab which has failed from top to bottom to discharge its official, national and moral obligations towards unfortunate brethren from East Punjab." The officials, he said were not only unsympathetic, but were positively cruel and heartless.

(Quoted in Singh 1995, 82)

Not surprisingly, with the emergence of the sun's first rays the next morning in Shahab's story, the horrors of the night too came to light. The girl had died, and her mother was seen clinging to her corpse. A thin film of moisture was visible on the mother's "half-closed eyes, as though her tears too had frozen with her blood" (Shahab 2005, 289). The news of these deaths brought some camp sweepers to the site, and they spread blankets on the corpses. In a bizarre move, they also kept covering the dead with woolen shrouds evoking envious stares from those who were still alive:

> ... if death did not involve a fear of the unseen and the unknown, they would all have been willing to die at that moment. Their bodies would also be wrapped in blankets and their shivering flesh and bones too would receive some warmth, some peace, some comfort.

(Shahab 2005, 290)

These lines, while acutely disturbing, also introduce an element of the macabre into the story.

As it happened, concerns over the condition of refugees in the grueling winter months had been raised in Pakistan more than once during that phase. Amtul Hasan in his book *Impact of Partition: Refugees in Pakistan: Struggle for Empowerment and State's Response* mentions the Deputy Commissioner of Lahore inaugurating a 'Quilt Week' in the city after the Partition, with the express objective of urging the residents to donate quilts. Liaquat Ali Khan, the first Prime Minister of Pakistan, too had requested other countries for assistance in this connection, stating that "two and a half million Muslim refugees will shortly have to face the rigors of Western Pakistan winter. It is of the utmost importance that they be provided with warm clothing and blankets" (quoted in Hasan 2006, 54). Even so, the contributions were pathetically scant for these languishing masses, and most of them had to fend for themselves in the later stages. While the men took up physical labor to earn a living, the women, particularly those without any male members with them, became extremely vulnerable. A number of such women ultimately ended up becoming victims of the flesh trade, a fate also befalling Dilshad in the third and final part of Shahab's story.

The Silver Lining

Not all tales of the Partition, though, end in such despair, and Mohinder Singh Sarna's[8] short story "Hope" is a testament to this. Written originally in Punjabi and subsequently translated into English by his son Navtej Sarna, it is the touching account of a bond developing between a refugee woman and her elderly neighbor. The unnamed narrator and her husband had reached Delhi after great difficulty and had found shelter in Lady Hardinge hostel which, till then, had been reserved for the attendants of patients admitted to Lady Hardinge Hospital. She was pregnant at that time, and the challenging circumstances had made her pensive: "Helpless as straws buffeted in the huge refugee wave that followed the dreadful aftermath of the country's partition, people had clung to whichever shore that came to hand" (Sarna 2013, 102). Her pregnancy, coupled with the surrounding turmoil, had filled her with a "strange restlessness" and "deep dejection" (Sarna 2013, 102). Since her husband was fortunate enough to secure a job after their migration, financial crisis had been averted; yet, the distressing sight of other refugees in the hostel had cast a pall of gloom over her. She was troubled by the thoughts of these people whose sole fault lay in that they were natives of parts of the subcontinent which had fallen "victim of an accursed political decision of departing rulers, and were left at the mercy of an angry fate" (Sarna 2013, 102).

The adjacent room was occupied by an old Sikh man who had arrived the day after this couple had started living in that hostel. He was an enigma, for he kept to himself and never spoke with others. The narrator had noticed that the aged man was without any family members and would "pass by quietly, eyes lowered, lost in faraway thoughts" (Sarna 2013, 103). Although he appeared distant to everyone else, she could visualize a father figure in him, and the fact that she had lost her own father while still a child may have strengthened this sentiment. One day the man did not emerge from his room in the morning, and the narrator began feeling anxious about his well-being. She went into his room to enquire about his health, and was upset to discover that her apprehension had proved correct. He was ill, lying curled up on a badly crushed blanket on an old string cot in the corner. His bloodshot eyes indicated that he had a high fever, and the narrator immediately grew worried. She felt his pulse and then covered him with the blanket before sending a young Sindhi boy next door to fetch the doctor. Realizing that his illness had caused him to remain without food or drink for hours, the narrator made tea for him. Having grown extremely weak, he had to remain bedridden for almost a week, and she tended to the ailing man despite the advanced stage of her pregnancy.

It was during this period of convalescence that the old man, a refugee from the northwestern part of the subcontinent, shared his tale of woe with the narrator. Both his son Navjot and daughter Navneet had lost their lives in the Partition frenzy, and the man was now merely a shell of his former self, resembling a person who had been drained of all vitality. Having chanced upon a newspaper piece carrying an announcement of the invention of "a bomb which is ten times more destructive than the atomic bomb" (Sarna 2013, 107), the man estimated that life on the planet would exist for "only six months from now" (Sarna 2013, 103). A chill ran down the spine of the narrator at his ominous words, more so since her thoughts immediately gravitated toward her unborn child. She realized that the blows of fate had caused the old man to become a cynic, and he now felt that humans did not deserve to live. Before long, she gave birth to twins – a girl and a boy – and in honor of the deceased children of the elderly Sikh, she decided to name her daughter and son Navneet and Navjot respectively. When the old man visited the narrator in the hospital and learned about this development, it warmed the cockles of his heart: "his eyes misted over" and he "kept smiling happily" (Sarna 2013, 108). The gesture had managed to tide over his erstwhile pessimism, and he expressed hope that people across the world would raise their voices against hydrogen bombs. His final declaration that "[l]ife cannot be defeated by atomic and hydrogen bombs" signals the optimistic note on which the author ends his tale.

Conclusion

Illness narratives have emerged in the postcolonial era as a distinct genre, particularly in the field of anthropology. These chronicles encompass illness experiences, and anthropologist Veena Das (2015, 28) characterizes them as "indexing the disorder of political and economic conditions in the postcolonial scenarios of civil wars" and "economic collapse". The three short stories discussed in this chapter may be considered under such a rubric as well, for although fictional in nature, they are not removed from reality, as borne by corresponding historical documents. The authors of these tales have related the agony of people who had to bear the dual brunt of being uprooted from their ancestral homes and getting afflicted by terrible diseases. Yet, it is pertinent to remember that religious rivalry spewing acute hatred proved to be the gravest malady gripping large chunks of the Indian public around this time. The rift between Muslims and non-Muslims (mainly Hindus and Sikhs) spawned pathogens of violence that went on to afflict the Indian subcontinent to an alarming extent. As with any major turbulent event, these disturbances caused a massive breakdown in the chain of command of both the civil and military wings of the government. The Partition-related division of assets had already weakened the existing official machinery, and the consequent transfer of officers and staff to the country of their choice further destabilized the administration. As such, the infrastructure of the recently independent India and the newly established Pakistan were grossly insufficient to cater to the needs of these suffering multitudes. This "dis-order" adversely affected the overall health of the body politic in several ways, and was not limited to the actual instances of ailments wreaking havoc on the physical well-being of the masses. It also resulted in a disruption in the sense of security that is associated with any stable society, causing a "dis-ease" in the minds of the commoners, including those who were not explicitly harmed by the Partition riots. This malaise seeped into other parts of the subcontinent and became all-pervasive in those tormenting years of the mid-twentieth century. Even the passage of three-quarters of a century has not been capable of fully healing its ravages – physical, psychological, or societal – although some instances of compassion witnessed during those dark times do allow us the latitude to envision a more humane future.

Notes

1 The provinces of Bengal in the eastern part and Punjab in the western part of British India were divided into two, taking into consideration their religious demographic. According to Sir Cyril Radcliffe's Partition Award, Muslim-majority North-West Frontier Province, Baluchistan, Sind and West Punjab were allotted to West Pakistan; eastern Bengal became East Pakistan, while Sylhet went to East Pakistan after the Sylhet Referendum of July 6–7, 1947. Historian Yasmin Khan (2007) provides a comprehensive account of this momentous event in the subcontinent's history in her book *The Great Partition: The Making of India and Pakistan*, shedding light on both the western and eastern sectors.

2 The Muslim League had given a call to observe August 16, 1946 as 'Direct Action Day' with the express objective of attaining a homeland for Indian Muslims. The unrests triggering after the public meeting held in Calcutta, the capital of Bengal province, in the wake of this explosive slogan went on for four days. Historian Sumit Sarkar (2000, 432), citing contemporary sources, has put the casualties in this riot at 4,000 deaths, while another 10,000 were injured.

3 This plan, formally known as the Indian Independence Act, was hailed as a crucial achievement of the last viceroy of colonial India, Lord Louis Mountbatten, but it initiated the chain of events which ultimately ended in unprecedented bloodbath.

4 The death toll associated with the Indian Partition has been put at diverse figures by different sources, and varies from 200,000 to 2 million (Pandey 2001).

5 Ghatak (1925–1976), better known as filmmaker extraordinaire for his Partition movies *Megha Dhaka Tara* (1960), *Komal Gandhar* (1961) and *Subarnarkeha* (1962), was a prolific writer in Bangla [Bengali] as well. He penned 40 odd short stories (though only 15 are extant), 2 novels, 6 plays, 25 screenplays and more than 80 film critiques. He was a native of Dhaka in eastern Bengal and had to relocate to Calcutta after the Partition. Apart from the story discussed in this chapter, translated from the Bengali original "Spatikpatra" (1949) into English by Rani Ray, [another English version (1979) has the title "Cocktail Glass"], some of his other Partition tales are "The Road" ["Sadak"] and "The Earthly Paradise Remains Unshaken" ["Bhuswarga Achanchal"].

6 Prafulla Chakrabarti has given the most comprehensive account of Bengali Partition refugees in his seminal book *The Marginal Men: The Refugees and The Left Political Syndrome in West Bengal*.

7 Shahab (1917–1986), a Pakistani civil servant by profession, was also an eminent Urdu writer, his best known work being the autobiography *Shahab Nama* (1987).

8 Sarna (1923–2001) was an Indian bureaucrat and Punjabi author of repute, having written scores of short stories, novels and poems over a six-decade long literary career. Born in Rawalpindi located in western Punjab, he moved to Delhi in the wake of the Partition disturbances, and the theme is handled from sundry perspectives in his short stories compiled in the anthology *Savage Harvest: Stories of Partition*.

References

Chakrabarti, Prafulla K. 1990. *The Marginal Men: The Refugees and The Left Political Syndrome in West Bengal*. Rahara: Lumiere.

Chatterji, Joya. 2007. "'Dispersal' and Failure of Rehabilitation: Refugees Camp-dwellers and Squatters in West Bengal." *Modern Asian Studies*, 41, no. 5 (September): 995–1032. Accessed February 19, 2022. doi: 10.101 7/S0026749X07002831.

Chattha, Ilyas. 2018. "After the Massacres: Nursing Survivors of Partition Violence in Pakistan Punjab Camps." *Journal of the Royal Asiatic Society, Series 3*, 28, no. 2: 273–293. Accessed February 6, 2022. doi:10.1017/S1356186317000694.

Das, Veena. 2015. *Afflictions: Health, Disease, Poverty.* New Delhi: Orient Blackswan.

Ghatak, Ritwik. 2012a. "The Crystal Goblet." In *Stories about the Partition of India,* edited by Alok Bhalla, 4:295–302. New Delhi: Manohar.

———. 2012b. "The Earthly Paradise Remains Unshaken." In *Stories about the Partition of India,* edited by Alok Bhalla, 4:133–141. New Delhi: Manohar.

———. 2012c. "The Road." In *Mapmaking: Partition Stories from Two Bengals,* edited by Debjani Sengupta, 1–15. New Delhi: Amaryllis.

Hasan, Amtul. 2006. *Impact of Partition: Refugees in Pakistan: Struggle for Empowerment and State's Response.* New Delhi: Manohar.

Hasan, Mushirul. 1997. "Partition: The Human Cost." *History Today,* 47, no. 9: 47–53. Accessed April 14, 2009. http://www.historytoday.com/mushirul-hasan/partition-human-cost.

Kaur, Ravinder. 2007. *Since 1947: Partition Narratives among Punjabi Migrants of Delhi.* New Delhi: Oxford University Press.

Khan, Yasmin. 2007. *The Great Partition: The Making of India and Pakistan.* New Delhi: Viking.

Pandey, Gyanendra. 1997. "Partition and Independence in Delhi: 1947–48." *Economic and Political Weekly,* 32, no. 36 (September 6–12): 2261–2272. Accessed April 6, 2010. http://www.jstor.org/stable/4405816.

———. 2001. *Remembering Partition: Violence, Nationalism and History of India.* London: Cambridge University Press.

Randhawa, Mohinder Singh. 1954. *Out of Ashes: An Account of the Rehabilitation of Refugees from West Pakistan in Rural Areas of East Punjab.* Chandigarh: Public Relations Department, Punjab.

Rao, U Bhaskar 1967. *The Story of Rehabilitation.* New Delhi: Publications Divisions, Ministry of Information and Broadcasting.

Sarkar, Sumit. 2000. *Modern India: 1885–1947.* New Delhi: Macmillan.

Sarna, Mohinder Singh. 2013. "Hope." In *Savage Harvest: Stories of Partition,* 102–108. New Delhi: Rupa.

Sengupta Chattejee, Swati. 2015. "Sanitation and Health at West Bengal Refugee Camps in the 1950s." *Vidyasagar University Journal of History,* III, 82–94. Accessed February 6, 2022. 8 West Bengal Camp Refugees in 1950.pdf (vidyasagar.ac.in).

Shahab, Qudrat Ullah. 1987. *Shahab Nama.* Lahore: Sang-e-Meel.

———. 2005. "Ya Khuda." In *Orphans of the Storm: Stories on the Partition of India,* edited by Saros Cowasjee and K. S. Duggal, 268–304. New Delhi: UBS.

Singh, Ganda. 1995. "A Diary of Partition Days." In *India Partitioned: The Other Face of Freedom,* edited by Mushirul Hasan, 2:27–86. Delhi: Roli.

Sinha, Avirup. 2015. "Refugee Influx, their Health and Hygiene Related Problems and Its Impact: A Case of Displaced Persons in Calcutta and Its Neighbourhood (1947–1952)." *Proceedings of the Indian History Congress,* 76: 822–829. Accessed February 6, 2022. https://www.jstor.org/stable/44156650.

14 Always in Search of her Ithaca

Women's Spiritual Well-being
in *Journey to Ithaca: A Pilgrimage in
Search of Identity* and *Eat, Pray, Love:
One Woman's Search for Everything*

Nibedita Mukherjee

Introduction

> Contemporary feminists have been the first to call attention to the exist-
> ence of a fundamental alliance between 'woman' and 'madness'. They have
> shown how women, within our dualistic systems of language and representa-
> tion, are typically situated on the side of irrationality, silence, nature, and
> body, while men are situated on the side of reason, discourse, culture, and
> mind.
>
> (Showalter 1987, 3–4)

Madness, like gender, is taken to be a constructed entity as in terms of behavio-
ral norms, it is patriarchy that decides what is 'normal' and hence acceptable in
society (Busfield 1996). Beauvoir has clearly stated "One is not born, but rather
becomes, woman" (2011, 330) and that

> woman has always been, if not man's slave, at least his vassal; the two sexes
> have never divided the world up equally; and still today, even though her
> condition is changing woman is heavily handicapped. In no country is
> her legal status identical to man's, and often it puts her at a considerable
> disadvantage.
>
> (2011, 29)

In the nineteenth century 'madness' began to be seen as a curable disease and the
'madman' of the earlier times lost his fearsome anomaly. The concept of 'mental
illness' came to be related to the fragile and dangerously seductive (as argued)
female character and it became a 'female malady' (Showalter 1987, 21). As per
psychiatry, the 'female madness' denoted

> depressive, hysterical, suicidal, and self-destructive behaviour thus became
> closely associated, from Victorian times, with stereotypes of womanhood in
> the writings of the psychiatric profession, in the public mind, and amongst
> women themselves. Freud himself classically asked: 'what do women want?',

DOI: 10.4324/9781003300762-16

and went on to diagnose penis envy. Classic hysteria, so common in Freud's day, may also have disappeared, but it has perhaps metamorphosed into new and primarily female conditions, notably anorexia nervosa, somatization disorder, and bulimia.

(Porter 2003, 88)

Showalter (1987, 61) discusses how in the late nineteenth century, unmarried middle-aged women were stigmatized by the use of terms like 'superfluous', 'redundant' and 'odd'. This feminization of mental health has been the subject of concern as *Sex and Seclusion* (Andrews and Digby 2004) and *Women's Voices in nineteenth Century Medical Discourse* (Theriot 1993) clearly pointed out. This trend continued even in the twentieth and twenty-first century and in *Women and Madness* (1972, 2005), Phyllis Chesler argued that women who dared to break traditional gender roles were skilfully designated as being mad or 'hysteric'. She writes, "What we consider 'madness',' whether it appears in women or in men, is either the acting out of the devalued female role, or the total or partial rejection of one's sex role stereotype" (Chesler 1972, 93).

Historical Perspective

The very word 'hysteria' was derived from the Greek word *hystera* which meant uterus. The Greeks conceived a notion that 'hysteria' was caused by unquenched physical desires. Plato in *Timaeus* stated that

the womb is an animal which longs to generate children. When it remains barren too long after puberty, it is distressed and sorely disturbed, and straying about in the body and cutting off the passages of the breath, it impedes respiration and brings the sufferer into the /extremist anguish and provokes all manner of diseases besides.

(Micale 2019, 19)

Nineteenth century onwards psychiatrists started linking gender to icons of insanity such as hysteria, anorexia nervosa, and neurasthenia. Treatment also came to be related to female physiognomy typically. Silas Weir Mitchell, an American physician, in his book *Fat and Blood* (1877) refers to the 'rest-cure' treatment wherein women were confined to their beds and were forced to consume an overwhelming diet of fattening food. This treatment led to the demeaning and darker perspective that the "rest-cure could be used to discipline women whose illness became a means of avoiding household duties" (Stiles, 4). Showalter argues that such anti-women treatment was caused by the fact that the psychiatry profession was male-dominated and female doctors were not allowed to join the Medico-Psychological Association (Showalter 1987, 127).

From the nineteenth century to the present, 'madness' and its symbolical cure has served as a trope in writings by women, which intends to present a counter-discourse to the male representation of women. Gilbert and Gubar posits "is a pen a metaphorical penis?" (1979, 3) and go on to discuss how patriarchy has always projected women's writing as a rebellion. The male narratives which romanticized the archetypes of madwomen through varied syndromes such as 'The Ophelia',[1] and 'The Lucia'[2]– all representing characters from literary works by men (Showalter 1987, 92), believed in projecting women as "The Angel in the House" (Patmore 1887) and this was completely as opposed to the female authors who started projecting women of inherent strength and indomitable spirit. Virginia Woolf spoke of the necessity of killing this image of "The Angel in the House" but she also pointed out how this led to the women author being perceived by patriarchy as the monster or the demonic self that cannot survive the societal imprisonment. She argues that a female writer "feels herself to be literally or figuratively crippled by the debilitating alternatives her culture offers her" (Gilbert and Gubar 1984, 57). This very perspective is named by Gilbert and Gubar as 'dis-ease' and it is this that leads to women's ultimate fragmentation. A study of Freud's *Dora: An Analysis of a Case of* Hysteria (1905) in the light of three literary texts belonging to different time frames, i.e., *Jane Eyre*, by Charlotte Brontë (1847), *Wide Sargasso Sea*, by Jean Rhys (1966) and *Grounded*, by George Brant (2013), proves that female mental suffering has always been perceived with societal lenses.

Mental Illness and Spirituality

There has been an ongoing debate regarding mental illness and spirituality. Researchers like Bergin (1983), Larson (1992), Hill and Pargament (2003), and Hatala (2013) have all argued that though mental illness and spirituality are dependent on multiple variables, in the majority of cases they depict a co-relation between spirituality, mental illness, and health promoting factors. The situation becomes even more complex when one considers the relation between women's illness and religion. Since the thirteenth century there has existed a link between religion, spirituality, and mental health. The earliest mental health hospital was built in 1247 called the Priory of St. Mary of Bethlehem which was supposed to provide shelter to 'distracted people'. Seventeenth century onwards there was a noticeable shift between religion and mental health. But psychoanalytical research of present times has depicted how spirituality is a multifaceted theoretical construct which enables an individual to rise above and beyond 'the real I' and be in a state transcendence which constitutes a state of peace, and harmony within the self (Boswell et al. 2006).

The female body is said to be a complex organism which suffers on account of multiple complex biological and psychological factors. Empirical research has been carried out to pinpoint how physiognomy and hormonal intervention leads to mental disorders in women (Andrews and Mathews 2004). The process of 'becoming and being' a mother aggravated the problem further as

> biology of becoming a mother and the psychology of being a mother entail complex processes which, even if things run smoothly in the best of all possible worlds, are marked by periods of susceptibility and fragility. In more

hostile and uneasy social environments they can be subjected to a range of pressures which make motherhood very difficult and mothers themselves vulnerable to a range of problems.

(Baistow 2007, 104)

So, the complex female physiognomy, in coursing through different stages of evolution (girlhood, motherhood, etc.) experiences emotional and hormonal upheaval which challenges their mental health which again may be real, or society induced (Butler 1993). Hence came the assertion that women were more susceptible to mental disorders on account of their gender, and it is spirituality which often granted a healing touch to the suffering female mind.

Spirituality is perceived as "a more general, unstructured, personalized, and naturally occurring phenomenon, where a person seeks closeness and/or connectedness between him/herself and a higher power or purpose" (Joseph et al. 2017, 506). Here, there exists a basic difference between religion and spirituality. Religion is based upon social beliefs and manifests itself through specific rituals whereas spirituality deals in the domain of personal experience and self-improvement through the creation of a being superior that the existing self (Thoresen 1998). Studies show how it leads to improvement of coping skills and positive outcomes for mental health related issues (Kharitonov 2012; Mueller et al. 2001).

Anita Desai and the Eastern Discourse of Spirituality

Journey to Ithaca by Anita Desai represents this quest of three different individuals hailing from three different places – Matteo is from Italy; Sophie is from Germany and Laila of Egypt. All three are disturbed souls who unknowingly desire to heal through their personal quests which again are varied and yet integrated. Matteo had always been a misfit and it is his travel to the East that finally led to his realization of his true identity, one which was linked to that of the Mother, his spiritual guide. His search takes him from Italy to India, from Bombay to Goa where he receives his moment of transcendence. Looking fixedly at a stone lodged in a tree trunk he perceives:

> Not a stone at all but a circle and it contained within it another circle, and another; that there was no beginning and no end to them, they were infinite, they were infinity. That circle was the universe itself, containing world within world, ring upon ring, sphere within sphere, and to his dazzled eyes they revolved within each other and yet remained perfectly static, maintaining a total balance and harmony that could only be divine.

(Desai 1995, 65)

Hermann Hesses's novel *Journey to the East* (1932) served as a model for Anita Desai's *Journey to Ithaca*. She here unites the essence of spiritual India manifested through the Vedantic philosophy as portrayed in the *Geeta*, the *Vedas*, and the *Upanishads*. Hindu worldview speaks of the healing of the wounded soul (the root cause of mental illness) through the understanding of the texts that preach the balance of the four elements – Earth, air, water, and fire – that constitute the human body. Matteo's search for mental peace and tranquility "to find India to understand India, and the mystery that is at the heart of India" (Desai 1995, 57) takes him to the Mother (Laila in her earlier life) who lives in an Ashram at the foothills of the Himalayas.

Sophie, Matteo's wife does not approve of Matteo's dedication to his eastern Guru. Her western pragmatism does not allow her to accept the concept of '*nish-kamkarma*' (work without desire for any worldly gains) as presented by The *Bhag-wad Geeta*. Sophie feels that "Work is work and should bear fruit" (Desai 1995, 125), but Matteo believes in, "a higher way of life … work without desiring the fruit from that work" (Desai 1995, 125). Sophie cannot accept this and with the tenacity of a wrestler who keeps on thrashing her bleeding wounds, she embarks upon a journey to reveal the truth about the Mother. The dictum of 'know thy-self' as preached by the Mother has unknowingly unleashed within Sophie a desire to know the unknown, the '*Paramananda*' (supreme joy). Her troubled spirit, her mental 'dis-ease' is similar to that experienced by searching souls who desire to discover their own "Ithaca" (by undertaking a spiritual journey of attainment.

Leaving her husband, her children, and her home behind, her 'troubled' mind follows the Mother's past which had spread across four continents; she moves from Cairo in Africa to France and Venice in Europe, then to America, and finally to India. This almost rollercoaster journey binds her as it reveals the strug-gle of another troubled soul Laila. She is the daughter of Hamid and Alma, who is a complete misfit in the house of her scholar parents. The extravagant compla-cency of her home in Alexandria makes her almost an eccentric. She condemned studies, and would "take a black pen and slash lines across a page of print, or even rip a page out of a book, crumple it and fling it out of the window in defiance" (Desai 1995, 160).

Her desperate parents send her to her aunt Francoise in Paris hoping that her mental 'dis-ease' would be cured there. But she grows even more disturbed, more unrestricted, and in such a restless mental condition she joins an oriental dance troupe for she felt that dancing would relieve the disjointed passions warring within her. But this dancing or methodical movement of limbs fails to provide her solace and she questions the purpose behind it all – "But why? Why must we do this?… What is the purpose? What is the meaning of these movements? Why do we perform them? For what reason? What cause?" (Desai 1995, 182).

In this disjointed frame of mind, she found the East calling out to her when in the decrepit shop of Madam Lacan she came upon the revered books like *Rig Veda, Samhita, Ratnavali, Brihadanayaka Upanishad, La Bhagavad Gita.*

Laila's feelings are further stirred when she joins Master Krishna as Lila (> Laila) for the dance presentation "Krishna Lila" and travels from France to America and then to Bombay. Through this dance presentation, she aimed to satisfy her eternal search for spiritual containment. But Master Krishna fails to satisfy her spiritual longing to mend her "dis-ease". Like a lost soul, she trav-eled from place to place, and from hill to hill in India. Her dissatisfaction, her eternal thirst for the Divine Lover (Lord Krishna) finally led her to the Master. Her final journey up a steep hill leads her to uncover her real self – She was Radha, the eternal beloved of her supreme Master Sri Krishna. Her dissatisfaction is quenched, her disturbed soul finds harbor and in the ecstatic joy she declares:

Arriving at last in the green valley,
My feet quickened their pace,
My Lord's voice in my ear, beckoning,
I know now my journey's ended,
I see now that mountain peak
That had been my true home
From which I was kept
And is now shown me
In a vision so radiant
I cry out in joy:
Love, I am come.
The Sun pours upon the abode of snow
It dazzles my eyes –
Everywhere is Brightness

(Desai 1995, 292)

The spiritual journey forms the leitmotif of this narrative of the quest of the dissatisfied soul for salvation and enlightenment. It is not a journey of the characters alone but that of the author too. By presenting the Mother as both the seeker and the provider of enlightenment and transcendence Desai represents a female figure who breaks all norms set by patriarchy to find her own Ithaca. Dance appears again and again in this text of divine pilgrimage for as per Eastern philosophy music is the unifying force that binds together the entire creation, the *Nadabrahma* of which rises the *Omkar*.

The Eastern Spiritual Discourse

Western psychology usually ignored the study of the self as a manifestation of the psyche or soul. James Hillman, a Jungian psychoanalyst has repeatedly argued that healing should be directed to serving the soul and include a transpersonal view which combines together the physical, emotional, and mental perspectives. The Vedantic philosophy, on the other hand, speaks of such a union and states, "know the body to be the chariot, the intellect the charioteer, the mind the reins, and the atman the controller of the chariot" (Bhattacharyya 2006, 139). The *Atman* or the Self which manifests itself through the body possesses the power to lead to supreme consciousness (Safaya 1975) and hence it is believed that knowledge of the *Atman* (Self) and the human psychology are mutually interdependent (Kulkarni 1978, 28). The *Jiva* which represents the mortal Self must pierce through the *Koshas* or sheaths that prevent the *Jiva* from becoming one with the

Atman and thereby achieving a state of *Paramananda* or transcendence. As the *Jiva* permeates these sheaths or Koshas (*annamaya kosha, pranamaya kosha, manomaya kosha, vijnanamaya kosha* and *anandamaya kosha*) it becomes one with the *Brahman* or the true Self (Chatterji 1992). This helps the mind to heal and achieve a status of transcendence. Applied Vedantic philosophy has come to be accepted as a means of cure for the unsettled mind and restless spirit and Chakkarath writes:

> For over 3000 years, Hinduism has provided a vast literature on various systems of philosophy that involves elaborate conceptual frameworks, critical thinking concerning the mind and the body, theoretical analyses of the human personality, introspective methods of observing psychological phenomena, various therapeutic techniques designed to help individuals cope with the difficulties of human life and reach higher levels of development, as well as broad range of social institutions that reflect, facilitate, and structure the kind of personality growth that Hindu culture regards as the basis for well-being and fulfilment.
>
> (2005, 34)

Other Eastern philosophies drawn from Buddhism, Confucianism and Taoism have also stressed upon the significance of spiritual thought as a cure for mental illness caused very often due to existential disorder. Buddha had preached the centrality of *'Dukha'* in human life. *Dukha*, interpreted as 'mental dysfunction' is at the root of mental illness in its varied forms, especially depression (Smith 1991, 101). Buddha had highlighted the eight-fold path or *astangika marga* as the means of winning over *Dukha* leading to mental disorders. Psychoanalysts and experts of Buddhism have looked upon the Buddhist way of life (stressing upon meditation) as a means of gaining mental tranquillity which became a linchpin in creating humanistic, cognitive, and existential schools of psychology (Aich 2013). On the other hand, Confucianism and Taoism, two schools of spiritual thought presented an equilibrium worldview model. It was derived from the rule of golden mean created by Confucius and helped to interpret the myths, folklores, and legends to present a world where harmony and balance prevail. This harmony can be at the level of nature, individual, or interpersonal. Self-reflection is perceived as a means of understanding and curing mental disorders (Hwang 2012). While Confucius had stressed upon self-cultivation and social collective responsibility (Feng et al. 2008), Taoism referred to dissatisfaction related to goal attainment as a cause of mental illness and stressed upon adaptive techniques which enabled the mind to attain peace and tranquillity (Young et al. 2008). It helped to eradicate psychological suffering and helped to stabilize the spirit.

The Female 'Writes Back' in Eat, Pray, Love

The female mental disorder was more specifically a gendered concept of 'othering' whose root lay within patriarchy. Hysteria was essentially perceived as 'a female disease' as it was believed "women are prone to Hysteria because of something fundamental in their nature, something innate, fixed or given that obviously requires interaction with environmental forces to become manifest but is still a primary and irremediable fate for the human female" (Chodoff 1982, 546). Elaine Showalter in 'Hysteria, Feminism and Gender' looked upon it as a means of protest against the oppression of Patriarchy and states that it is "a specifically feminine protolanguage, communicating through the body messages that cannot be verbalized" (1993, 286). Susan Gubar in "The Blank Page and the Issues of Female Creativity" (1981) argues how the female has always been the 'sculpture', 'the written word' or 'the painting' but never the sculptor, the author, or the painter. According to her, "if the creator is a man, the creation itself is the female, who, like Pygmalion's ivory girl, has no name or identity or voice of her own" (Gubar 1981, 250). She compares a 'text' to a 'female body' or 'corpus' by referring to Barthes' words, "There are those who want a text (an art, a painting) without a shadow, without the 'dominant ideology'; but this is to want a text without fecundity, without productivity, a sterile text" (1975, 32). It is for this reason that Jacques Derrida, as per Gubar, refers to the concept of the 'pen penis' used to write upon the 'virgin page'. She argues,

> This model of the pen-penis writing on the virgin page participates in a long tradition identifying the author as a male who is primary and the female as his passive creation—a secondary object lacking autonomy, endowed with often contradictory meaning but denied intentionality. Clearly this tradition excludes woman from the creation of culture, even as it reifies her as an artifact within culture. It is therefore particularly problematic for those women who want to appropriate the pen by becoming women writers. Especially in the nineteenth-century, writers, who feared their attempts at the pen were presumptuous, castrating, or even monstrous, engaged in a variety of strategies to deal with their anxiety about authorship.
>
> (1981, 253)

So 'articulate hysteria' (cited by Showalter 1993, 333) becomes a means by which female authors use hysteria as a language of 'writing back', as a 'cure' for "the dis-ease of women in patriarchal culture" (Kahane 1985, 31). The French feminist critics, especially Hélène Cixous and Luce Irigaray in advocating the concept of écriture feminine presented how hysterical themes and metaphors were common in the writings of women and

> writing the disordered body represents a textual performance of identity; a renegotiation of female subjectivity previously defined by patriarchal parameters. Such texts can undoubtedly be considered a continuation of many of the goals of 1970s writing projects that sought to overcome the position of silence culturally ascribed to the feminine and enact a deliberate deconstruction of socially constructed taboos concerning the female body.
>
> (Felman 1975, 2)

Thus, writings representing women as hysterics can be segregated in two groups, one that highlights illness as the consequence and punishment meted out to women who dared to break the patriarchal dictum, and another where hysteria/ madness/ the female malady is looked upon as an agency; as a means of empowerment through which women gain control over their own body (Ramsey-Portolano 2018). This debate has been conclusively argued by Gubar when she states,

> no woman is a blank page: every woman is author of the page and author of the page's author. The art of producing essentials—children, food, cloth—is woman's ultimate creativity. If it is taken as absence in the context of patriarchal culture, it is celebrated within the female community by the matrilineal traditions of oral storytelling. The veiled, brown, illiterate old woman who sits outside the city gates in Dinesen's tale therefore represents her grandmother and her grandmother's grandmother: "they and I have become one." Existing before man-made books, their stories let us "hear the voice of silence".
>
> (1981, 266)

It is this power of 'writing back' through not just representation of the female malady as an agency, but also beyond and above it, in searching for a spiritual state of transcendence, does Anita Desai represent her female characters in *Journey to Ithaca*. They might or might not attain 'Ithaca' but the journey itself is rewarding enough and raises the feminine to a level of almost unattainable supremacy.

Elizabeth Gilbert seeks for a similar state of transcendence in her memoir *Eat, Pray, Love: One Woman's Search for Everything Across Italy, India and Indonesia*. Throughout literary history, it is the male hero who enjoys the right to undertake a journey of self-development. In *Beyond Feminist Aesthetics: Feminist Literature and Social Change* (1989) Rita Felski observes how unlike her male counterpart who launches upon journeys of self-exploration and adventure, the female protagonist's "... trajectory remains limited to the journey from the parental to the marital home and... [her] destiny remains permanently linked to that of her male companion" (125). Any violation of this norm ends in suffering and self-destruction. So, *Eat Pray Love* questions the established norms of a work of self-exploration by challenging the gender role as it is a text written by a female author about a female protagonist. She begins her journey after a troubled divorce in the middle stage of her life. The protagonist is not spiritual in any sense, in fact, she prays to God for the first time when she faces an existential crisis. Torn by feelings of guilt, regret, and despair she talks to the "creator of the universe as though [they] had just been introduced at a cocktail party" (Gilbert 2006, 16), and her only prayer is "Please tell me what to do" (Gilbert 2006, 17). She does not seek transcendence at the expense of self-deprivation, rather she desired "worldly enjoyment and divine transcendence which is the glory of human life and the singular balance of the good and the beautiful" (Gilbert 2006, 22).

The novel begins with Liz, the narrator-protagonist highlighting her dissatisfaction and hence depression with the way her life is. She has accumulated worldly pleasures and yet is unhappy. She expresses her sense of not belonging,

> Wasn't I proud of all I'd accumulated — the prestigious home in the Hudson Valley, the apartment in Manhattan, the eight phone lines, the friends and the picnics and the parties, the weekends spent roaming the aisles of some box-shaped superstore of our choice, buying ever more appliances on credit? I had actively participated in every moment of the creation of this life—so why did I feel like none of it resembled me?
>
> (Gilbert 2006, 18)

This dissatisfaction is the root cause of *dukhya* or as per Buddhism 'mental dysfunction' which leads to mental illness like depression. And to overcome this Liz begins on a journey which she later realizes is a quest for self-exploration through spiritual healing:

> It wasn't so much that I wanted to thoroughly explore the countries themselves. This has been done. It was more that I wanted to thoroughly explore one aspect of myself set against the backdrop of each country...I wanted to explore the art of pleasure in Italy, the art of devotion in India and, in Indonesia, the art of balancing the two. It was only later...that I noticed... it seemed [like] a voyage of self-discovery.
>
> (Gilbert 2006, 31)

Her spiritual quest carries her to the far East or more specifically to India. Her quest is certainly not easy. Like Laila, Sophie, and Matteo in *Journey to Ithaca* she encounters one false saint after another but the battle to conquer the self goes on, for as the monk at the Ashram pointed out,

> The resting place of the mind is the heart. The only thing the mind hears all day is clanging bells and noise and argument, and all it wants is quietude. The only place the mind will ever find peace is inside the silence of the heart. That's where you need to go.
>
> (Gilbert 2006, 152)

The battle is not easy, Liz struggles and struggles, realizing that spiritual experience is greater than the dogmatic study of religion and it is not specific to one faith. In a moment of illumination, she realizes that the

> union with God occurs in a meditative state, and is delivered through an energy source that fills the entire body with euphoric, electric light. The Japanese call this energy ki, the Chinese Buddhists call it chi, the Balinese call it taksu, the Christians call it The Holy Spirit, the Kalahari Bushmen call it n/um (their holy men describe it as a snakelike power that ascends

the spine and blows a hole in the head through which the gods then enter). The Islamic Sufi poets called that God-energy "The Beloved," and wrote devotional poems to it. The Australian aborigines describe a serpent in the sky that descends into the medicine man and gives him intense, otherworldly powers. In the Jewish tradition of Kabbalah this union with the divine is said to occur through stages of spiritual ascension, with energy that runs up the spine along a series of invisible meridians.

(Gilbert 2006, 154)

Liz realizes that to find true happiness one has to select one's own thoughts and gain supreme mastery over the Id. By developing such inner strength and a positive attitude can one emerge victorious over one's own self. Through Praying ('talking to God') and Meditation ('listening to God') Liz achieves her transcendence, her moment of liberation, and thus victory over her 'mental dis-ease', her depression. Like Laila's moment of self-realization in Desai's narrative, here Liz relates her enlightenment with that achieved by Lord Budha after 39 days of meditation. It is a moment of supreme joy, of liberation not only her own self but also the self of all female creator artists who seek this moment of enlightenment. The ultimate truth was,

> I got pulled through the wormhole of the Absolute, and in that rush I suddenly understood the workings of the universe completely. I left my body, I left the room, I left the planet, I stepped through time and I entered the void. I was inside the void, but I also was the void and I was looking at the void, all at the same time. The void was a place of limitless peace and wisdom. The void was conscious and it was intelligent. The void was God, which means that I was inside God. But not in a gross, physical way—not like I was Liz Gilbert stuck inside a chunk of God's thigh muscle. I just was part of God. In addition to being God. I was both a tiny piece of the universe and exactly the same size as the universe.

(Gilbert 2006, 215)

Notes

1 The Ophelia syndrome is usually associated to women who suffer from memory loss and Hodgkin's lymphoma in association to Ophelia, a tragic character in Shakespeare's *Hamlet*.
2 Scott, Sir Walter. 1886. *The Bride of Lammermoor*. Adam & Charles Black. *Lucia di Lammermoor* (1835) is an opera by Gaetano Donizetti where Lucia the female protagonist is in love with Edgardo who belongs to a rival family in seventeenth Century Scotland. She is forced to marry Arturo, but her fragile mind cannot sustain the pressure and on her marriage night she murders her husband and herself dies.

References

Aich, Tapas Kumar. 2013 January. "Buddha Philosophy and Western Psychology". *Indian Journal of Psychiatry*, 55 (2), 165–170.

Andrews, Jonathan and Digby, Anne, Eds. 2004. *Sex and Seclusion, Class and Custody: Perspectives on Gender and Class in the History of British and Irish Psychiatry* (*Clio Medica 73*). New York: Rodopi.

Andrews, Marcus H. and Mathews, Stephen G. 2004. "Programming of the Hypthalamo-pituitary Adrenal Axis and Serotonergic Involvement". *Stress*, 7 (10), 15–27.

Baistow, Karen. 2007. "'On Being a Mother': Motherhood and Mental Health". In *The Female Body in Mind: The Interface between the Female Body and the Mind*. Edited by Mervat Nasser, Karen Baistow, and Janet Treasure. London and New York: Routledge, 104–118.

Barthes, Roland. 1975. *The Pleasure of the Text*. Trans. Richard Miller. New York: Hill and Wang.

Beauvoir, Simone de et al. 2011. *The Second Sex*. New York: Vintage.

Bhattacharyya, A. K. 2006. *Hindu Dharma: Introduction to Scriptures and Theology*. Lincoln, NE: iUniverse.

Boswell, G. H., Kahana, E., and Dilworth-Anderson, P. 2006. "Spirituality and Healthy Lifestyle Behaviors: Stress Counter-balancing Effects on the Well-being of Older Adults". *Journal of Religion & Health*, 45, 587–602. doi: 10.1007/s10943-006-9060-7.

Brant, George. 2013. *Grounded*. London: Oberon Books Ltd.

Brontë, Charlotte. 1847. *Jane Eyre*. Peterborough, ON: Broadview Press.

Busfield, Joan. 1996. *Men, Women, and Madness: Understanding Gender and Mental Disorder*. New York: New York University Press.

Butler, J. 1993. *Bodies that Matter: On the Discursive Limits of Sex*. New York: Routledge.

Chakkarath, P. 2005. "What Can Western Psychology Learn from Indigenous Psychologies? Lessons from Hindu Psychology". In *Culture and Human Development: The Importance of Cross-cultural Research for the Social Sciences*. Edited by W. Friedlmeier, P. Chakkarath, & B. Schwarz. Erlbaum: Psychology Press and Taylor & Francis.

Chatterji, J. C. 1992. *The Wisdom of the Vedas*. Wheaton, IL: Quest Books Theosophical Publishing House.

Chesler, P. 2005. *Women and Madness*. New York: Palgrave Macmillan.

Chodoff, Paul. 1982. "Hysteria and Women". *American Journal of Psychiatry*, 139(5), 545–551.

Desai, Anita. 1995. *Journey to Ithaca*. New Delhi: Penguin Random House.

Felman, Shoshana. 1975. "Woman and Madness: The Critical Phallacy". *Diacritics*, 5, 2–10.

Felski, Rita. 1989. *Beyond Feminist Aesthetics: Feminist Literature and Social Change*. Cambridge, MA: Harvard University Press.

Feng, L., Cao, Y. P., Zhang, Y., Wee, S.-T., & Kua, E.-H. 2011. "Psychological Therapy with Chinese Patients". *Asia-Pacific Psychiatry*, 3, 167–172.

Freud, Sigmund. 1905. *Dora: An Analysis of a Case of Hysteria*. Springfield, OH: Collier Books.

Gilbert, S. M., & Gubar, S. 1984. *The Madwoman in The Attic: The Woman Writer and the Nineteenth-Century Literary Imagination*. New Haven, CT and London: Yale University Press.

Gubar, Susan. 1981. "'The Blank Page' and the Issues of Female Creativity". *Critical Inquiry*, 8 (2), Writing and Sexual Difference, 243–263.

Hesse, Hermann. 1956. *The Journey to the East*. Trans. Hilda Rosner. New York: Picador.

Hwang, K. K. 2012. *Foundations of Chinese Psychology: Confucian Social Relations*. New York: Springer.

Joseph, R. P., Ainsworth, B. E., Mathis, L., Hooker, S. P., & Keller, C. 2017. "Incorporating Religion and Spirituality into the Design of Community-based Physical Activity

Programs for-African American Women: A Qualitative Inquiry". *BMC Research Notes*, 10, 506.

Kahane, Claire. 1985. "Introduction. Part 2". In *Dora's Case: Freud-Hysteria-Feminism*. Edited by Charles Bernheimer and Claire Kahane. New York: Columbia University Press, 19–32.

Kharitonov, S. A. 2012. "Religious and Spiritual Biomarkers in both Health and Disease". *Religion*, 3, 467–497. Doi: 10.3390/rel3020467.

Kulkarni, T. R. 1978. "Psychology: The Indian Point of View". *Journal of Indian Psychology*, 1 (1/2), 22–39.

Micale, Mark S. 2019. "A Short 'History' of Hysteria". In *Approaching Hysteria: Disease and Its Interpretations*. Princeton, NJ: Princeton University Press, 19–30.

Mitchell, S. Weir. 1877. *Fat and Blood: and How to Make Them*. Philadelphia, PA: J.B. Lippincott.

Mueller, P. S., Plevak, D. J., & Rummans, T. A. 2001. "Religious Involvement, Spirituality, and Medicine: Implications for Clinical Practice". *Mayo Clinic Proceedings*, 76, 1225–1235. Doi: 10.4065/76.12.1225.

Patmore, Coventry. 1887. *The Angel in the House*. London: Cassell and Co.

Porter, Roy, Nicholson, Helen, and Bennett, Bridget, Eds. 2003. *Women, Madness and Spiritualism*, 3 vols. London and New York: Routledge.

Ramsey-Portolano, Catherine. 2018. *Performing Bodies: Female Illness in Italian Literature and Cinema* (1860–1920). Vancouver-Madison-Teaneck-Wroxton: Fairleigh Dickinson University Press.

Rhys, Jean. 1966. *Wide Sargasso Sea*. New York: W.W. Norton & Company.

Safaya, R. 1975. *Indian Psychology*. Shahdara and Delhi: Munshiram Manoharlal.

Showalter, Elaine. 1987. *The Female Malady: Women, Madness, and English Culture, 1890– 1980*. London: Penguin Books.

———. 1993. "Hysteria, Feminism, and Gender". In *Hysteria Beyond Freud*. Edited by Sander L. Gilman, Helen King, Roy Porter, G.S. Rousseau, and Elaine Showalter. Berkeley, CA, Los Angeles, CA, and London: University of California Press, 286–344.

Stiles, Anne. "The Rest Cure, 1873–1925". BRANCH: Britain, Representation and Nineteenth-Century History. Edited by Dino Franco Felluga. Extension of Romanticism and Victorianism. Retrieved December 20, 2021. http://www.branchcollective. org/?ps_articles=anne-stiles-the-rest-cure-1873-1925.

Theriot, Nancy M. 1993. "Women's Voices in Nineteenth-Century Medical Discourse: A Step Toward Deconstructing Science". *Signs*, 19, 1–31.

Thoresen, C. E. 1998. "Spirituality, Health and Science". In *The Emerging Role of Counseling Psychology in Health Care*. Edited by S. Roth-Roemer, S. R. Kurpius, and C. Carmin. New York: Norton, 409–431.

Young, D., Zhou, L., Zhu, J. F. 2008. "Daoistic Cognitive Psychotherapy: Philosophical Foundation and Basic Procedure". *World Cultural Psychiatry Research Review*, 3, 32–36.

15 Disjunctured Subjectivities and Corporeal Well-being

Issues of Mobility and Health in Select Transgender Life Narratives from India

Rajesh V. Nair and Lekshmi R. Nair

Introduction

The post-structuralist discourse on gender attempts a revaluation of the hegemonic sex/gender dichotomy and brings into perspective the contingent nature of gender. Gender is perceived as flexible, fluid, shifting, and non-normative, defying cataloging into binary heteropatriarchal standards. Trans people occupy a social space that is largely defined by their bodies, bodies that challenge and defy social structuring. The transbody assumes centrality by virtue of its liminality and disjuncture. This chapter places in perspective select transgender life narratives from India in an attempt to trace the trajectory of the mental, physical, and spiritual well-being of trans people, as they negotiate the transition from the cisgender normative towards a gender-fluid existence. The impact of the COVID-19 pandemic on their emotional and physical health is also investigated with the help of three case studies to understand the extent to which the state, the trans community, and the general public have functioned as support systems to stabilize trans lives. Analyzing the concepts of gender dysphoria and bodily transition, space, and mobility, and the depathologization of trans subjectivity, this chapter examines the multifarious aspects of trans identity and establishes that the pathological positioning of gender inconsistent subjects has undergone a transformation in the postmodernist discourse, where the sexed body exercises agency in a chosen gender, resisting and managing social and medical stigmatization (Hines 2010, 3).

Bodies in transition

Transgender subjectivity renders problematic assumptions regarding gender identity. As bodies in transition, the transgendered body refuses to adhere to the heteronormative definitions of sex, gender, and embodiment. The social illegibility of these sexed bodies defies the systemic gender codes and serves "as a cleaving point of abstruseness and unease – separating, pathologizing, and psychologizing trans subjectivity" (Phillips 2014, 20). Placing in context Kristeva's notion of abjection, Robert Phillips argues that trans activism regards abjection as a constructive political strategy that dismantles power structures sustained by the methodical exclusion, repression, and silencing of other subjectivities (20). As a marginal group, transgenders are reclaiming their abjection by articulating the distinctive

DOI: 10.4324/9781003300762-17

nature of their gendered identity. In her seminal work *Powers of Horror: An Essay on Abjection*, Kristeva wrote that abjection draws her "toward the place where meaning collapses" (1982, 2). In this liminal space, the gendered subject experiences "a crisis of meaning in which transformation is possible – the difference between internal and external becomes unclear, and in the process, conditional identity is stripped away to reveal a queer object" (Phillips 2014, 20). Transgenders problematize their gender nonconformity by embracing abjection, challenging and dislodging systemically constructed notions of gender and identity.

"Transsexuality consists in entering into a lengthy, formalized, and normally substantive transition: a correlated set of corporeal, psychic, and social changes" (Prosser 1998, 4). The gender ambivalent subject finds the process of transition to their felt gender as a means of belonging to the systemic order. Gender dysphoria, or the notion of being entrapped in the wrong body, triggers the desire to restructure the nature of their biological bodies and seek conformity to their felt gender through the bodily transition. The "unnatural and constructed" (Garner 2014, 30) nature of transbodies destabilizes the notion of being and the attendant gendered power structures. Nikki Sullivan notes: "all bodies mark and are marked" (2006, 561). The transbody situated at the opposite end of the gender spectrum is a marked body, an estranged body that defies boundaries. The explicit transformation of transbodies is an attempt to conform to the bodily parameters of the cisgender normative. The socially constructed heteronormative categories of personhood coordinate a particular physical body with a birth-assigned gender.

> Transgender phenomena-anything that calls our attention to the contingency and unnaturalness of gender normativity– appear at the margins of the biopolitically operated-upon body, at those fleeting and variable points at which particular bodies exceed or elude capture within the gender apparatus.
>
> (Stryker 1998, 40)

David Getsy designates, transgender capacity as the ability or the potential for making visible, bringing into experience, or knowing genders as mutable, successive, and multiple; as the various modes of gender nonconformity underscore accounts of gender's dynamism, plurality, and expansiveness (2014, 47). The reductive, static, dimorphic nature of sex and gender collapses and deconstructs itself to accommodate transgender fluidity, divergence, and survival strategies. Getsy argues that transgender epistemologies and theoretical models fundamentally remap the study of human cultures. "That is, once gender is understood to be temporal, successive, or transformable, all accounts of human lives look different and more complex" (Getsy 2014, 48). Rithu Meher (2022), a transwoman gave us a detailed account of the experiences during her surgery:

> I had to flee my home in 2016 because I was being persecuted there. During my stay with a group of hijras in Bangaluru, I was physically and mentally abused. I had to do sex work because I had to. Finally, I ran away to Kadappa, Hyderabad, where I met a nani who was very kind. When I told

her I wanted to change my gender through sex reassignment surgery, the ill woman helped me pay for it. In 2017, I went to a hospital in a remote area to have surgery. The surgery was painful, and I had a lot of bleeding when I was taken back to our place. I lived alone for 41 days, going through all the rituals and taking holy baths, until I became a real woman.

Transgressing gender norms in childhood is an early manifestation of gender dysphoria. The unwillingness to participate in childhood games with children of their own sex, the enthusiasm to imitate the dressing and bodily mannerisms of the opposite sex, and the eagerness to spend time with people of their own kind are practices that echo their nonconformity to the naturalness of the cisgender norm. However, transgender childhood carries the mark of a fixed, normalizing gender template, conflicting with the innate gender sensibilities of the child. The caged body seeks release from its assigned gender and all its associated power and privilege. In *Me Hijra, Me Laxmi*, Laxmitalks about her adoption of the hijra lifestyle as a liberating experience, though she never opted for the sex reassignment surgery: "When I became a hijra, a great burden was lifted off my head. I felt relaxed. I was now neither a man nor a woman. I was a hijra. I had my own identity. No longer did I feel like an alien" (43).

Family and society are dominant power systems that enforce the hierarchical and pervasive nature of cisgenderism; any deviation from the expected standards or modes of gender behavior is regarded as immoral and deviant, justifying discrimination and punishment. Gender identities that do not align with the assigned gender at birth are pathologized and denigrated. Trans people are exposed to widespread stigmatization, social exclusion, and violence; their claims to recognition and acceptance are often met with mockery and rejection. Revathi, in her autobiography, describes the physical violence that she had been subjected to in her home whenever she dressed up as a girl or danced like a woman in public. Laxmi recollects how traumatized her parents were upon learning the truth about their only son's gender identity. Families feared the shame, ridicule, and exclusion they would invite upon themselves, once their child's gender identity became public knowledge. Hence, every attempt to suppress the child's naturally felt gender began at home, often taking the form of violent beatings and emotional abuse. Families find it difficult to come to terms with the child's sexuality, which is a clear deviance from standard gender behavior. The alienation that trans people suffer inside their homes and in their immediate community initiates a movement out of the familiar domestic and social space in search of a new space inhabited by 'their own kind'. Transgender mobility spirals from this overtly emotional need to seek a space where they can articulate their experiences of gender, manifested as gender practices and rituals in queer communities.

Attempts at visibility and proclaiming one's gender identity begin at an earlier age for trans individuals. Transgender life narratives offer ample instances of conflicting emotions experienced by parents and siblings, and family interventions to curtail a sexual identity that had evolved outside the patriarchal norm of heterosexuality. Awareness of one's difference from same-sex peers translates into inner turmoil and identity confusion. Rithu Meher gave a highly emotional account of her childhood days:

> I had a forgettable childhood in Vypin, Kochi. As a child, I used to play with the girls in my locality. When my identity was revealed, I faced harsh treatment from my father and brother. My mother was a silent witness, and she was sympathetic. One day, my brother started beating me violently. I cried aloud in pain, but no one could help me. I passed through fits of trauma. I was a big embarrassment to my family before the public. Eventually, they threw me out of the house....

Exploration of sexuality leads to stigmatization, shame, and oppression. Commitment to the unique but ambivalent gender experience is reinforced with exposure to and interaction with similar identities. A sense of community and oneness is imperative to attaining the much-desired congruence between the assigned gender and the felt gender. Self-disclosure is significant in identity construction, and the gendered mind proves to be the key factor influencing and determining the reformulation of the gendered self. The body is the agency that generates meaning in discord and functions as the site of power and repositioning. As Butler argues, the body takes on new or alternative meanings – termed as resignification – the body functioning as the site of radical subversion (1993).

Space and mobility

Theoreticians such as Henri Lefebvre have extrapolated on the constructedness of space and the implication of power within it . When we look at the case of sexual minorities, particularly transgender people, this postulation becomes even more complicated and problematic, as gender minorities' mobility is influenced by power, identity, and broader social dynamics (Lubitow et al. 2017, 4). *The Truth About Me: A Hijra Life Story* (2010), A. Revathi's life narrative, assists her in identifying and locating herself: "Every morning, the pottais would leave to ask for money from shopkeepers. They went in a group to different areas called bazaars. After they were done with collecting money from a bazaar, they divided the collection amongst themselves…" (44). Indeed, even in the twenty-first century, transgender people, a group that is socially excluded, still make money by begging, performing sex work, and giving blessings at important events like weddings and childbirths. Revathi elaborates on this aspect:

> In this Delhi, for centuries, they've treated us like gods. They fall at our feet and seek our blessings. Our word is considered all powerful and whatever we say comes true. When we go to shops, we clap hands and say "Ramramji! Namaste babu!" and they give us money, a rupee or 5 rupees, or whatever they want to give. We accept this money, place our palms on the shopkeeper's head and say "Be well! We hope your business goes well.

(44)

The traditional profession of sex work exacerbates transgender mobility. The majority of this population is involved in this profession for a variety of reasons. They face physical violence and other forms of abuse from their clients, rowdies, and even the police authorities, who are supposed to protect them. Manjami Prameesh (2022), a transwoman studying BA English at a college in Kochi, Kerala revealed in a recent discussion with the authors:

> I don't personally want to do sex work, and till now, I have not been in that profession. Unfortunately, many of my friends are doing sex work for a host of reasons: they do not have money for food; they do not have a place to stay because of high rent; and more importantly, they need to save money for their transition surgery and the subsequent medical treatment, which is pretty expensive. Even if they get clients, they can earn only Rs. 400 or 500 per day, which is very inadequate. I hope my education will empower me from indulging in sex work in the future...

Prameesh added that they rarely had independence within their group due to harassment and intervention by senior members. Many people feel as if they are being imprisoned within their community, with little freedom of choice or movement. Rithu Meher, another transwoman from Kochi, told the authors in a telephone interview that she had a terrible time living with her group in Bangalore in 2016; they coerced her into sex work against her will and even physically assaulted her when she protested. Meher was eventually forced to flee to Kerala, leaving behind all her certificates.

In her autobiography, Revathi narrates the inhuman physical abuse she had to endure at home once her true identity was revealed. In order to escape the sheer pain inflicted on her body, Revathi declares: "I swear I won't do this again! I'm willing to plead at your feet! But please keep my father and brothers away from me. I don't want to get beaten again. I can't bear the pain" (56). Revathi reveals that she had initially chosen to do sex work, not for money but because she could not repress her sexual feelings. But she soon discovered the "horror and violence of this choice" (110) and yearned to return to her parental home. Indeed, space is founded on vulnerability and precarity in an environment fraught with danger, and the case of transgender people is particularly significant in this context (Nayar 2017, xiii). The transgender body is more vulnerable, as it is easily targeted and subjected to violence by the public. The spatial positioning of transgendered bodies is determined by the social reaction. Life within the hijra community is also fraught with jealousy, fights, treachery, and rivalry. Transgender people are targets of public scrutiny and face physical violence from both within and outside their families. Revathi continues:

> Men and even women stared at us and laughed, and heckled us. I realized what a burden a hijra's daily life is. Do people harass those who are men and women when they go out with their families? Why, a crippled person, a blind person—even they attract pity and people help them. If someone

has experienced physical hurt, they are cared for both by the family and by outsiders who come to know of it. But we—we are not considered human.

(83)

During our interactions with Arjun Geetha, a Kochi-based transman who is presently working in a product insurance department confides:

It is a pity that society still looks at transgender people as sex objects, and wherever such a person goes, he/she has to face verbal abuse and very often physical attack from people around them... Sometimes, even police officers don't spare us! However, the condition of transmen like me is much better in the sense that we are relatively 'invisible' and not easy to recognise, unlike transwomen..."

Education possibly empowers the group, providing them visibility and mobility, but within the educational institutions, transgenders are ignored and sidelined by their peer group. Prameesh's words highlight this aspect:

I should admit that, I am a lonely person on my college campus... and I face discrimination from my own classmates and some teachers. Not many friends even talk to me, and they refuse to sit on the same bench with me. Yet, some teachers and students are very supportive by giving me emotional support, which motivates me to continue my studies.

Many transgender autobiographical narratives share a common pattern regarding their mobility; once their sexual orientation is revealed to family members and the wider public, they are frequently subjected to mental and physical torture, forcing them to leave their homes, join their groups, and adopt the hijra lifestyle. Their outward mobility is compounded further by their collective dissatisfaction. Self-realisation ultimately proves to be a dreadful experience for them.

Immobility intensifies a persons fragility, as it restricts an individuals freedom and prevents them from freely expressing their personalities (Nayar 2017, 3). Immobility regimes seek to undermine the bodys sovereignty, one of which is mobility (2). During the state-imposed lockdown period following the Covid epidemic, citizens' freedom of movement was curtailed, with thousands losing jobs and receiving inadequate medical care. Sexual minorities, such as transgenders, fared poorly in that many were left jobless, without access to adequate medical treatment, and those suffering from chronic conditions suffered the worst. Transgender sex workers struggled immensely to make a living during the pandemic. Prostitutes and hijras, for example, battled to live because they had no way to make ends meet due to their invisibility in public space and received virtually no support from the state. Further, sex hormones are short-lived chemicals that change the physical attributes of the body which in turn demonstrates how sex and gender categories are fluid and subject to transformation.

It has been demonstrated that gender nonconforming individuals create their identities through their mobility in public spaces, regardless of the resistance they encounter. "Transmobilities" (Lubitow) were severely restricted in India during the Covid epidemic. Sharing their harrowing experiences during that time period, a couple from Kochi, Kerala, claimed that at one point, they were unable to obtain even basic necessities due to shop closures. Speaking on the issue of mobility, Geetha revealed how movement empowers his community:

> My identity as a transman was not revealed, till my post-graduation period. Ever since, I have been sidelined and ignored by my parents and friends. I passed through a phase of terrible mental stress and depression. The pandemic made the situation worse. Luckily for me, I managed to get connected to a few people in my group when the lockdown was relaxed. I felt a sense of belonging and could travel and meet people in my community. Now, I am an activist, working for an NGO for transmen in Thiruvananthapuram. Mobility gives me freedom to express my identity without any inhibition.

Fortunately for them, the food packages given by the Kerala government were a blessing. The majority of them lost their jobs, owners increased rent, and no sex work, not even begging, was feasible to survive. As usual, civil society was insensitive. Meher's comment was quite shocking: "During the lockdown time, seven members of our community committed suicide due to emotional distress caused by being locked in their places without food, work, or adequate health care, and the media made no mention of this at all".

Physical health

Transgender people struggle to reconcile their identities with their bodies. Gender reassignment is a long, gradual process. They are subjected to a thorough mental, endocrinologic, and surgical assessment prior to the hormone therapy that precedes surgical transition. The hormone therapy itself carries risks of thrombosis, liver problems, and the uncommon development of a pituitary prolactinoma. Androgen therapy increases the risk of heart disease, endometrial hyperplasia, and endometrial cancer in transgender women. However, insufficient long-term research exists to examine transgender medication's long-term consequences (Mail and Safford 2003, 196).

Transgenders face violent situations in their own households once their sexual preference is revealed to family members and others. Manjami Prameesh's words are significant here:

> When my father and brothers came to know that I was a girl instead of a boy, they targeted me cruelly. I went through extreme mental harassment and was on the verge of depression. One day, my father (who had very high expectations of me), tied me to a rubber tree and beat me mercilessly. Had

it not been for the intervention of my helpless mother, I would have died of physical injuries...

Similarly, Revathi recounts her experience of transition, which translates itself into an experience of intense pain, suffering, and shame:

He beat me hard mindlessly, yelling that he wanted to kill me, I who had dared to run away. I tried to protect my face and head with my hands to keep the blows from falling. But nevertheless they came down hard, and I felt my hands swell. I was beaten on my legs, on my back, and finally my brother brought the bat down heavily on my head. My skull cracked and there was blood all over, flowing, warm.

(55)

Hijras are often victims of violence, and some form groups to take care of their members. Revathi elaborates:

I tried to make people understand our predicament. Everyone knows about the violence we suffer, but we do not speak of this in public out of fear. Don't different groups of people have their own sangams[1] which fight for their rights? Do we hijras have such a sangam? How many of us are even conscious that there is a social group called hijra? Since people are not even aware of our existence, they think ill of us. It is our duty to dispel such ignorance.

(246–247)

Indulging in sex work invites many health hazards for transgender people, including sexually transmitted diseases. Violent sexual acts also cause body problems and great physical pain. Revathi comments on this angle:

(He wanted me to have anal sex with him). He spat abuse at me and forced me into the act. When I screamed in pain and yelled for my guru, he shut my mouth with one of his hands, whipped out a knife with the other and threatened to take it to my throat.

(108)

Very often, the post-surgery phase for a transgender person is very painful. Meher observes:

After my surgery, I had to walk down from the second floor of the hospital as there was no lift facility. Once I got into an autorikshaw, it started bleeding, and it took a few days to be alright. One has to stay away from the other for 41 days until the whole ceremony gets over... After transition, regular check-ups are important, including the consumption of hormone tablets...

Laxmi worked in a dance bar but never encouraged sex in exchange for money: "I have always considered myself to be monarch of my own body" (2015, 35).

She was routinely molested by her older cousins in her younger days. Dancing feminized her body, making her the object of sexual interest: "My body was a playhouse and a plaything, and any man could do anything with it" (27).

Mental and emotional health

Childhood abuse, homophobia, psychological and physical abuse, and substance abuse are among the major mental health issues. Teenagers who had been sexually abused had a higher chance of needing mental health help or ending up in a mental health center or hospital (Mail and Safford 2003, 189). Hormone imbalance leads to psychological problems. Many transgenders are not in a position to buy expensive tablets and consult doctors for their health issues due to the severe financial crisis. A hormone tablet costs around Rs. 1,200, and laser treatment for hair removal is charged at Rs. 2,000. Meher adds: "During the pandemic, I could not purchase medicine for 6 months, and consequently, I suffered from stress and other related ailments." Anxiety, depression, suicide, and alcoholism are all manifestations of mental illness. As mentioned earlier, out of stress, many transgenders resorted to suicide during the pandemic. Revathi's words corroborate the poor state of affairs: "As I have said repeatedly, my work was hard. I faced all sorts of problems, I endured physical violence and torture of the mind. I had to fight every day with police and rowdies". Overall, we may observe that emotional health is a composite of a sense of self-worth, combined with strong social and/or spiritual support, and access to expressive or creative outlets. (Mail and Safford 2003, 191).

Spiritual health

It is a fact that the LGBT community faces emotional estrangement and stress due to the antagonistic attitude of the straight people around them, and the spiritual well-being of the former is a pertinent aspect to be discussed along with physical and mental health. However, they face conflicts from many quarters, including "denominational teachings, scriptural passages, shame, depression, and suicidal ideation (89)" (qtd. in Mail and Safford 2003, 192). Revathi's Guru advises her that since hijras are thought of as godly beings and hence treated with respect, they should behave in a manner worthy of that respect:

> We must not desire men, and seek to misbehave with them. Those who think we are divine and give us money to earn our blessings should never think we have gone bad. When you go to ask for money, the seths[2] are bound to be nice to you. Some will tease you, but you must not to flirt with them. Understood?

(45)

Spirituality "provides personal growth, value and direction which in turn, relates to healthier emotional well being" (Mail and Safford 2003, 192) and Prameesh revealed to us that she is still deeply religious and visits temples. Furthermore, the devastating impact of AIDS has underlined the critical significance of spiritual wellness.

Spirituality, for them, is a means of finding meaning in their liminal existence as they relentlessly struggle to achieve congruence between their perceived gendered self and their birth-assigned corporeal body. Revathi recounts the elaborate rituals associated with the *nirvaanam*, the surgical transition procedure, which is regarded as nothing short of a veritable rebirth. Those who undergo *nirvaanam* are treated with great respect and are taken special care of during the healing period. They have to abide by the rules laid down by the community with regard to their diet and physical well-being. On the 40th-day the transitioned hijras are allowed to look at themselves in the mirror after puja and other ritualistic practices. Revathi says that she was in an elated state of mind as she glanced at her own image alongside the face of the goddess in the mirror: "Beguiled by her rich beauty, I could not recognize myself. My face had changed! I felt like a flower that had just blossomed. It seemed to me that my earlier male form had disappeared and in its place was a woman. I felt exultant" (88). Her autobiography recounts the many instances where Revathi had celebrated festivals and performed pujas with her family back in her hometown of Namakkal. In fact, she was praised for her disguise as the 'kurathi'[3] at the Mariamman temple festival in her village. For Revathi those were moments she had "given form" to her real feelings:

> I was unwilling to shed my female clothe and stood for several minutes in front of the mirror …Reluctantly, I changed into my regular clothes. As I re-emerged in my man's garb, I felt that I was in disguise, and that I had left my real self behind.
>
> (16)

Transgender narratives in India reveal a deep spiritual affinity towards community rituals as well as institutionalized religious practices. This act of conforming and partaking in the religious rituals is part of the coming-out process and the subsequent adoption of the felt gender. It is in these spiritual spaces that the felt gender is often manifested, explored and revealed.

Depathologising trans subjectivity

McNay observes that it embodies the carnal dimensions of subjectivity (1999). Redrawing the contours of the body through reconstructive surgery defies the Freudian dictum that anatomy is destiny. Trans subjectivity is precariously positioned between the sexed body and the gendered mind. Gender dysphoria implies an intrinsic discord or incongruence between the body and the mind, and transformative surgery is deemed as a means to harmonize the self with the body. As a trans agency, surgery redefines the contours of the body and rewrites the normative scripting of gender and sexuality based on dichotomous models. There is a continual struggle to strike a balance between their perceived self and their assigned bodies. Corie J. Hammers points out that queer sex and queer sexual subcultures signify non-normative sexual economies, "a resistance to heterosexual hegemony and the celebration of diversity" (226). The trans body, as a corporal and sexual agency, thus becomes a key site of mobilization, and generative in meaning-making (Hammers 2010, 231).

Sex reassignment surgeries have become imperative to ensure trans mobility as the body is considered the most potent marker of gender identity. The physical self is aligned with the gender self-image to embody gendered experiences and express their preferred gender identity. Apart from this need to align their morphological sex with their visible gender, surgical transformation is required in order to legalize the change in gender marker in identity documents so as to facilitate social, spatial, and economic mobility. It proved to be extremely difficult to obtain a ration card, voter's ID, and open bank accounts as a transgender. A. Revathi recounts her exhausting experience of trying to get her driver's license issued in her name and how she had to settle for one that referred to her as "Revathy who is Doraisamy" (226). In *A Life in Transactivism*, she narrates the ordeal of having undergone medical examination in a hospital where she was reduced to "a freak; an object of curiosity" (xxvii). She put up with the embarrassment in order to get her passport as a trans woman.

Medicines and hormone therapy to enhance bodily characteristics help conform to the perceived gender standards. Transformative surgeries were accompanied by elaborate rituals and practices in the hijra community. On the 40th day, after her surgery, Revathi is finally allowed to look at herself in the mirror. She could hardly recognize the transformation that had come upon her: "My face had changed! I felt like a flower that had just blossomed. It seemed to me that my earlier male form had disappeared and in its place was a woman. I felt exultant" (88). Born as Laxminarayan Tripati, transwoman Laxmi never underwent sex-change surgery. Having disclosed her gender identity very early in life, like Revathi, Laxmi defied the upper caste restrictive systemic order to embrace her destiny as a woman. Vivienne Cass noted that the psychological process of confronting personal information that relates to membership in a stigmatized social category is a generic one (1996, 233). When transgender people declare their identities in defiance of society's rules, they gain a sense of self-awareness and control over their own lives.

Pathologizing self-identified gender identities and stigmatizing nonconforming people strengthened the hierarchical cisgender normative. The "trans depathologization framework introduces a paradigm shift in the conceptualization of gender identities from conceiving gender transition as a mental disorder to recognizing it as a human right and expression of human diversity" (Suess et al. 2014, 74). The binary model of gender classification is deconstructed to accommodate fluid sexualities. Gender inscribes itself as a lived embodiment, transcending its materiality and operating and performing through the body. Susan Stryker argues that lived experience "provide[s] a site for grappling with the problematic relationship between principles of performativity and a materiality that, while inescapable, defies stable representation" (147). The illegible, unstable transgender body is objectified and pathologized in the heteronormative order. In the depathologization framework, the constructed body is regarded as a social assemblage that generates new meanings, as it negotiates the fluidity and variability of gender across space and culture.

Conclusion

The discussion of select trans-life narratives shows us that transgender activism and mobility are inextricably linked. Activism helps the liminal sexual groups by raising awareness about their rights and grievances, as well as breaking the social stigma against them, though to different degrees. Moving in groups ensures their mobility and freedom, and Revathi, Laxmi, or even Arjun Geetha, have been constantly in a state of mobility, coordinating activities on behalf of their communities. Though the lockdown during the surge of Covid has curtailed the free movement of transgenders in search of their jobs, including sex work, begging, dancing, etc. the situation is slowly improving, and they are now in a position to take care of their health requirements. The government is also funding them, giving them reserved seats in educational institutions, reassignment surgery to a few, and so on. The fact remains to be addressed that gender transformation surgery continues to be very expensive and the expenses after surgery remain costly. It is high time that the state addresses this serious issue and allocates funds for the health and well-being of this sexual minority, who are also citizens of this country. Many transgender people are subjected to physical violence while working in sex work; many have admitted to the authors that they are forced to have sex because they need money for surgery. So, it becomes imperative that a special fund be allotted to them for this cause. Though there is a need for strict laws, the proper implementation of the existing ones is even more important. Above all, social apathy towards this group needs to be changed, and creative interventions from all sections of society, including the academics, are the need of the hour as transgenders are no more to be excluded from mainstream society. Thus, the mental health and wellness of the transgender community in general and India in particular depends on the reframing of social mindset and the culture of exclusion should be done away. Let the existing laws be more transparent and stress-free for them, including procuring a passport, ration card, or driving license. Third gender status is a welcome sign to begin with. The derailment of the world during the high point of the pandemic is slowly becoming a nightmare, as the entire world is back on track in this period of the new normal, and transgenders should not be an exception.

Acknowledgements

The authors wish to thank Manjami Prameesh, Rithu Meher, and Arjun Geetha for their valuable inputs about the lives of transgenders in India, particularly during the Covid phase in the preparation of this chapter.

Notes

1 **Sangams:** associations.
2 **Seths:** Merchants or rich men.
3 **Kurathi:** A woman fortune-teller.

References

Butler, Judith. *Bodies that Matter*. Routledge, 1993.

Cass, Vivienne. "Sexual Orientation Identity Formation: A Western Phenomenon". In *Textbook of Homosexuality and Mental Health*, edited by Robert P. Cabaj and Terry S. Stein, American Psychiatric Press, 1996, pp. 227–251.

Garner, T. "Becoming". *Transgender Studies Quarterly*, vol. 1, no. 1–2 (May). Duke University Press, 2014, pp. 30–32.

Geetha, Arjun. Telephone interview with the authors. 24 February 2022.

Getsy, David J. "Capacity". *Traivinsgender Studies Quarterly*, vol. 1, no. 1–2 (May). Duke University Press, 2014, pp. 47–49.

Hammers, Corie J. "Corporeal Silences and Bodies that Speak: The Promises and Limiations of Queer in Lesbian/Queer Sexual Spaces". In *Transgender Identities: Towards a Social Analysis of Gender Diversity*, edited by Sally Hines and Tom Sanger, Routledge, 2010, pp. 224–242.

Hines, Sally and Tom Sanger. Editors. *Transgender Identities: Towards a Social Analysis of Gender Diversity*. Routledge, 2010.

Kristeva, Julia. *Powers of Horror: An Essay on Abjection*. Translated by Leon S. Roudiez. Columbia University Press, 1982.

Lubitow, Amy, et al. "Transmobilities: Mobility, Harassment, and Violence Experienced by Transgender and Gender Nonconforming Public Transit Riders in Portland, Oregon". *Gender, Place & Culture A Journal of Feminist Geography*, 28 September 2017, pp. 1–21 http://dx.doi.org/10.1080/0966369X.2017.1382451.

Mail, Patricia D. and Lauretta Safford. "LGBT Disease Prevention and Health Promotion: Wellness for Gay, Lesbian, Bisexual, and Transgender Individuals and Communities". *Clinical Research and Regulatory Affairs*, vol. 20, no. 2, 2003, pp. 183–204.

McNay, Lois. "Gender, Habitus and the Field: Pierre Bourdieu and the Limits of Reflexivity". *Theory, Culture and Society*, vol. 16, no. 1, 1999, pp. 95–117.

Meher, Rithu. Telephone interview with the authors. 21 February 2022.

Nayar, Pramod K. *The Extreme in Contemporary Culture: States of Vulnerability*. Rowman and Littlefield, 2017.

Phillips, Robert. "Abjection". *Transgender Studies Quarterly*, vol. 1, no. 1–2 (May). Duke University Press, 2014, pp. 19–21.

Prameesh, Manjami. Telephone interview with the authors. 20 February 2022.

Prosser, Jay. *Second Skins: The Body Narratives of Transsexuality*. Columbia University Press, 1998.

Revathi, A. *The Truth About Me: A Hijra Life Story*. Translated by V. Geetha. Penguin Books, 2010.

———. *A Life in Trans Activism*. Zubaan, 2016.

Stryker, Susan. "The Transgender Issue: An Introduction". *A Journal of Lesbian and Gay Studies*, vol. 4. no. 2, 1998, pp. 145–158.

———. "Biopolitics". *Transgender Studies Quarterly*, vol. 1, no. 1–2 (May). Duke University Press, 2014, pp. 38–42.

Suess, Amets, et al. "Depathologisation". *Transgender Studies Quarterly*, vol. 1, no. 1–2 (May). Duke University Press, 2014, pp. 73–77.

Sullivan, Nikki. "Transmogrification: (Un)Becominig Other(s)." In *The Transgender Studies Reader*, edited by Susan Stryker and Stephen Whittle, Routledge, 2006, pp. 552–564.

Tripathi, Laxminarayan. *Me Hijra, Me Laxmi*, translated by R. Raj Rao and P. G. Joshi, Oxford University Press, 2015.

16 Sustainable Eating and Wellness

Examining Nutrition Strategies
in Barbara Kingsolver's *Animal,
Vegetable, Miracle: Our Year of
Seasonal Eating* and Ruth Ozeki's
A Year of Meats

Shymasree Basu

Eating with the fullest pleasure – pleasure, that is, that does not depend on ignorance – is perhaps the profoundest enactment of our connection with the world. Wendell Berry (1990, 152).

Understanding Food Ethics and Sustainability

The discourse on food is increasingly addressing issues of sustainability as eating right becomes an environmentally conscious act. As issues of climate change become more and more urgent, our society is at a crossroad where individuals, groups, communities and governments have to restructure food systems to preserve the planet. Sustainability, is not just a buzzword today, it is the most vital aspect of the food systems we inhabit. A simplistic view of food systems will not suffice if one has to understand the need for sustainability and the need to evolve nutrition strategies based on sustainability. Ronald L. Sandler in *Food Ethics: The Basics* defines food systems and global food systems in the following manner:

> *Food system* refers to the complex network of processes, infrastructures and actors that produce the food we eat and deliver it to where we eat it. Most of the food movements that we hear about—slow foods, local foods, organic foods and food justice—have emerged as a response to ethical concerns regarding the increasingly dominant food system often referred to as the *global food system*.
>
> (Sandler 2015, 3)

While elaborating on global food systems Sandler emphasizes its 'transnational and industrial' (2015, 4) character and observes that despite its dynamic and decentralized nature, some of its salient characteristics makes such systems problematic as their comprehensive operations come into direct conflict with issues of food ethics and food security. Among its manifold drawbacks, global food systems endanger food sovereignty and food autonomy, adversely affects communal

DOI: 10.4324/9781003300762-18

and cultural diversity practices. Food systems have widespread ecological impact because of their agricultural practices and it negatively impacts animal welfare through its meat processing standards. Sustainability advocates desire policy change and a reform in global food systems based on a respect for biodiversity and food justice whereby independent farmers and farming operations would be saved and not have to succumb to vested interests of large corporations who are routinely rewarded by national and international agricultural laws. The 2006 Sustainable Consumption Roundtable Report "I will if you will: Towards Sustainable Consumption" observes that sustainability as a long-term goal can be achieved through 'sustainable habits and choices' (2006, 1) but such a change will come through a 'supportive framework' (2006, 1) consisting of 'people, business and government' (2006, 1) which forms the 'triangle of change' (2006, 1).

Addressing Sustainability Activism in Fiction and Non-Fiction

Debating the food ethics of the global food systems one must realise that 'living within ecological limits is the non-negotiable basis for our social and economic development' (2006, 1) and sustainability advocates must address the issue of consumption while making allowances for the abovementioned ecological limits. The Sustainable Consumption Report identifies that the real challenge for implementing sustainable consumption at a global level must consist in breaking consumption patterns which are "locked in" (2006, 6) and perpetuate cycles of unsustainable choices which are determined by a variety of socio-cultural factors. Nutrition is one of the key discourses where unsustainable consumption patterns need to be broken. Ruth Ozeki's *My Year of Meats* and Barbara Kingsolver's *Animal, Vegetable, Miracle* address the food ethics debate and advocate sustainable nutrition choices through fiction and actual farming experiment. Ozeki and Kingsolver understand that nutrition strategies are based on certain culinary habits which unwittingly adhere to the "locked in" paradigm of unsustainable choices. These texts seem to suggest that a change in sustainable consumption habits will require people, governments, and businesses ("the triangle of change") to act in unison and replace conventional patterns of growing, cultivating, cooking, eating, and sharing food. Ozeki and Kingsolver's texts provide a blueprint for implementing such a change and in the process suggest an alternative to the 'locked in' model of social behavior which when practiced effectively might put an end to the unfair practices of global food system networks and empower the independent farmers and local food growers and ensure 'food justice' (Sandler 2015, 27) at the grassroots level.

Ruth Ozeki's novel *My Year of Meats*, published in 1998 exposes the global beef industry and its malpractices especially the widespread use of a synthetic hormone DES in livestock. The novel examines the role of media in popularizing a food culture which is based on eating habits that back large meat processing corporations. Akiko, a Japanese housewife, and Jane Takagi-Little, a Japanese-American television script writer are remotely situated characters but a certain television documentary called "My American Wife" deeply affects their lives and compels a change in the way they think about food and nutrition. Jane is more intrinsically connected to the documentary as she is at the helm of the creative team filming the documentary. Jane Takagi writes the brief for "My American Wife" in the following manner:

Meat is the Message. Each weekly half-hour episode of "My American Wife" must culminate in the celebration of a featured meat, climaxing in its glorious consumption. It's the meat (not the Mrs.) who is the star of the show! Of course, the "Wife of the Week" is important too. She must be attractive, appetizing, and all-American. She is the Meat Made Manifest: ample, robust yet never tough, or hard to digest. Through her, "the Japanese housewives will feel the hearty sense of warmth, of comfort, of hearth and home-the traditional family values symbolized by the red meat in rural America" (Ozeki 1998, 12).

At the outset of the novel, when Jane is planning the show, she is aware of the corporate funding for "My American Wife" but what begins as a promising professional project soon transforms into a rite of passage. At the end of the novel, Jane Takagi knows the truth about the politics of the meat market in America and plans to publish her expose based on the data she procured while filming the documentary in the feedlot of a cattle ranch.

Monoculture and Feedlot Livestock farming: Threats to Sustainability

The monoculture farming tradition has been rightfully seen as an evil which empowers big business houses and does not safeguard the interests of the farmers. Meat production in America is monopolized by business houses which promotes monoculture. Vandana Shiva in "The Hijacking of the Global Food Supply" calls this the "emergence of food totalitarianism" (Shiva 2014a, 52). Ken Midkiff and Wendell Berry in "The Meat We Eat" have been unequivocal about the need to change the practices of the United States Department of Agriculture (USDA) which has jeopardized food security by favoring corporate business houses. Midkiff and Berry observe:

> This concentration of our food supply is also a national security threat…The giant companies own it all, from feed mills, to nurseries, to finishing operations, to slaughterhouses, to delivery, to retailers…Their goal is uniformity of product, the better to maximize volume, efficiency, and the speed of the so-called disassembly line, where the cadavers are carved up. The products that land on the store shelves are dismally uniform; every pork chop looks and tastes like every other pork chop. What they also have in common is that the animal from which they have been taken has been raised on a diet of antibiotics. As a result, the meat is now laden with pathogens—disease—causing bacteria— that have grown resistant to those antibiotics, as well as with heavy metals used as appetite enhancers. No wonder the meat tastes lousy.
>
> (2004, 14–15)

Jane's journey through the heartland of America acquaints her with the politics of the meat industry and the operations of Concentrated Animal Feeding Operation (CAFO) which have endangered the diversity and the ecosystems associated with animal husbandry and farming.

While filming her show Jane acquires insights about farming and cattle raising in America as well as eating traditions. Cultures of consumption were changing in places to accommodate vegan diets and organic produce-based nutrition plans. Yet the threat to the food security system remained with the widespread use of hormone-enhanced meat which in turn was responsible for the alarming rate of obesity among adult Americans. While interviewing one of her participants Jane learns about DES and its widespread use in the meat industry. About DES, Jane observes:

Using DES and other drugs, like antibiotics, farmers could process animals on an assembly line, like cars or computer chips. Open-field grazing for cattle became unnecessary and inefficient and soon gave way to confinement feedlot operations, or factory farms, where thousands upon thousands of penned cattle could be fattened at troughs. This was an economy of scale. It was happening everywhere, the wave of the future, the marriage of science and big business (Ozeki 1998, 149).

Later in the novel, she encounters the horrors of a feedlot facility in Michigan and the operations at the slaughter house are equally nightmarish. Jane's cameraman Suzuki, captures the heifers feeding on a bunker on what turns out to be "an aborted fetus, almost fully grown, with matted fur, a delicate skull, and grotesquely bulging eyes" (1998, 314). The feedlot horror gives way to the brutality of the slaughterhouse. Jane observes:

Stepping into the slaughterhouse was like walking through an invisible wall into hell. Sight, sound, smell-every sense I thought I owned, that was mine, the slaughterhouse stripped from me, overpowered, and assaulted. Steam hissed, metal screeched against metal, clanging and clamoring, splitting the ear, relentless. Chains, pulleys, and iron hooks whipped around us with unbelievable speed, and as far as the eye could see, conveyors sneaked into the distance, heaped with skinned heads and steaming hearts…

Blood was everywhere: bright red, brick red, shades of brown and black, flowing, splattering, encrusting the walls, the men. The floors were graded toward central drains for easy cleaning, yet the place was caked with a dee, rotting filth (1998, 330).

Ozeki's description of the slaughterhouse serves as an objective correlative of the consequences of using hormones widely in feedlot operations and raises concerns about food security. At the end of the novel, Jane's decision to turn vegetarian and publish a book on her findings about the meat industry is Ozeki's attempt to introduce a corrective eco justice model into global food discourse. The novel anticipates debates on sustainability which would gain ground at the turn of the millennium. Jane's evolving understanding of nutrition and food is complemented by the sexual awakening of Akiko, a Japanese housewife. Watching Jane's documentary, she revises her own culture's conceptions about food and later overcomes an eating disorder to escape an oppressive marriage in the wake of giving up meat. Ozeki's text in making a plea for a more evolved understanding of food and a revision of the Western diet is introducing the ecological frame of reference into food discourse. Cheryl J. Fish remarks that Ozeki's novel

> suggests the importance of environmental justice and ecofeminism as social movements and interrelated critiques that have the power to bring together seemingly disparate individuals in a global economy; the novel also makes a claim for a kind of environmental and social justice citizenship.
>
> (Fish 2009, 44)

But more importantly, Ozeki's novel hints at the need to dismantle global food systems to make way for the local by suggesting an alternate discourse to rectify Western food diets which because of its excessive reliance on global food systems and synthetically enhanced produce was losing sight of the ecological imperatives of inhabiting a food chain.

This is what Barbara Kingsolver calls the "obligate symbiosis" (2007, 126) which should inform our eating choices and our nutrition plans. Her locavore experiment is as much a return to nature as also a concerted effort to acquire a deeper understanding of the ecology of food. What Ozeki explores in the realm of fiction, Kingsolver makes real with a life experiment in seasonal eating as a locavore. Kingsolver's text engages with the sustainability question as each step of her farm operations – from choosing seeds to slaughtering chicken to making cheese – her food choices are ecologically informed and aimed to change the Western diet with a movement away from processed to organic. Kingsolver's work gives us a blueprint to suggest that "sustainable networks" (SDC 1) of change are possible and it is possible to subvert traditions of sustainable consumption by reconstituting the sustainability triangle of people, business, and government along ecological lines.

Locavore Experiment with Kingsolver: Eating Seasonal and Growing your own Food

In *Animal, Vegetable, Miracle* Kingsolver spends a considerable part of her introduction discussing the implications of her decision to undertake a locavore experiment which was, in her words, "the adventure of realigning our lives with the food chain" (2007, 6). Kingsolver's experiment was the model for a farming culture which would in a small way counter the evils of industrial farming but more importantly because it was ecologically motivated it would also construct a healthy food culture where sustainability would also determine nutrition by promoting mindful food choices prioritizing seasonal produce. She defines food culture in the following manner:

At its heart, a genuine food culture is an affinity between people and the land that feeds them. Step one, probably, is to live on the land that feeds them, or at least on the same continent, ideally the same region. Step two is to be able to countenance the ideas of "food" and "dirt" in the same sentence, and three is to start poking into one's supply chain to learn where things are coming from. In the spirit of this adventure, our family set out to find ourselves a real American culture of food, or at least the piece of it that worked for us and to describe it to anyone who might be looking for something similar (2007, 20).

She also mentions that food cultures are both "aesthetic" and "functional" (2007,15) and allows the mindful citizen to balance the quantity and quality and move towards a more ecologically informed nutrition plan where the food is sourced locally and is seasonal. Knowledge about seasonal fruits and vegetables would empower anyone to follow a nutrition plan which would try to do away with fossil fuels that are present in industrial agriculture-based produce and substantially reduce the ecological footprint. The functional aspect of a strong food culture becomes evident when knowledge about ecology, biodiversity, and sustainability motivates our food purchases. Mindful eaters would obviously source their food from local farmers which would integrate community-centered farms into the economy and challenge the global food system which obviously favors industrial farming backed by corporate organizations.

In order to liberate our palates from the bane of processed or refined food knowledge about farming should be complemented by a desire to keep to home-cooked food. The paper earlier noted the inevitability of falling into certain 'locked' (SDC 2006, 6) patterns of consumption which discouraged sustainable habits of farming and eating. Kingsolver holds culture responsible for promoting a perception among the urban citizens that cooking was a time-consuming and dreary job and such a mindset encouraged the affinity towards packaged and processed food. She observes that a reliance on "packaged" and "takeout" food indicates an "obligate symbiosis" (2007, 126) and people feel it frees them from the kitchen. What it does in the long drive is create a "pathological food culture" (2007, 126).

Individual Responsibility Begins with Resisting Food Culture

Julian Dastar in his Tedtalk on "Sustainable nutrition without thinking" also mentions our autopilot mode of shopping from supermarkets where a "context" influences our food choices and we choose to buy impulsively rather than mindfully. He advocates psychological nudges to reform our consumption patterns by suggesting supermarkets to give us more information on the product labels and also give us feedback on our ecological footprints. But such reform measures are unrealistic as supermarket chains favour industrially farmed produce. Until a more supportive context emerges and gives us our psychological nudge we must plan our nutrition by prioritizing the food we get rather than the food we want (Dastar 2021). Kingsolver proposes a return to the kitchen for a similar reason by using seasonal and local produce and by putting them into innovative menus. Family recipes, and shared wisdom on food all come into play when one is cooking to feed a family. It is here, in the kitchen, that a strong food culture is consolidated and there is a fair chance that we are able to embrace sustainability. Speaking in favor of such a food tradition, Kingsolver remarks:

Cooking is the great divide between good eating and bad. The gains are quantifiable: cooking and eating at home, even with quality ingredients, costs pennies on the dollar compared with meals prepared by a restaurant or factory. Shoppers who are most daunted by the high price of organics may be looking at bar codes on boutique- organic prepared foods, not actual vegetables. A quality diet is not an elitist option for the do-it-yourselfer. Globally speaking, people consume more soft drinks and packaged foods as they grow more affluent; home-cooked meals with fresh ingredients are the mainstay of rural, less affluent people. This link between economic success and nutritional failure has become so widespread, that it has a name: the nutrition transition (2007, 127).

A lifestyle change is imperative to embrace sustainability as a nutritional goal, and a food culture to be aesthetically and economically viable the cooking paradigms need to be reworked to accommodate what we get instead of what we want. Kingsolver's text is punctuated with recipes which suggest various ways to cook seasonal ingredients like zucchini, squash, tomatoes, and local mushrooms.

"Animal, Vegetable, Miracle" also focuses on the ways government legislation has not mandated sustainability as a farming goal. More importantly, conglomerates cashing in on the cult of organic food "follow the letter of organic regulations while violating their spirit" (2007, 123). Kingsolver believes that a better way to preserve food security is by patronizing local farms which specialize in sustainable farming and "organic agri-forestry" (Dastar 2021). When Kingsolver is advocating for the locals she seems to be answering Michael Pollan's concern in his book 'In Defense of Food' that the need of the hour was to create a "broader, more ecological-more cultural-view of food" (2007, 102). Like home-cooking, investing in sustainable local farms is an affirmative step towards building a strong food tradition. Kingsolver defends her promotion of the local in the following manner:

> Local food is a handshake deal in a community gathering place. It involves farmers with first names, who show up week after week. It means an open-door policy on the fields, where neighborhood buyers are welcome to come have a look, and pick their food from the vine. Local is farmers growing trust.

> (2007,123)

The sustainable local farm is a return to the food chain but also celebrates the legacy of farmers. Living off the produce of the land we start to value the role of the farmer in the food chain. Moreover, it makes us responsible custodians of biodiversity, food ethics, and food justice. It also gives one the knowledge to combat "food totalitarianism" and ensure "food democracy" (Shiva 2014a, 52). Both Ozeki and Kingsolver have shown how a move towards sustainable nutrition is a micro-narrative which involves an intimate knowledge about the sources of the food which finds its place on our plate. In Ozeki's *My Year of Meats* Takagi showcases a lesbian couple who have turned vegetarian after coming to know about the prevalence of hormones in meat. They describe this nutrition choice as an "ethical one" (1998, 243). Seeing them, a viewer in Japan starts using organic vegetables more copiously in her stews and sauces, giving her meat dishes depth and flavor (220). Becoming mindful about what we eat is the first step towards sustainable nutrition and ecologically run agri-farms can help motivate us towards mindful and sustainable nutrition.

The quest for a sustainable diet involves ecologically involved dietary choices. Not everyone needs to become vegetarian and take recourse to a plant-based eating regime. Kingsolver observes that animal harvesting is essential as it balances vegetable but one should choose free-range livestock raised on manual grazing. She remarks perceptively:

> I respect every diner who makes morally motivated choices about consumption…But I've come to different conclusions about livestock. The ve-vangelical pamphlets showing jam- packed chickens and sick downer- cows usually declare, as their first principle, that all meat is factory- farmed. That is false, and an affront to those of us you can't run away on harvest day who work to raise animals humanely, or who support such practices with our buying power…But meat, poultry, and eggs from animals raised on open pasture are the traditional winter fare of my grandparents, and they serve us well here in the months when it would cost a lot of fossil fuels to keep us in tofu…A hundred different paths may lighten the world's load of suffering. Giving up meat is one path; giving up bananas is another. The more we know about our food system, the more we are called into complex choices. It seems facile to declare one single forbidden fruit, when humans live under so many different kinds of trees.
>
> (2007, 224–225)

Thus, Kingsolver admits, that our nutrition choices are subject to the ecological limits within which we operate. If we refer back to the triangle of people-business and government as an agent of sustainable change as proposed by the SCR (Sustainable Consumption Roundtable) and try to come up with evolved consumer choice patterns based on the three "E"s of "Engage, Enable, Exemplify and Encourage" (2006, 12–13) we have to make changes at the individual level by breaking unhealthy habits and learning about agriculture and ecosystems to promote sustainability as a food goal.

The Indian Context: Legacy of Vandana Shiva

In India, the work of Vandana Shiva to promote sustainable farming and seed-sharing to combat monocultures of farming through Navdanya is an effective implementation of the four E patterns. Shiva, writing on the new agricultural paradigm that Navdanya embodies, remarks:

Navdanya's "Health per Acre" shows that a shift to biodiverse organic farming and ecological intensification increases the output of nutrition while reducing input costs. When agriculture output is measured in "health per acre" and "nutrition per acre" instead of "yield per acre", biodiverse ecological systems have a much higher output. This should be the strategy for protecting the livelihoods of farmers as well as the right to food and the right to health of all our people. The paradigm shift we propose is a shift from monocultures to diversity; from chemical-intensive agriculture to ecologically intensive, biodiversity-intensive agriculture; from external inputs to internal inputs; from yield per acre to health and nutrition per acre; from food as a commodity to food as nourishment and nutrition (2014b, 117).

How the Pandemic Impacted Our Food Culture and Our Food Chain

The urgency to implement sustainability and create a food culture around it has never been so vital as in this our post-pandemic new reality. The pandemic has adversely affected the global food system and due to the closure of borders the food supply chain has also been compromised. Hunger and the availability of food have become very real concerns. Dipa Sinha in her paper "Hunger and Food Security in the Times of Covid-19" has remarked on the food crisis which India had faced during the 2020 lockdown:

The global novel coronavirus pandemic and the ensuing economic slowdown have led to rising concerns of food insecurity across the world. Quarantine requirements, social distancing norms, lockdowns, border closing, etc., have disrupted supply and distribution networks making the availability and accessibility of food uncertain. Loss of livelihoods due to the associated economic distress has made it more difficult for people in the informal sectors and in precarious occupations to meet their basic needs. The World Bank has estimated that 71 million people will fall be pushed into extreme poverty across the globe as a result of the pandemic (World Bank 2020). The UN has stated that we are facing an impending food emergency and the World Food Programme estimates that an additional 130 million people could fall into the category of being food insecure over and above the 820 million who were so classified by the State of Food Insecurity in the World Report, 2019 (United Nations 2020). In India too, the Covid-19 pandemic and the national lockdown have led to a loss of livelihoods and have added to the demand depression that the country was already facing (5320).

In the conclusion to her paper, she has noted that the government public distribution schemes to help address the food crisis have only been moderately successful what with "quotas" of distribution being limited (5329). The Committee on World Food Security High-Level Panel of Experts on Food Security and Nutrition Rome, September 2020 in their HLPE issues Paper "Impacts of COVID-19 on food security and nutrition: developing effective policy responses to address the hunger and malnutrition pandemic" has studied the food and nutrition problem more comprehensively. It states:

The COVID-19 pandemic that has spread rapidly and extensively around the world since late 2019 has had profound implications for food security and nutrition. The unfolding crisis has affected food systems1 and threatened people's access to food via multiple dynamics. We have witnessed not only a major disruption to food supply chains in the wake of lockdowns triggered by the global health crisis but also a major global economic slowdown. These crises have resulted in lower incomes and higher prices of some foods, putting food out of reach for many, undermining the right to food, and stalling efforts to meet Sustainable Development Goal (SDG) 2: "Zero hunger". The situation is fluid and dynamic, characterized by a high degree of uncertainty. According to the World Health Organization, the worst effects are yet to come (Ghebreyesus 2020; Khorsandi 2020). Most health analysts predict that this virus will continue to circulate for a least one or two more years (Scudellari 2020) (HLPE1).

According to the HLPE Report on of the major issues affecting food security during the lockdown was the disruptions in the food chain brought about by the stringent lockdown measures. The report states:

There have been major disruptions to food supply chains in the wake of lockdown measures, which have affected the availability, pricing, and quality of food (Barrett 2020). The closure of restaurants and other food service facilities led to a sharp decline in demand for certain perishable foods, including dairy products, potatoes, and fresh fruits, as well as specialty goods such as chocolate and some high-value cuts of meat (Lewis 2020; Terazono and Munshi 2020). As the pandemic-related lockdowns took hold in many countries in March-May of 2020, there were widespread media reports of food items being dumped or plowed back into the fields because of either collapsed demand or difficulties in getting these foods to markets (Yaffe-Bellany and Corkery 2020). Farmers without adequate storage facilities, including cold storage, found themselves with food that they could not sell. The movement of food through the channels of international trade was especially affected by lockdown measures. As borders closed and demand for certain food items dropped, food producers reliant on selling their crops via distant export markets were highly vulnerable, particularly those producers focused on perishable food and agricultural products, such as fresh fruits and vegetables, or specialty crops, such as cocoa (Clapp and Moseley 2020). In the early months of the outbreak of COVID-19, some food-exporting countries also imposed export restrictions on key staple food items like rice and wheat, which led to some disruptions in the global movement of these staples as well as higher prices of these crops relative to others (Laborde et al. 2020). Certain countries, including those with a high prevalence of food insecurity, are highly dependent on imported food and on commodity exports (FAO et al., 2019), which may make them particularly vulnerable to these types of supply chain disruptions. Many of these export restrictions were lifted by August 2020, *"although the risk remains that such restrictions might be re-imposed, depending on the severity of any future spikes in the disease and the reimposition of lockdown measures"* (Italics mine) (HLPE 3).

Conclusion: Sustaining the Sustainability Movement on Our Plates

Now on the verge of a probable third wave, we need to implement the lessons we learnt about food security and start practicing a sustainable food culture where the sustainability triangle of people of "people, business and government" (SDC

2006) will work together to redress the food shortage which will inevitably affect the food supply chain if restrictions are levied once more. For those of us who live in India, we have always had a strong community-centric food tradition which might be easily adapted to sustainability goals. Chef Vikas Khanna in his latest book *Barkat* which documents the FEED INDIA campaign that he spearheaded during the pandemic has written about food ethics as integral to Indian existence. He speaks about Maa Annapurna in the Hindu tradition as the nurturer-deity and the festival of Ramadan which celebrates 'unity through food' (2021, 107). Thus, the ideal of food justice has already been enshrined in the Hindu way of life. Chef Khanna writes about how different sections of the Indian community came together to feed the migrant workers during the lockdown proving the resilience of the Indian food tradition. Individuals like Khanna have implemented other channels of food supply and have brought in local communities to feed millions. Wendell Berry in his book "What are People for?" had observed:

Eaters, that is, must understand that eating takes place inescapably in the world, that it is inescapably an agricultural act and that how we eat determines, to a considerable extent how the world is used. This is a simple way of describing a relationship that is inexpressibly complex. To eat responsibly is to understand and enact, so far as one can, this complex relationship (1990, 149).

Berry asks each individual to participate in the food production, to try to cook their own food, to ensure the origin of their food, and also try to buy produce and meat from local farmers (149–50). Sustainability advocates are also urging city dwellers to invest in permaculture and grow their own food. "Smell of the Earth" a sustainable farming initiative located in Bolpur, West Bengal holds regular farming courses to educate people on farming methods. They have taken it upon themselves to teach self-reliance in food production as well as water and energy management for they believe that that is the most important lesson the pandemic has taught us all (Fb post 20th October 2020). Their motto is: "Let's learn to heal our planet ecosystem-by-ecosystem" (Fb Post 10th November 2021).

The need of the hour is trying to invest in a sustainable nutrition plan and a food culture where the consumer or the eater would know 'eating is an agricultural act' (Berry 1990, 146) and thereby rectify the "cultural amnesia" (Berry 1990, 146) that industrial farming has promoted. We need to design a "transition from the globalization paradigm to the localization paradigm" (Shiva 2014b, 136). We need to prioritize "decommodification of food, the reclamation of food as our being, our nourishment, our identity, and our human right" (Shiva 2014b, 136). The future need not be bleak if we can make the right choices and as Kingsolver states "Food is the rare moral arena in which the ethical choice is generally the one more likely to make you groan with pleasure" (2007, 22). Let us have our pleasure by eating responsibly.

References

Berry, Wendell. 1990. "The Pleasures of Eating." In *What are People For: Essays by Wendell Berry*, 145–152. San Francisco: North Point Press.

CFS (Committee on World Food Security). 2020. *Impacts of COVID-19 on Food Security and Nutrition: Developing Effective Policy Responses to Address the Hunger and Malnutrition Pandemic.* Italy: HLPE Joint Steering Committee.

Dastar, Julian. 2021. "Sustainable Nutrition without Thinking." *TEDxHWZ*, December 18, 2021. https://www.youtube.com/watch?v=bgCtGqLEZdA

Fish, Cheryl J. 2009. "The Toxic Body Politic: Ethnicity, Gender, and Corrective Eco-Justice in Ruth Ozeki's 'My Year of Meats' and Judith Helfand and Daniel Gold's 'Blue Vinyl.'" *Melus* 34(2): 43–62.

Khanna, Vikas. 2021. *Barkat: The Inspiration and Story behind One of the World's Largest Food Drives, FEED INDIA.* New Delhi: Penguin Random House.

Kingsolver, Barbara, Steven L. Hopp and Camille Kingsolver. 2007. *Animal, Vegetable, Miracle: A Year of Food Life.* New York: Harper Collins.

Midkiff, Ken and Wendell Berry. 2004. *The Meat You Eat: How Corporate Farming Has Endangered America's Food Supply.* New York: St.Martin's Griffin.

Ozeki, Ruth. 1998. *My Year of Meats.* Edinburgh: Picador.

Pollan, Michael. 2008. *In Defense of Food.* New York: Penguin.

Sandler, Ronald L. 2015. *Food Ethics: The Basics.* Abingdon: Routledge.

Shiva, Vandana. 2014a. "Hijacking of the Global Food Supply." In *The Vandana Shiva Reader*, foreword by Wendell Berry, 41–54. Kentucky: University Press of Kentucky.

Shiva, Vandana. 2014b. "Toward a New Agriculture Paradigm: Health per Acre." In *The Vandana Shiva Reader*, foreword by Wendell Berry, 113–138. Kentucky: University Press of Kentucky.

Sinha, Dipa. 2021. "Hunger and Food Security in the Times of Covid 19." *Journal of Social and Economic Development* 23(Suppl. 2): 5320–5331.

Sustainable Development Commission and National Consumer Council. May 2006. *Sustainable Consumption Roundtable I Will if You Will: Towards Sustainable Consumption.*

17 Disease, Wellbeing, and the Idea of Health in Select Cinematic Representations of the Macbeth Metaphor

Anuradha Mazumder

Composed in the first decade of the seventeenth century, and replete with images of disease and illness, *Macbeth* shows a sustained engagement with the motif of illness that, in turn, underscores its underlying concern with health. However, 'health' is not delineated in the play as a biomedical condition but as a socio-cultural concept, in which individual and communal health and wellbeing are imbricated: as inordinate ambition leads Macbeth on the path of murder and violence, he progressively displays signs of paranoia and 'madness;' as his sickness intensifies, his oppression of Scotland reaches a feverish pitch. Conversely, the more Scotland bleeds, the more friends turn into enemies and desert the royal couple, the worse the manifestations of their disease become. Through such a holistic coalescing of the health of the body and that of the body politic, Shakespeare examines the correlation between disease and violence: for Macbeth's murder of King Duncan spirals into a series of violent murders and bloodshed that disrupt his sanity and his country's health. Shakespeare, thus, locates disease not within the body nor outside it, but in the complex exchanges between an individual and his environment; if the interaction is violent in nature, attainment of health remains an impossible dream. In charting such an intricate trajectory of disease, the play anticipates the biopsychosocial model of health advanced by Engel in 1977, which recognizes the complex interactions of biological, psychological, and social factors in understanding health and illness; a concept that has gained wide acceptance in the scientific community in the last two decades (Fava and Sonino 2017). This chapter will study two contemporary film adaptations of the play vis-à-vis such holistic ideas of health and wellbeing – Vishal Bhardwaj's *Maqbool* (2004) and Justin Kurzel's *Macbeth* (2015) – to analyze how recent adaptations reimagine Shakespeare's *Macbeth*, and re-contextualize its themes of peace and health, violence and disease in the present day. The films take the disease-violence association a step further by locating the former within the cultural construct of violent masculinity that was widely in circulation in Shakespeare's time and survives to this day. This chapter will thus explore how the adaptations compel us to re-think health and disease from a cultural perspective and examine the prospect of health and wellness in our historical moment, fraught as it is with ceaseless violence.

For all its blood and violence, *Macbeth* portrays the contrasting forces of peace and harmony with equal emphasis through its imagery and symbolism; the

DOI: 10.4324/9781003300762-19

playwright wishes to impress upon our minds the state of grace that the eponymous hero sacrifices at the altar of power and personal ambition. Through the repetition of such keywords as "honour", "duty", and "service" in the first section of the play, Shakespeare evokes the image of an ordered and well-knit society, where the personal and the political exist in a complementary and symbiotic relationship with each other. When the country's territorial integrity is threatened by foreign attacks, brave Macbeth successfully overpowers the enemy on behalf of his king. However, when the same valiant warrior – driven by ambition, emboldened by the witches' prophecy, and goaded by an ambitious wife – murders Duncan for the throne, the violence of the act unsettles him and his country. Order, stability, and peace – the measures of health in any society – desert the kingdom and its new king. Henceforth, images of disease dominate the play – Macbeth hallucinates and sees daggers in the air; Lady Macbeth's doctor diagnoses her disease as spiritual, and beyond the scope of his medical knowledge; while Rosse mournfully narrates Scotland's "violent sorrow" (Muir 2013, 132) under Macbeth's reign to Malcolm, in Act IV, Scene iii. All through, the royal couple's descent into "madness" is portrayed against the backdrop of a Scotland bleeding to death, thereby portraying personal and communal health as mutually inclusive states of being. Besides, though Macbeth displays symptoms of melancholy (as the disease was outlined by the prevalent humoral theories of health in Shakespeare's time), the play does not name his illness as such, thereby avoiding the delimiting of the disease within the body of the protagonist: instead, "madness", "thick-coming fancies", "heat-oppressed brain" are some of the abstract images it employs to refer to Macbeth's sickness. Shakespeare thus clearly portrays Macbeth's disease as more than a biomedical disorder, implying its psychological, spiritual, and social dimensions. As Suparna Roychoudhury (2013) observes:

> With its melancholy remaining unmarked, and its hallucinations not easily interpreted as such, the play's portrayal of pathological imagination is situated outside, or alongside, the terms of contemporary medical discourse. It forces its audience to consider the nature of imaginative disease more abstractly, in terms of the relation between mind and world.
>
> (Roychoudhury 2013, 219)

The fact that Macbeth begins to hallucinate as soon as the couple agrees on regicide offers ample evidence of the protagonist's acute awareness of this coalescing of the "microcosm" (man) and the "macrocosm" (world/the body politic), and of the repercussions of disturbing the balance. As Bernard McElroy (2003, n. p.) maintains, the play "presents us with a man who has a clear conception of the universe and his proper place in it"; and what differentiates "such villains as Claudius, Angelo, and Macbeth from Richard III, Iago and Edmund is that the former fully admit the validity and worth of the moral laws they violate." Macbeth banishes sleep and peace with the first "unnatural" act itself – Duncan having been a saintly King at that, "so clear in his great office" (Muir 2013, 39), by Macbeth's own admission. Ironically, all his other crimes proceed from his desperation to secure his peace of mind, which continues to elude him, in the same way as peace and health continue to elude Scotland under his tyranny. Insomnia, the disease that nearly kills Macbeth, reflects the diseased state of his body, mind, and soul as well as the diseased state of Scotland during his reign.

In the context of the intertwining of man and world in the play, Act IV Scene iii, commonly referred to as the scene of "Malcolm's testing of Macduff," assumes special significance. As noted by Muir, it is the only scene in the play to provide vivid images of a suffering Scotland under Macbeth's misrule. Shortly before the scene, the trouble-torn tyrant seeks out the Weird Sisters in the desperate hope of calming his inner demons; while in the scene that immediately follows Scene iii, Lady Macbeth is discovered sleepwalking at night, disheveled and disoriented, trying to cleanse her hands of invisible bloodstains. Nowhere else in Shakespeare's oeuvre is the interdependence of individual and communal health stated more clearly and persuasively as in *Macbeth*. However, Shakespeare also promises a cure for Scotland's disease in the figure of Malcolm, who will restore the country "to a sound and pristine health" (Muir 2013, 148). The play, thus, finally endorses not the valiant, violent masculinity of Macbeth but an alternative version of manhood that is evident in Malcolm – one who is less glorious a warrior, but who possesses the "King-becoming graces" (Muir 2013, 127) of patience, temperance, stableness and humble service to the state; virtues that ensure the holistic health of man and his world.

It is, therefore, somewhat surprising that popular twenty-first-century film adaptations of *Macbeth*, whether in the East or the West, focus single-mindedly on the mental discord and suffering of Macbeth and his wife, understating the play's holistic melding of private and communal health. In doing so, they temper down the central concern that catalyzes the anti-Macbeth movement in the latter half of the play and establishes the moral dominance of Malcolm and Macduff. Of course, film adaptations of literary texts have no aesthetic obligation to be 'faithful' to their literary sources; film criticism has moved beyond the fidelity/betrayal discourse. Nonetheless, adaptations that concentrate on the personal crime-and-remorse story of the Macbeth couple at the expense of the play's lamentation over a diseased land present a reductionist reading of the play. Both *Maqbool* and *Macbeth*, the films selected for this study, seem to fall into the familiar trap of valorizing the inner discord of the "villain-hero" in a near-total omission of the land and its suffering. They also stay silent on the possibility of a final cure for the land's ailment, in a marked departure from their dramatic source.

It is important to note how Bhardwaj and Kurzel magnify the violence inherent in Shakespeare's protagonist by portraying their heroes as irascible, and cold-blooded in the execution of bloody deeds. Kurzel stages battle scenes, left offstage by Shakespeare, in which he depicts Macbeth's lust for violence and victory on the field by bathing the screen in bold, luxurious red. Bhardwaj similarly includes a bloody prologue to the film with close-up shots of the corrupt police officers Pandit and Purohit – "Bollywood" counterparts of the Weird Sisters – frolicking with a petty criminal of a rival gang before shooting him dead in a police vehicle, smearing the car windows, and the screen with blood. A dabbler in astrology,

Pandit ominously predicts Miya Maqbool bathing Mumbai in blood in the near narrative future. In the next scene, Mughal – archrival of Maqbool's mentor, the ganglord Jahangir Khan/Abba Ji – is disposed of under Maqbool's supervision, following the ruthless laws of gang-rivalry in modern urban metropoles. While Bhardwaj situates his film in the twenty-first century Mumbai underworld, a world obsessed with murder, violence, and power through political patronage, Kurzel sets his film in medieval Scotland, a world of war, gore, death, and glory. Both directors accentuate the bloody, violent aspect of their protagonists and the worlds they inhabit.

While there is no denying that violence is commercially viable for filmmakers, this chapter reads such directorial choices as a reflection of the overly individualistic and machoistic culture of the present day. Our culture celebrates the individual (even the idiosyncratic, the violent, and the dysfunctional individual) at the expense of the communal, equating heroism with aggression; man-versus-society, as opposed to man-in-society, is the dominant cultural trope of our times. This chapter argues that in their amplification of the play's latent violence and chaos the adaptations are the products of their times; they call into question the possibility of holistic wellness in a world suffused with violence. Through creative improvisations, the films recycle the Macbeth metaphor to scrutinize the relationship of violence with the cultural construct of heroic masculinity – traditionally associated with aggression and paternity – and explore the implications of the association for personal and communal wellbeing in the contemporary world. Bhardwaj's Maqbool and Kurzel's Macbeth are haunted by the question of heirs and succession; they display a lust for power and a propensity to inflict violence that places them unequivocally within the centuries-old cultural discourse on heroic masculinity. Interpreted in the context of the all-pervading violence in our lives – acts of violence induced by religious intolerance, terrorism, and xenophobia; and aggressive, machoistic rhetoric in politics and media – these adaptations are a comment on our times by informed and sensitive artist-interpreters.

Such a study, however, demands that an important question concerning film adaptations of literary texts is first addressed; a question aptly phrased by Morris Beja (1979, 80): "What relationship should a film have to the original source? Should it be 'faithful'? Can it be? To what?" Considering how poststructuralist criticism has dislodged the very idea of the "originality" of texts, can we afford to continue the valorization of the literary source, tacitly suggesting the inferiority of the adaptation? Given the critical consensus that a "text is a multidimensional space in which a variety of writings, none of them original, blend and clash" (Barthes 1977, 146), could any literary text render up to the intelligent reader "a single, correct 'meaning' which the filmmaker has either adhered to or in some sense violated or tampered with" (McFarlane 1996, 3)? The answers are, unsurprisingly, in the negative; because all texts, consciously or otherwise, refer to and borrow from other pre-existing texts. Julia Kristeva (1986, 37) coined the term "intertextuality" to refer to this relational dynamic among texts that make them part of a larger matrix of cultural discourse: "any text is constructed as a mosaic of quotations; any text is the absorption and transformation of another." Thus, with the concept of "originality" having been challenged and destabilized, questions of "fidelity" and "betrayal" have lost currency and legitimacy in adaptation criticism. "Bakhtin's conception of the author as orchestrator of a pre-existing discourse, along with Foucault's downgrading of the author in favor of a pervasive anonymity of discourse, opened the way to a non-originary approach to all arts" (Stam and Raengo 2005, 9).

Recent film criticism, therefore, focuses on an intertextual approach to onscreen adaptations of literary texts. Such an approach studies how a cinematic text relates to its literary source – which images and symbols from its literary source the adaptation retains and which ones it leaves out and why – and how it enters into a dialogue with previous genres and historical contexts. An intertextual approach also studies how the filmic text builds upon and reinterprets themes that may have been latent, or hinted at in the literary source to create new meanings for contemporary audiences. It is chiefly through such a critical lens that this chapter analyzes the adaptations by Bhardwaj and Kurzel. It explores how the adaptations reformulate the Macbeth metaphor by bringing the cultural construct of valiant masculinity in dialogue with the motifs of peace and health. It argues that the ambiguous endings of both adaptations, unlike the neat conclusion of the Shakespearean play, reflect the directors' uncertainty regarding the possibility of health and wellness in our conflicted times.

Bhardwaj transplants Shakespeare's *Macbeth* into the criminal world of Mumbai, with its distinct ethos. While the play mourns the collapse of law and order and "slides imperceptibly from a picture of defilement of nature … into lamentation over a land" (Biswas 2006, n. p.), there is no "defilement" or "violation" to lament over in the Bhardwaj adaptation, since the action unfolds in the crime world, which exists beneath the legal and moral ground. Besides, the film blurs the legal/illegal and moral/immoral boundaries by showing the state machinery to be as corrupt as the crime world it is supposed to keep in check. As Pandit and Purohit discuss the subtle strategies of police encounters in Mumbai, the audience understands that corruption and violence are the diseases that plague Mumbai; and that there is no difference between the scourge and the purge. However, despite these outward differences with its dramatic source, Bhardwaj's film explores the motif of dis-ease and illness within a similar interpretative framework, i.e. within the cultural construct of virile manhood. Members of the criminal underworld are shown as bound by unwritten, but firmly entrenched, codes of loyalty and brotherhood that closely resemble the spirit of the comitatus held sacred in old, heroic societies. Maqbool himself is aware of the inviolable nature of these bonds, and the ripples of repercussion and retribution that an act of betrayal would cause. This is why, despite his love for Nimmi, Abba Ji's mistress, and Lady Macbeth's Indian counterpart, he is not easily convinced of murdering his mentor. When he agrees to it, love for Nimmi does not appear to be the sole reason to stir him to action; Maqbool considers murder seriously, only when Nimmi hints that the young Guddu, son of Kaka/Banquo and Abba Ji's son-in-law-to-be, would soon inherit the underworld empire, thwarting Maqbool's ambitions.

Maqbool commits the murder soon after, his act clearly propelled by the conventional patriarchal anxiety regarding paternity and succession, in addition to his desire for Nimmi. In an unmistakable paralleling of the play, while the violence of the act throws the criminal world into a state of chaotic confusion, the perpetrator too suffers swift retribution. However, unlike in the play, the film focuses on the disease within its protagonist's mental hell in which guilt, fear, and anxiety rage unchecked. Maqbool's doubts about the paternity of Nimmi's child and his fear of Guddu/Fleance's revenge add to his madness and make him hallucinate, while Nimmi struggles to calm him down. His paranoia is soon followed by Nimmi's own swift decline into madness – in an ironic reversal of roles, as the insomniac and delirious Nimmi complains of her unborn child crying inconsolably over the murder of its father, the helpless Maqbool fails to convince her that the child is his. Though Nimmi's newborn is later found safe in the hands of Sameera and Guddu in the hospital the safety appears tentative; the film ends on an inconclusive note, as if unconvinced of the prospect of peace and health returning to a world so out of joint. The audience is left wondering if the apparent joy at the birth of an heir in the underworld ironically points toward a future saga of love, betrayal, revenge, and deadly intrigue. In his deft transposition of the spirit of the dramatic source into the Bollywood movie, Bhardwaj, thus, asks pertinent questions about the relationship between disease and violence, underscoring how health and wellness, at the personal and the collective level, remain a far cry when violent masculinity becomes ascendant.

James I published a short piece called *A Counter Blaste to Tobacco*, anonymously, in 1604 (its authorship was disclosed 12 years after its publication). Instigated by a concern for public health, and assuming his kingship to be divinely sanctioned, he attempts to curb the widespread smoking habit among the English population in this document. In his analysis of the relationship between King and country, while suggesting remedies for curing a diseased commonwealth, James compares the ruler of the kingdom with a physician:

> For remedie whereof, it is the Kings (as the proper Phisician of his politicke-body) to purge it of all those diseases, by Medicines meete for the same: as by a certaine milde, and yet just form of government to maintaine the Publicke quietnesse, and prevent all occasions of Commotions by the example of his owne Person and Court....
>
> (James I 1954, 8)

Critical of the narratives of masculine valor and soldierly virtues in his day, James advocates a different set of values and qualities in a King, endorsing a milder, more prudent manhood as being fit to govern the country and lead it to prosperity and health. Macbeth and Maqbool fail precisely in this respect; they are both ineffectual in purging "the gentle weal" (Muir 2013, 93) and cleansing the burden of misdeeds from their minds when they find themselves at the helm of their respective "kingdoms". Diseased in body and mind, they fail to be the physicians to the world they inhabit, becoming the scourge instead.

The same excess of violence marks Kurzel's adaptation, indicating its similar predisposition of situating dis-ease in the complex interaction between man and world, and specifically within the referential framework of violent manhood. Kurzel begins his filmic narration not with the scene of the three witches planning to meet Macbeth, portending moral confusion as in the play, but with that of Macbeth and his Lady cremating their dead baby son. A violent battle scene immediately follows; as if Macbeth's own misery drives him to unleash hell on his enemies. In the battle, we encounter the fearsome image of Macbeth the warrior, a merciless slayer on the field. The violence in Kurzel's Macbeth is visceral and overwhelming.

The sophisticated, civil world of Shakespeare and his contemporaries was different from the world of the Homeric epics that celebrated the menacing force of violent heroism and war without limitations. Shakespeare's Macbeth is a glorious warrior, but not in the same sense as Achilles is in *The Iliad*. Achilles is the child of an ancient world that glorified rage and violence and sang epic songs in celebration of them; Achilles is completely consumed by his passionate fury and unapologetic of the violence that he unleashes in the world (Sloterdijk 2012). Shakespeare's Macbeth, on the other hand, is modern in his temperament – he has a complex inner life hidden away from the rest of the world, he suffers pangs of guilt and conscience and fear, thereby becoming more comprehensible to twenty-first-century audiences. Kurzel's Macbeth, however, looks even more tormented from the beginning: he is not the usual war hero, beloved of King and country, motivated by the heroic ideals of war that lead to the formation of character and nations. He is withdrawn, insular and violent. He fights fiercely but mechanically – his bloody sword slashing his enemies indiscriminately – all the while appearing to burn in the fires of his private hell. Through a series of close-up shots of his protagonist's face Kurzel "psychologizes" the character to such an extent that his Macbeth, played by Michael Fassbender, appears to be suffering from battle fatigue. As Ari Mattes (2015) notes:

> Fassbender's Macbeth is the clear product of the age of modern warfare, an embodiment of the psychological damage of warfare under conditions of modern armament. [His Macbeth] appears from the outset more like an Iraq veteran suffering from Post Traumatic Stress Disorder than a glorious, triumphant hero, as in the play.
>
> (Mattes 2015, n. p.)

Even after winning the decisive Battle of Ellon, Macbeth responds to the warmth of Duncan's welcome in the royal camp with terse courtesy, further accentuating his insular nature. The audience knows that seeds of betrayal have been sown in his heart by the Weird Sisters already: as they touch Macbeth's face while delivering their mysterious prophecy in a previous scene, Kurzel's Macbeth visualizes his coronation in an ambitious leap of the imagination. However, Macbeth worries that his crown would be a fruitless one; for he has cremated a baby boy before, and lost a young son in the war – Kurzel's improvisations on Shakespeare, both – while the witches have promised Banquo that, the latter's sons will be kings. Kurzel, thus, significantly heightens Macbeth's anxiety about his barren scepter, portraying it as the mainspring of his violence; he connects the themes of violence, paternity, and succession – the time-honored concerns of heroic manhood – in this visually magnificent film.

In fact, both directors provide strong psychological motivations for the reckless pursuit of violence by their protagonists – motivations that are either absent or latent in the play. The violence perpetrated by the title characters in both films is shown to stem from their anxieties related to power and its retention through successors. While Maqbool sacrifices his peace of mind at the altar of illicit love and strives to ensure his control of Abba Ji's gangland through his infant son, Kurzel's Macbeth is bruised by war and grief-stricken at the loss of his two sons. Both protagonists brood over questions of paternity and succession – one doubting his paternity initially, the other lamenting its tragic loss endlessly. Both directors, thus, weave the scripts of violence and masculinity together to examine their role in disrupting personal and communal health, thereby thematically linking violence not with heroism, but disease.

Indeed, the constituent attributes of masculinity and their implications for peace and wellness are implicit in the play itself; one can never forget Macbeth's reproach to his wife when she invokes his manliness to instigate him to murder in Act I, Sc. vii: "Pr'ythee, peace. I dare do all that may become a man; / Who dares do more is none" (Muir 2013, 41). As Philippa Sheppard (2018, n. p.) observes in her insightful essay on the dominant definitions of manhood in Western Europe at the time of the composition of *Macbeth*:

> The street sense of manhood was inextricably linked to the ability to inflict violence. This had been culturally entrenched by conduct books, from Castiglione's *The Courtier* onwards, long before the composition of these plays. These books codify manliness as chiefly exhibited through military prowess and paternity.

The adaptations by Bhardwaj and Kurzel offer a critique of this 500-year-old culture of violent, machoistic masculinity that forces individuals and communities to live diseased, dysfunctional, restless lives.

Kurzel exploits the cinematic possibilities of the grey, rugged landscapes of the Isle of Skye, the location where the film is shot, brilliantly; the somber landscape lends the film a grimness of tone that aptly parallels the moral confusion and corruption of the opening scenes of Shakespeare's play. Yet, instead of using the barren, brooding landscape to symbolize the diseased state of Scotland, he uses the Scottish scenery literally, as a magnificent canvas against which the saga of Macbeth's personal suffering is played out. Except for the single scene of the burning of Macduff's wife and children at stake, the horrors of the land stay muted in the film. Kurzel also redacts certain scenes and dialogues – such as the episode of Malcolm's testing of Macduff, and Macbeth's poetic lines on the balm of sleep being crucial to health – that significantly compromises the play's exploration of the themes of disease and health. While in Shakespeare's *Macbeth* the villain-hero's insomnia is central to his existential state, Kurzel leaves out the most beautiful passage in Act II Scene ii, where the hero laments his inability to enjoy "the innocent Sleep" and cries out in anguish, "Macbeth does murther Sleep" (Muir 2013, 53). Such omissions take away from Macbeth his tragic stature and emphasize the bestiality of his violence.

Ironically, as in the original, so in the screen adaptation, peace is achieved through violence when battles are fought for king and country – rebels are felled and rebellions are quelled right at the play's beginning by "valiant" Macbeth's brute force – but when the protagonist takes recourse to violence for personal gain hell breaks loose within and around him. Almost imperceptibly, Macbeth slides down the moral scale by choosing mindless violence as his way of life. However, unlike in the play, the stress in the film invariably falls on the mental agony of the royal couple, in near-total exclusion of the lament over the land that they contaminate with their violence. In fact, in both adaptations, the camera zooms in on the theatre of the protagonist's mind, the land and its suffering being secondary concerns.

While military prowess and paternity constituted one register of manliness in Shakespeare's time, Sheppard also talks about a large number of books and pamphlets written during the time that extolled "the masculine virtue of self-control" and decried bestial violence. King James himself promoted an image of manhood in which "manly strength is exemplified by peaceful and prudent service to the state" (Sheppard). Shakespeare's *Macbeth* records the transition from the first to the second kind of manhood; it opens with a celebration of heroic manhood, demonstrates the failure of the warrior as a peacetime ruler, and ends with the hope of the diseased land's return to health under Malcolm's prudent leadership. The cure to the disease is identified, and a return to healthy normalcy is promised at its end.

It is, therefore, pertinent to ponder why the adaptations under study fail to end with such an unambiguous message of hope and health. Maqbool's baby boy snuggling in Guddu's arms may hint at a temporary respite, but his birth could also suggest the continuity of the violent bloodline. Kurzel's film ends with a stronger sense of uncertainty – Banquo's young son Fleance grabs dead Macbeth's sword and runs away, while Malcolm storms out of the throne room in Dunsinane Castle after staring long and hard at the throne and his sword. We do not know if he runs in pursuit of Fleance. Kurzel leaves his film open-ended and ambiguous, perhaps suggesting an unending cycle in the struggle for the throne and thus, an eternal deferment of peace, stability, and health.

Questions of health and wellbeing have intrigued humans since time immemorial. Ancient societies struggled against fatal diseases and epidemics and feared contagion since the latter threatened to wipe out entire populations. Understandably, literature too has had an abiding interest in disease and health and has explored various dimensions of these since classical antiquity. An epidemic, for instance, serves the theatrical economy of Sophocles' *Oedipus Rex* by forming the background for the evolution of its plot. Despite this, however, knowledge of medicine was sparse; even in Shakespeare's England "it was expounded by numerous charlatans and quacks as well as by honest physicians" (Sett 1962, 185). Shakespeare's plays are significant in the history of medicine not merely for their numerous references to disease and its treatment but because, running deep into their imagery and characterization, such references reflect the playwright's more than a casual interest in health.

Living in the midst of an ongoing pandemic as we are now, the importance of finding a cure for illness and bringing the world back to a state of health could not be lost on us. However, the definition of health is a much-debated topic, since health means different things to different peoples and cultures. According to the Constitution of the World Health Organization, health is "a state of complete physical, mental and social well-being, and not merely the absence of disease and infirmity". Though health experts around the world have pointed out its limitations, especially lately, the definition is nevertheless significant in its inclusion of the mental and social domains, in addition to the physical, within the bracket of health. Emerging academic disciplines such as the medical humanities similarly underscore the urgency of recognizing health as an interdisciplinary concept, inviting considerations of the psychological, emotional, and spiritual states of human beings, along with their physical and biomedical condition, in studies on illness, health and wellbeing.

In the context of these new ways of looking at health and disease, the selected adaptations of Shakespeare's *Macbeth* could be read as contemporary critiques of the biomedical narrative of health, in which the diagnosis and treatment of an illness are based solely on biological and physical factors. The films inherently acknowledge the psychological, social, spiritual, environmental, and cultural aspects of disease, and attribute the hero's illness to a violent, self-serving, and dysfunctional culture among other things. They depict the attainment of health as being contingent upon the absence of violence, while simultaneously recognizing the acrimonious truth that contemporary societies are inconceivable without violence. As countries and communities are torn apart by wars, as governments and non-state actors indulge in unapologetic displays of violence, health, indeed, appears to be deferred to an indefinite future in our times. Even after the mutant variants of the Coronavirus have lost their potency, even after the "waves" of the pandemic have receded, the return of health and normalcy in the world remains, at best, a conjecture. In this context, the selected adaptations of *Macbeth*, with their exploration of health and disease from a cultural perspective, become ever so relevant.

References

Barthes, Roland. 1977. *Image-Music-Text*. London: Fontana.
Beja, Morris. 1979. *Film and Literature: An Introduction*. New York: Longman.
Biswas, Moinak. 2006. "Mourning and Blood-Ties: Macbeth in Mumbai." *Journal of the Moving Image*. Accessed January 27, 2016. https://jmionline.org/articles/2006/mourning_and_blood_ties_macbeth_in_mumbai.pdf.

Fava, Giovanni A. and Nicoletta Sonino. 2017. "From the Lesson of George Engel to Current Knowledge: The Biopsychosocial Model 40 Years Later." *Psychotherapy and Psychosomatics*, 257–259. Karger. Accessed January 12, 2022. https://www.karger.com/Article/FullText/478808.

James I. 1954. *A Counter-Blaste to Tobacco.* Foreword by Ann Hill. London: The Rodale Press.

Kristeva, Julia. 1986. "Word, Dialogue and the Novel." In *The Kristeva Reader*, edited by Toril Moi, 34–61. New York: Columbia University Press.

Mattes, Ari. 2015. "Justin Kurzel's Macbeth: Visually Magnificent but Dramatically Unsatisfying." *The Conversation.* Accessed December 20, 2021. https://theconversation.com/justin-kurzels-macbeth-visually-magnificent-but-dramatically-unsatisfying-48004.

McElroy, Bernard. 2003. "Macbeth: The Torture of the Mind." *EXPLORING Shakespeare. Gale Student Resources in Context.* Accessed January 19, 2018. https://bolosbritlit.weebly.com/uploads/4/8/5/7/4857234/macbethsmindsecondary.pdf.

McFarlane, Brian. 1996. *Novel to Film: An Introduction to the Theory of Adaptation.* Oxford: Clarendon Press.

Muir, Kenneth, ed. 2013. *Macbeth.* India: Bloomsbury.

Roychoudhury, Suparna. 2013. "Melancholy, Ecstasy, Phantasma: The Pathologies of Macbeth." *Modern Philology* 111, no. 2: 205–230. Accessed December 13, 2021. https://www.jstor.org/stable/10.1086/673309.

Sett, Ralph F. 1962. "Dunsinane Revisited: Medicine in Shakespeare's Macbeth." *The Linacre Quarterly* 29, no. 4: 185–189. Accessed December 11, 2021. https://epublications.marquette.edu/lnq/vol29/iss4/5/?utm_source=epublications.marquette.edu%2Flnq%2Fvol29%2Fiss4%2F5&utm_medium=PDF&utm_campaign=PDFCoverPages.

Sheppard, Philippa. 2018. "Humbling the Soldier in Kurzel's Macbeth and Parker's Othello." *Literature/Film Quarterly* 46, no. 1. Accessed October 22, 2021. https://lfq.salisbury.edu/_issues/46_1/humbling_the_soldier_in_kurzels_macbeth_and_parkers_othello.html.

Sloterdijk, Peter. 2012. *Rage and Time.* Translated by Mario Wenning. New York: Columbia University Press.

Stam, Robert and Alessandra Raengo. 2005. *Literature and Film: A Guide to the Theory and Practice of Film Adaptation.* Malden, MA: Blackwell.

Index

abjection 207, 208, 219
aboriginal 14, 23–31, 33, 34, 35, 180
afflictions 7, 34, 193
Ahuja, Neel 33
alienation 209
amebiasis 186
American Psychiatric Association's
    Diagnostic and Statistical Manual of
    Mental Disorders 51
Archer, Seth 34
Artemis 122
artificial intelligence 68
astangikamarga 200
asthma 186
asylum 14, 15, 50–61, 101

Bakr, Abu 38
Bashford, Alison 32, 34
Basu, Moushumi 178, 180
Bates, Daisy 34
Bedford 53, 155
Bennett, Michael J. 27, 31, 32, 34
Bhardwaj, Vishal 233, 235, 236, 237, 238,
    240
biomedical 1, 10, 168, 169, 170, 234, 242
biopsychosocial 3, 233, 243
Bollywood 235, 238
Borderless Journal 69, 70
Brahman 200
Buddhism 200, 203
Butler, Judith 197, 205, 210, 219

Cameron, Catherine M., Paul Keltom and
    Alan C. Swedlund eds. 34
Campbell, Judy 26, 27, 28, 29, 34
cancer 7, 8, 12, 64, 213
Carpenter, Mary Wilson 51, 52, 57, 59
Castiglioni 137, 155
Chakrabarty, Dipesh 19

Chatterjee, Subhasish 180
Chatterji, Joya 192
cholera 8, 9, 23, 64, 175, 179, 184, 185,
    186, 187
Chomsky, Noam 19
city-makers 15, 72, 84
Collins, David 27, 30, 34
colonisation 4
Columbian Exchange 23, 24, 26, 34, 35
communal 110, 159, 185, 221, 233–236,
    240
Comprehensive Primary Health Care 131
Confederation of Indian Industry (CII)
    121, 129
Confucianism 200
constitution 4, 16, 20, 57, 87, 89, 90, 92,
    95, 96, 242
contagion 16, 27, 32, 66, 67, 98, 99, 109,
    111, 112, 115, 138, 139, 141, 144,
    149–151, 155, 184, 241
Covid-19 pandemic 1, 11, 12, 15, 18, 19,
    32, 46–48, 58, 62, 64–66, 70, 72–75,
    77–79, 81, 83–89, 91, 94, 99, 111, 113,
    116, 153, 157, 166–167, 181, 207, 229
Cox, Frank 34
Crosby, Alfred 23, 26, 30, 34
cure by touch 154

Das, Suranjan 65
Defoe, Daniel 8, 19
dengue 9, 23, 64
depathologisation 220
diarrhoea 187
digital divide 65, 70
diphtheria 23, 186
Directive Principles of State Policy 91
Disability Adjusted Life Years (DALY's)
    122
Donkin, Major Robert 34

Douglous, Brown and Nic Latulippe 96
Duffy, J. 26, 34
Duncan Gleneagles 122
dysentery 23, 186

Ebola 9, 11
Elizabethan England 146, 153, 155
epidemiology 6, 46
esoteric 17, 157, 168–181
etiology 7, 43, 46

fatigue 65, 174, 184, 239
FDI 118, 120
federalism 15, 87, 88, 90, 92, 94, 95, 96, 97
Federation of Indian Chambers of
    Commerce and Industry (FICCI) 121, 129
Fenn, Elizabeth A. 34
finance 81, 84, 85, 120, 122, 124, 130,
    133, 186
Finley, Lana Louise 180
first wave 12, 13, 47, 65, 70, 74, 88, 91
Foucault, Michel 19, 60

Geetha, Arjun 212, 218, 219
gender dysphoria 207, 208, 209, 216
gender identity 207, 209, 217
gender nonconformity 208
germ theory 38, 153
Ghatak, Ritwik 17, 182, 184, 185, 192, 193
Ghebreyesus, Tedros Adhanom 32, 34, 230
Gilbert and Gubar 195, 196
Gott, Richard 180
The Great Plague of London 158, 167
Grieves, Vicki 180

Hasan, Amtul 193
Hasan, Mushirul 193
healing 1, 10, 17, 53, 61, 95, 140–141,
    145–148, 150–151, 157–159, 162–169,
    174, 178–181, 191, 197, 199, 203, 216
Health and Wellness Centres (HWCs) 131
Hewa, Soma 23, 31, 34
Hindus 191
Hines, Sally 220
Historical Records 34
Hobbesian 185
hysteria 195, 196, 200–202, 205, 206

immunity 13, 14, 33, 37, 39, 42, 46, 47,
    48, 154, 155
Indian Public Health Standards (IPHS) 126
indigenous 1, 14, 16, 17, 23, 24, 25, 26, 29,
    170, 173, 174, 175, 176, 178, 179, 180,
    181, 205

informal sector 72, 229
inoculation 31, 32, 35, 37, 38, 39, 41, 42,
    48, 49, 184
intertextuality 236
isolation 1, 13, 14, 43, 47, 58, 67, 68, 95,
    160
ithaca 18, 155, 194, 195, 197, 198, 199,
    201, 202, 203, 205

Jacobean immunity politics 154
Jakovljevic, Miro 172, 181
James, Lovely Awomi 181
Jiva 199
Jones, D. S. 24, 34
Jones, Kathleen 15, 55, 56, 60
Julius Caesar 142, 153

Karki, Rebecca 181
Kaur, Ravinder 192
Kechutzar, Sashikaba 173, 180, 181
Khan, Liaquat Ali 189
Khan, Yasmin 192, 193
King George III 52, 59
Kire, Easterine 17, 168–181
Kirkpatrick, James 29, 35
Kristeva, Julia 207, 208, 219, 236, 243
Kumbh mela 99, 100, 101, 106, 107, 108,
    113, 114
Kurzel, Justin 233, 235, 236, 237, 239,
    240, 241, 243

Lefebvre, Henri 210
Lindsay, B. C. 35
lockdown 63, 65, 66, 67, 70, 72, 73, 74,
    77–80, 84, 92, 93, 94, 95, 100

Macbeth 16, 18, 137–159, 161, 163, 165,
    167, 233–243
Madley, B. 29, 35
malaria 8, 9, 23, 26, 64, 123, 139, 174,
    186, 187
malnutrition 184, 186, 229, 232
masks 63, 78, 88
maternal health 12, 19
McMillen, C. W. 9, 19, 35
media 12, 13, 16, 63, 97–101, 103,
    105–116, 187, 190, 201, 209, 213, 222,
    230, 235, 236, 239
Meher, Rithu 211, 218, 219
mental health 5, 6, 19, 50, 51, 53, 170,
    195–197, 205, 215, 218–219
migrants 15, 33, 72–86, 98, 101, 187, 193
misinformation 16, 98, 99, 111, 115
Modicare 126, 127

Mohajir' 186
motherhood 17, 157, 159, 162–163, 165, 197, 205
Muir, Kenneth 234, 235, 238, 240, 241, 243
multicultural 72, 98, 178
Muslims 16, 98, 99, 100, 101, 102, 106, 109, 110, 111, 113, 114, 186, 187, 191, 192

Naga 17, 168, 169, 170, 171, 172, 173, 174, 175, 176, 177, 178, 179, 180, 181
Namocare 126
National Democratic Alliance (NDA) 124
National Health Bill 124
National Health Policy Draft (2015) 121
The National Institute of Wellness 2
new normal 13, 15, 62, 63, 65–69, 71, 218
9/11 syndrome 11, 19
Nottingham 53
NRHM 124, 125, 130, 132
Nunn, Nathan and Nancy Quian 23, 35

occult 1, 180
oil crisis 118
online 65, 66, 68, 69, 70, 85, 110, 113, 115, 154, 181, 242
Ottawa Charter 2, 3, 20, 57
Ozeki, Ruth 18, 221, 222, 223, 224, 225, 227, 232

panic 8, 13, 55, 62, 64, 65, 66, 185
Pasteur, Louis 9, 38, 39
pathogen 3, 4, 23, 24, 26, 37, 38, 191, 223
Phillips, Robert 219
physical distancing 67
plague 8, 10, 19, 23, 26, 29, 35, 37, 64, 98, 116, 138, 139, 141, 144, 145, 147, 149, 151, 152, 154, 155, 158–161, 163, 164, 167, 175, 237, 238
pneumonia 98, 186
Portea 122
Porter, Roy 49, 206
Pradhan Mantri Jan Arogya Yojana 126
Prameesh, Manjami 211, 212, 213, 218, 219
Prosser, Jay 208, 219
Public Health Foundation of India (PHFI) 125
public playhouse 151, 152, 155
Public-Private Partnership (PPP) 45, 122, 123, 125, 130

Qudrat Ullah Shahab 17, 182, 186

Randhawa, Mohinder Singh 193
Rashtriya Swasthya Bima Yojana (RSBY) 124, 130, 132
reasons for migration 76
refugee 17, 182, 183, 184, 185, 186, 187, 189, 190, 191, 192, 193
rehabilitation 5, 17, 182, 192, 193
The Retreat 53, 54, 117
Revathi, A. 219
Ritskes, Eric 181
Rockefeller Foundation 125
Rural Health Statistics Bulletin 119, 128, 133

Sarkar, Sumit 193
Sarna, Mohinder Singh 193
SARS 11, 98
Saxena, Rekha 97
second wave 12, 13, 15, 18, 66, 94, 100, 102, 112, 113
sexuality 158, 160, 163, 208, 209, 210, 216, 219
sex-worker 71
Shelley, Mary 11
shortage 66, 78, 119, 231
smallpox 8, 14, 23–32, 33, 35, 38–39, 40–41, 98, 139, 175, 179
Smith, Leonard 53, 60
Sontag, Susan 4, 7, 8, 11, 19, 47, 50, 71
starvation 78, 79, 174, 186
stranded 47, 73, 78–81, 83, 85
Szwed, J.F. 35

Tablighi 99–104, 107, 109–112, 115
Taoism 200
Taylor, Gray 156
Tench, Watkin 28, 30, 32, 35
theory of the humours 153
Tidswell, F. 25, 35
Tillin, Louise 92, 97
topic analysis 103
transbodies 208
transgender activism 218
transgender fluidity 208
transgender life narratives 18, 207, 209
transgender subjectivity 207
transmobilities 213, 219
Tripathi, Laxminarayan 220
tuberculosis 7, 9, 12, 26, 35, 185
typhoid 8, 23

unemployment 64, 78, 82, 89, 91
Universal Health Coverage 125, 126, 128, 130, 131, 132, 133
Upanishads 197

vaccination 14, 24, 31, 32, 33, 34, 35, 38, 39, 40, 41, 42, 43, 44, 45, 46, 47, 48, 49, 92, 95
vaccine 1, 12, 13, 14, 32, 33, 37–40, 42–47, 49, 66, 94, 120
Vedantic Philosophy 197
Versluis, Arthur 181
violence 11, 16, 24, 53, 54, 60, 68, 71, 98, 109, 112, 115, 157–158, 166–167, 182, 185, 186, 191–193, 209, 211, 214, 215, 218, 219, 233–242
viral 20, 26, 29, 38, 47, 62, 64, 66, 99, 109, 110, 111, 112
virgin soil 24, 25, 33, 34

Walton John, K. 52, 53, 61
Warren, Christopher 29, 30, 31, 35
weaponization 24, 29
wellbeing 2–5, 14–15, 17–20, 73–74, 78, 80–81, 84, 106, 111, 168–169, 179, 195, 197, 199, 201, 203, 205, 233, 235–237, 239, 241, 243

West Bengal 70, 81, 85, 92, 95, 113, 123, 129–130, 131, 184–185, 192–193, 231
Willaert, Rita 175, 179, 181
witchcraft 141, 152, 158, 160, 163, 167
Wockhardt Hospitals 122
women 12, 17, 18, 38–39, 43–44, 55, 65, 68, 73, 80, 130, 133, 137, 151, 157–161, 163–167, 179, 182, 186, 189, 194–197, 199, 201–206, 211–213
Woolf, Virginia 34, 196
working from home 68
World Bank 78, 85, 118, 122–124, 129, 130, 133, 229
World Health Organisation 20
Wright, B. 28, 35

"Ya Khuda" 17, 182, 186, 193

Žižek, Slavoj 11, 13, 15, 20, 62, 63–64, 67–71